Two Decades of
Health Services

Two Decades of Health Services:

Social Survey Trends in Use and Expenditure

Ronald Andersen
Associate Professor
Center for Health Administration Studies
University of Chicago

Joanna Lion
Director of Information Services
Massachusetts Hospital Association

Odin W. Anderson
Professor and Director
Center for Health Administration Studies
University of Chicago

Ballinger Publishing Company • Cambridge, Massachusetts
A Subsidiary of J.B. Lippincott Company

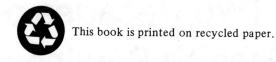 This book is printed on recycled paper.

International Standard Book Number: 0-88410-117-7

Library of Congress Catalog Card Number: 76-14785

Printed in the United States of America

Library of Congress Cataloging in Publication Data

Andersen, Ronald.
  Two decades of health services.

  Bibliography:
  Includes index.
  1. Medical care—United States—Utilization.
2. Medical care, Cost of—United States.
3. Insurance, Health—United States. 4. Health surveys—United States. I. Lion, Joanna, 1939 joint author. II. Anderson, Odin Waldemar, 1914- joint author. III. Title. (DNLM: 1. Health and welfare planning—United States. 2. Economics, Medical—United States. 3. Health services—Utilization—United States.
W84 AA1 A49t]
RA410.53.A7   362.1'0973   76-14785
ISBN 0-88410-117-7

Contents

✳

List of Tables

✳

Foreword

For ten years, the confidence of Americans in their leaders has been declining. Every sector of economic, political, and intellectual life has been affected: organized labor and big business, Congress and the executive office, the press and higher education. It is ironic that medicine, the one major sector in which leadership still inspires substantial public confidence, is the target of politicians, labor leaders, and journalists who inspire very little.* It is described as chaotic in its organization, inadequate to the immense task of preserving and improving the nation's health, inequitable in its method of distributing services, and unresponsive to the needs of the public. Numerous plans for fundamental reform of medicine are before the Congress and the likelihood that medicine can long resist significant further government intervention is extremely small.

We trust leaders whose rhetoric fits their actions and whose actions are rooted in the sound analysis of objective facts. Those who wish to reform medicine and by so doing, to inspire confidence in their own ability to lead, will find in this volume exactly what they need. Four surveys, conducted by the Center for Health Administration Studies and the National Opinion Research Center, covering the years 1953, 1958, 1963 and 1970, trace a period of major change in the technology, organization, and financing of medical care. The analysis bears not only on the performance of medicine, but on the

---

*A Harris Survey conducted between February 23 and March 4, 1976 shows that the leadership of medicine inspires a great deal of confidence in 42% of those questioned. Congress, organized labor, and the press had the confidence of 9%, 10%, and 20% respectively.

way in which it adapts to change and innovation. In its objectivity and rigor, this volume conforms to and contributes to the scholarly reputation of the Center for Health Administration Studies and the Graduate School of Business at The University of Chicago. I commend its authors for an outstanding achievement.

Richard N. Rosett
Dean, Graduate School of Business
University of Chicago
April 4, 1976

※

Acknowledgments

This book would not have been possible without the talents and close working relationships of a large number of people. Any social survey the size of this one requires numerous individuals behind the scenes long before the final data are ever put into book form.

Complex sampling needs were ably overseen by Benjamin King. In the stage of data collection we are grateful to Ruthe Nepon, who coordinated all of the interviewing and verification through the National Opinion Research Center. Her excellent field staff was spearheaded by Ann Roberts, Ann Nelson and Susan Firestone. Of course, no social survey is better than the quality of the interviews. We are grateful to the NORC interviewers for a job well done using a complicated schedule. In verification, Peter Kurz, Dervan Pullar and Ruth Kellam accomplished some ingenious field work while securing information from doctors, hospitals and insurers.

This study required lengthy and meticulous programming. We are particularly thankful for the talents at various times of Scott Harrison, Jarvis Rich, Nelson Co and Robert Cripe. George Yates had the intricate task of putting all of the programming together into a coherent system. He did this with competence and humor.

Research assistants formed the backbone of the study from its inception to its completion. No one but a research assistant can explain exactly what a research assistant does, but the study could not have been completed without them. We wish to thank Rachel Greeley, Barbara Nausieda, Joan Daley, Elinor Socholitzsky, Robert Mackler, Cynthia Romagnoli and Charles Brown.

In the final stages of the project, expertise on a broader scale came into play in the form of comments on the final form that the manuscript should take. Help was received from Lee Benham, Stephen Shortell, Lu Ann Aday, Joel May and many other colleagues at the Center for Health Administration Studies (CHAS). When Joanna Lion left CHAS in December 1974, much of the "onsite" coordination necessary to complete the project was competently assumed by Judith Kasper and Virginia Daughety. Lloyd Ferguson and, after his death, John Schneider were invaluable as medical consultants at various stages of the project.

Voluminous typing is necessary to prepare a manuscript such as this for the publisher. We wish to acknowledge the fine efforts of Linda Randall and Evelyn Friedman in completing this task. The analysis of sampling error, so important in a descriptive volume of this type, was ably prepared by Martha Banks, who is a co-author of the methodological appendix. Peter Weil and Richard Foster were major contributors to the analyses of price and use changes presented in Chapter 3.

This work was made possible by contracts HSM-110-70-392 and HRA-106-74-24 with the National Center for Health Services Research. We are grateful for the continuous and vigorous support of the directors and associate directors of the National Center who held office through the duration of this project including Paul Sanazaro, Robert Van Hoek, Gerald Rosenthal, Robert Huntley and Robert Eichhorn. We also feel fortunate to have worked with a series of interested and supportive project officers who have devoted much time and energy to the study, including Jack Clark, Bonnie Owen, William Kitching and Daniel Walden.

Finally, we take pleasure in acknowledging the role played by George Bugbee, director of CHAS at the time this project was conceived and initiated. Without his encouragement and enthusiastic backing of the study, particularly during some periods when the undertaking was in doubt, it is unlikely the project would have begun.

Ronald Andersen
Joanna Lion
Odin W. Anderson
February 5, 1976

✳

Introduction

This is a book about the public's use of and expenditures for health services in the United States. It documents trends in health services using four parallel surveys of the nation's families spanning almost 20 years.[1]

Particular emphasis is given to changes taking place between the last two studies, conducted in 1964 and 1971. In the interval, the Medicare and Medicaid laws went into effect. The data from these studies thus provide an opportunity to examine improvements in health services utilization for the elderly and the poor, who were the target groups for the legislation.

Another impetus for the most recent study was the pending passage of additional major health legislation. It was felt that a detailed examination of the health service utilization and expenditure patterns of groups of special concern to policymakers, including the inner city poor, the rural population and the elderly, would provide useful background information when formulating and implementing national health insurance legislation.[2]

1. The previous studies were published as: Anderson and Feldman (1956); Anderson, Collette and Feldman (1963); and Andersen and Anderson (1967).
2. The data presented in this final report from four relatively comprehensive national surveys must necessarily be selective. In general, this book includes trend data on the most basic measures of use, expenditures and health insurance coverage used in the earlier studies. In some instances, data from the 1958 study have been omitted for the sake of brevity when, in the authors' judgment, trends for the entire period could be adequately described by reference to the 1953, 1963 and 1970 data alone. In other instances, comparisons excluded the first study. This usually means that comparable data from the 1953 study were not available or were not relevant (as in the case of major medical insurance

This volume and a companion volume (Andersen, Kravits and Anderson, 1975) comprise the final reports from this project. This volume describes the basic findings of the project concerning health service utilization and expenditures for various groups in the population and documents significant changes taking place over time.[3] The companion volume attempts to use a more analytical approach and more elaborate statistical techniques to explain the utilization patterns observed.[4]

CURRENT SURVEY

In the latest survey 3,880 families were interviewed in their homes in early 1971. One or more members of each family provided information regarding use of health services, the cost of these services and how this cost was met for the calendar year 1970. In addition to data provided by the sample families, information has been collected from physicians, clinics, hospitals, insuring organizations and employers about the families' medical care and health insurance for the survey year. This additional information serves to verify the family information as well as to provide additional details about medical care that many families are unable to give.

In the earlier studies, verifications were carried out for inpatient hospital services and health insurance coverage. Verifications were not attempted in the earlier studies for reported physician services, outpatient hospital services and claims paid by health insurance as was done in the latest study.

When verification data were available, the general procedure was

coverage). Finally, a considerable part of the analysis is limited to 1963–1970 comparisons or to cross-sectional analysis of the 1970 data alone. In some instances comparable data are not available from the earlier studies. In other instances the earlier data were omitted because the authors judged the most pertinent inferences could be drawn by focusing on the later data.

3. In the final reports of earlier studies an attempt was made to trace the development in the field of health survey utilization studies up to the time the report was written. See, for example, Andersen and Anderson (1967: 5-9). No such effort will be made in this work because of the recent publication of a number of comprehensive surveys of the field. See Aday and Eichhorn (1972); Flook and Sanazaro (1973); and Aday and Andersen (1975).

4. In addition to the companion volume, data from the most recent survey were also released in a series of preliminary reports: Andersen and Kravits (1971); Andersen et al. (1972); and Andersen et al. (1973). Data from the study are currently available for secondary analysis through the National Archives, 1970 Survey of Health Services Utilization and Expenditure, Center for Health Administration Studies, University of Chicago; Records of the United States Public Health Service, Records Group No. 90, Acc. No. NN-375-174, Attention: Charles M. Dollar, Director, Machine Readable Archives Division, National Archives and Record Service, Washington, D.C. 20408. Secondary analyses which were completed or in progress in March 1976 are documented in Appendix V.

to combine it with the family data (social survey) to arrive at what we call our "best estimate" data. In general, when both respondent and verification data were available, the verification data were accepted. There were exceptions when, for example, respondents had well-documented records of their medical care or there was special reason to believe the verification data might be incomplete or inaccurate. When verification data were not available, what the respondent reported was accepted as our best estimate.

In trend analyses, this volume uses best estimate data when it is available for all years. To maximize comparability among the studies, respondent data will be used for all years in cases where best estimate data are available only for 1970, as is the case for physician services. Best estimates for physician and hospital outpatient care are, however, provided in Chapter Five, which compares social survey estimates with best estimates using 1970 data only.

The sample for the latest study was designed so that the inner city poor, the aged and rural residents were overrepresented. This design allows for more detailed analyses of these special groups than would a self-weighting probability sample. All tables in this report are based on weighted distributions to correct for the oversampling of the above groups and to allow estimates to be made for the total noninstitutionalized population of the United States.

Since the statistics in this report are based on a sample, they are subject to sampling variability. Particular care must be exercised where the unweighted number of observations is small. Consequently, no estimates based on fewer than 25 observations are published in the text tables. Also, certain observations with extreme values that were judged to have an excessive influence on mean estimates are excluded from some text tables. In all tables where observations were excluded, the criteria for exclusion and the estimate including the extreme values are provided in the methodology appendix. Further, this appendix contains sampling error estimates which can be used to judge the stability of estimates provided in the text.

PLAN OF VOLUME

The findings are divided into seven chapters. All deal with the health care of the noninstitutionalized population of the United States according to its utilization, expenditure and health insurance experience. Further, differences in that experience for various subgroups defined according to age, sex, income, race, education and residence are examined.

The first two chapters address questions concerning utilization: (1) Where and why do people receive health services? and (2) What kinds and how much of these services do they receive? The kinds of services considered are physician and dental visits, hospitalization, surgery, and medical care associated with pregnancy.

The third and fourth chapters consider the financing of health services. The magnitude and rate of increase of health service expenditures are examined at the individual and family level. Trends are considered for total expenditures as well as for components of the "medical care dollar" including hospital, physician, drug and dental expenditures. Also treated are the sources of payment for medical care with emphasis given to Medicaid and welfare, Medicare, voluntary insurance, and out-of-pocket payments by consumers.

Chapter Five is devoted to comparing 1970 estimates of utilization and expenditure based only on the social survey data with the "best estimates," which include information from the verification studies. Since considerable effort went into the verification process, the impact of the verification of the final estimates of the study is of considerable methodological interest. Also, some of the best estimates, particularly concerning physician services, are not found elsewhere in the volume. Prior chapters utilize social survey estimates from the latest study because they are most comparable to estimates from earlier studies which did not verify physician services.

Chapter Six provides a picture of the utilization and expenditure experience of people with no health insurance and varying types of health insurance. The tables in this chapter provide some control for age and income level and show differences in people's medical care experience according to the presence of insurance and whether it is basic insurance, major medical or prepaid group practice. In addition, comparisons are made between people with drug, dental and doctor visit insurance and those without these types of coverage. Many of the optional coverages examined in this chapter are proposed in one or another of the national health insurance bills. Documentation of the experience of people who already have such coverage, and comparing these experiences with those of people who do not, might prove of assistance when attempting to assess the impacts of the various proposals.

A final chapter highlights the main findings of the study and suggests what their policy implications might be. A series of appendixes describe the methodology, define the key terms used throughout the volume, and reproduce the interview schedules and questionnaires used in the latest study.

Chapter 1

Where and Why People Receive Health Services

This chapter examines where people usually go for their medical care. Also considered are some reasons for seeking medical care. These include physical examinations, symptoms of illness, severity of diagnoses and days when people are unable to perform their usual activities.

REGULAR SOURCES OF MEDICAL CARE

Where people usually seek care when they are sick influences whether or not they will obtain care on a preventive basis. More importantly, once the decision to seek care is made, the regular source largely determines the type, amount and continuity of care the patient receives.

The proportion of the population who name a place—such as a hospital or health center—rather than a particular doctor as their regular source of care increased considerably between 1963 and 1970 (Table 1–1). In contrast, the proportion that named a particular physician declined. Those claiming no regular source of care decreased slightly.

The trends for the population as a whole generally held for both sexes and all age groups (Table 1–1). Males in 1970, as in 1963, were somewhat less likely to report a regular source of care than were females. Children were more likely to have a clinic as their regular source of care and less likely to have no source of care than adults. Young and middle-aged adults appeared most likely to report no regular source of care in both periods.

5

Changes in regular source of care between 1963 and 1970 varied according to family income (Table 1-1). The proportion of the population in the low and middle income groups that named a particular MD as the regular source of care decreased considerably while remaining the same for the high income group. The proportion naming a clinic as the regular source of care increased for all groups. Only for the highest income group did the proportion reporting no regular source of care decrease. Thus, the differences according to income in the 1963 study have become more extreme, with the poor less likely to have a regular MD and more likely to have no regular source of care.

The changes taking place for the nonwhite population between 1963 and 1970 parallel those for the low income group (Table 1-1). Compared to whites, the proportion of nonwhites reporting an MD as their usual source of care decreased, but there was no corresponding decrease in the percent of nonwhites reporting no regular care. Nonwhites, then, can be characterized as the population group least likely to have any regular source and most likely to use a clinic, if indeed they report a source at all.

People living in families in which the family head had not completed high school were less likely to name a physician as their regular source of care and more likely to name a clinic or report no regular source at all than were people in families headed by someone who had at least completed high school (Table 1-1). In the interval between 1963 and 1970, changes in regular source of care for all educational levels were similar to those for the total population: decreases in the proportion reporting no regular source or a particular MD and an increase in the proportion mentioning a clinic. Thus, while the sources of regular care for the less educated appear similar to those with low incomes and the nonwhites, the differences between the less educated and the rest of the population were not magnified with the passage of time as they were for the poor and nonwhites.

The residence data in Table 1-1 point up similarities in regular source of care between the most urban and the most rural populations. Those people living in the central city of Standard Metropolitan Statistical Areas (SMSAs) were least likely to report an MD as their regular source of care and most likely to have no regular source. In both respects, the group most like them is the rural farm population. Between 1963 and 1970, the reporting of no regular source of care decreased for urban and rural nonfarm residents but not for the farm residents.

Table 1-2 presents data concerning the regular sources of care people have according to various combinations of age, income and place of residence. Having a low income and living in a central city results in the greatest proportion of people who report no regular source of care for every age group. Those most likely to have a regular source of care are high income children regardless of residence. People living in the central city with a low family income are more likely than most others to report a clinic as a regular source of care. This finding is particularly pronounced for low income children. In fact, over half of these children who live in a central city report a clinic as their regular source of care. Middle and high income groups in every age and residence category report an MD as their regular source of care more often than do low income people.

The meaning of "clinic" as a regular source of care varies considerably. Persons who use a hospital outpatient department or even an emergency room as their regular source of care will report that they use a "clinic" as will members of a large prepaid group practice plan such as Kaiser or Health Insurance Plan of Greater New York (HIP) or users of a group of doctors in specialty practice. One way of differentiating care received by people who say they use a "clinic" is to ask if, within the institution where they obtain their regular care, they usually see the same doctor. Such information might be of particular value in assessing whether the patient feels comfortable about seeking care and the degree of continuity of care that he might receive.

Table 1-3 shows that there are considerable differences in the portions of people with a clinic as a regular source of care who see a particular doctor, according to basic social and demographic variables. About two-thirds of the whites who use a clinic have a particular doctor at that clinic compared to only one-third of the nonwhites. Higher income clinic users are more likely to name a particular doctor at their "clinic" than are clinic users with less income. Old people are considerably more likely to have a particular doctor at their "clinic" than are younger people and women are somewhat more likely than men. Finally, city dwellers, where most of the emergency rooms and large outpatient departments are concentrated, are much less likely to have a particular doctor that they see.

These findings suggest that much of the "clinic" care reported by the well-off white segment of the sample is provided by prepaid group practice or private doctors incorporated into nonprepaid clinics, while the "clinic" care reported by less advantaged portions of the population is more depersonalized service provided in out-patient departments and emergency rooms. The fact that old people are much more apt to have a regular doctor when they use a clinic might be related to the financial impact of Medicare, which makes a private doctor possible.

PHYSICAL EXAMINATIONS

While health professionals channel much of the patient's care once the patient enters the medical care system, the patient must initiate the contact in most instances. One reason for such contacts is the general physical examination. While the contribution of the regular checkup to the health level of a population has not been empirically established, the frequency of physical examinations is still a commonly accepted measure of preventive health care.

Within a year's period, over one-half of the U.S. population has a physical examination or checkup. Between 1963 and 1970 the proportion reporting yearly physical examinations appeared to increase while the proportion reporting they had never had an examination decreased from 10 percent to 5 percent (Table 1-4).

Females appeared slightly more likely than males to have had an examination within a year in the 1963 study and this discrepancy increased by 1970 (Table 1-4). Young children 1 to 5 years of age are more likely to have had a recent examination than people in any other age group. However, this group, along with older children 6 to 17, is also most likely *never* to have had a physical examination. However, between 1963 and 1970 children generally experienced the biggest gain in proportion having an exam within a year and also had the biggest percentage point decrease in the proportion reported never to have had a physical examination.

In 1963 the low income population was least likely to have had a physical within a year and most likely to report never having had an examination (Table 1-4). In 1970 this was still true, but the gaps had. narrowed considerably so that the frequency of exams was more similar across income groups.

Table 1-4 indicates that exams are becoming more frequent for both whites and nonwhites. In both years exams within a year were actually reported as frequently by nonwhites as by whites. However, nonwhites were also more likely to report never having had a physical exam in both time periods.

The relationship between education and frequency of exams is similar to that for income and exams (Table 1-4). The least educated (and lowest income) groups are least likely to have had a recent examination and most likely never to have had one. However, the trend data show the least educated group increased the frequency of examinations while the behavior of those with more education remained relatively constant. Consequently, differences according to education level (and income) decreased over time.

In 1963 the rural farm population was much less likely to have had an examination within a year and much more likely never to have had an examination than the rest of the population (Table 1-4). Over the next seven years the frequency of exams for the farm group increased considerably. Thus, by 1970, while the urban and rural nonfarm population were still receiving more physical examinations than the farm population, the differences were much less than they had been in 1963. In 1970 the physical examination behavior of central city residents was very similar to that of other urban dwellers.

Table 1-5 shows the relationship between regular source of care and length of time since the person's last physical examination. People using specialists as their regular source of care are most likely to have had an examination within a year and persons without a regular source least likely. Further, in the period between 1963 and 1970, the proportion of people with a specialist who had an exam within a year increased while the proportion of people with no regular source of care who had an exam within the year actually decreased—thus widening the gap. Table 1-5, then, suggests that over time the discrepancy in terms of exam frequency between those without a regular source of care and the rest of the population is increasing. In this period the frequency of exams for those seeing general practitioners or going to a clinic as their regular source increased slightly.

In the last two studies the reason for the last physical examination for every person reporting an examination was elicited. The reason was selected from a card including the following alternatives: (1) Symptom: "wasn't feeling good, was bothered by some symptom or condition"; (2) Required: "examination was required for a job, school, insurance, armed forces, or something like that"; and (3) Preventive exam: "there was nothing particularly wrong and the examination wasn't required—it was just time for a checkup or physical examination."

Table 1-6 shows that the most common reason given for the last physical exam changed from going for a symptom in 1963 to going for a preventive exam in 1970. The proportion reporting that the exam was required remained about the same. Overall, the proportion reporting each of the three reasons was near one-third of all those having examinations in 1970.

The most prevalent reason for males having a physical examination was that it was required (Table 1–6). More examinations for men are apparently given for purposes of work and insurance. Women are more likely to have examinations in response to symptoms or as preventive measures. The shift from symptoms to prevention as a reason for the exam appeared stronger for women than for men.

Preventive exams are most common among young children of 1 to 5 of both sexes (Table 1–6). Required exams are more frequent among adolescents and young adults, particularly males. For older adults symptoms become a more important reason for exams. However, the biggest shift between 1963 and 1970 from symptoms to prevention was among the older age groups. Consequently, the distribution of reasons for exams for older adults was more similar to that for the rest of the population in 1970 than was the case in 1963.

In 1963, the lowest income group was most likely to mention a symptom as the reason for their last physical exam while the higher income groups were more likely to report required or preventive exams (Table 1–6). In 1970 this general pattern still held, but all income groups reported symptoms as a reason less often and preventive exams more often than seven years earlier. However, while the proportion of required exams had increased for the low income groups it had decreased for the higher income levels.

The nonwhite population reported a larger proportion of exams in response to illness and a smaller proportion as preventive than did the white population in 1963 (Table 1–6). By 1970 nonwhites were as likely to report a preventive exam as were whites.

The relationships between reason for exam and education are similar to those previously described for income. People with less education were more likely to give symptoms as a reason for exams and less likely to report preventive exams in 1963. By 1970 these relationships still held but were much weaker than they had been earlier.

The farm population was similar to low income and education groups in 1963 in the sense that a symptom was a more important reason for exams and prevention was mentioned less often than was true for the rest of the population (Table 1–6). However, the shift toward prevention in 1970 was not stronger but actually appears weaker than for the rest of the population. Consequently, large differences in reason for exam by residence remain in 1970. It should also be noted that in 1970 preventive exams were less common for central city residents than for other urban persons.

RESPONSE TO SYMPTOMS OF ILLNESS

Symptoms of illness are a frequent reason for people seeing a physician. In this section some data are provided on the type of symptoms that brought people to doctors in 1963 and 1970. In addition, a few of the symptoms are examined in more detail to see how different types of people react to them. The data presented here are based on a checklist of 20 symptoms. The respondents or their proxies were asked if they had had the symptom during the survey year or up to the time of the interview in the following year. If a symptom was reported, information was collected regarding if, and when, a physician had been seen about the symptom.

Table 1–7 shows that the symptoms for which people were most likely to see a doctor within a year included infection in the eyes and ears, pains in the heart, abdominal pains, sore throat and fever, and unexplained loss of ten pounds. In contrast, getting up tired and waking up with stiff and aching joints are symptoms for which the majority of people have never seen a physician. The symptoms responded to most often tend to be acute conditions involving infection or pain and/or symptoms that might be signs of serious chronic disease. Those responded to least often may seem more like a way of life than conditions necessitating treatment to some people, especially older people.

Between 1963 and 1970 there appeared to be no dramatic shifts in the population's differential response to the symptoms on the list (Table 1–7). That is, those symptoms which people were most likely to see a doctor for in 1963 generally continued to be the ones responded to most often in 1970. Conversely, symptoms which were least likely to result in a doctor visit also tended to be the same in 1963 and 1970.

However, there did appear to be an increase in the tendency of people to see a doctor for most symptoms over the seven year period (Table 1–7). Of the 20 symptoms on the list, people were more likely to have seen a doctor for 13 of them in 1970 than in 1963, less likely for four and there was no change in response for three.

In Table 1–8 we have taken the six most commonly reported symptoms to contrast how response differs according to demographic and social characteristics. In both 1963 and 1970 females were generally more likely to see a physician than were males. However, males appeared to become relatively more responsive over time. For each of the five symptoms for which people were more likely to see a doctor in 1970 than in 1963, the percentage point increase in response over the time period appeared greater for males than females.[1]

Children or the aged are most likely to see a doctor for the most

1. For the symptom sore throat and fever, there was an overall decrease in response between 1963 and 1970. The decrease for males and females was similar.

common symptoms (Table 1–8). For sore throats and backaches children are most responsive while for stiff joints and headaches those 65 and over are most responsive. Further, in the interval between 1963 and 1970 it was children and/or the aged who posted the biggest percentage point increase in percent seeing a doctor for these six commonly experienced symptoms (Table 1–8).

In 1963 whites were more likely than nonwhites to see a doctor (Table 1–8). However, the gap narrowed by 1970 as the nonwhite response became more like that for whites.

People in families headed by a person with eight years or less of formal schooling were usually less likely to see a doctor than those in families headed by someone with at least some college education in 1963 (Table 1–8). However, many of these differences were small. The picture had not changed much, relatively, by 1970. Again, those with the most education seemed more responsive than those with less education, but the overall relationship between education and seeing a doctor for symptoms continued to appear weak.

In both 1963 and 1970 (Table 1–8), the rural farm population appeared less likely to see a physician than those living elsewhere. The general magnitude of discrepancies in response between the farm population and the rest of the population did not appear to change much in this time period. The differences between central city residents and other urban dwellers were not consistent for these six symptoms according to the 1970 data.

RESPONSE TO DISABILITY DAYS

Of central concern for policy purposes is the population's use of medical care in relationship to some measure of illness level or "need" for health services. While it is extremely difficult to define and measure "need," one gross measure is the presence of symptoms, considered in the previous section. Another that has been used in social surveys is disability days—days during which people reported they stayed in bed or were otherwise unable to carry on their usual activities because of illness or injury. This section considers disability days and physician contacts during the two weeks immediately preceding the interviews of the latest study.

Table 1–9 suggests that whites are more likely to report disability than blacks regardless of residence or income. Detailed tables from a preliminary report showing disability according to age indicate that the percent reporting disability is much higher for white children than it is for black children (Andersen and Kravits, 1971). For example, 16.3 percent of white children aged one to five were reported to have experienced disability compared to only 9.5 percent of the blacks, and for those aged six to 17 the percentages are 19.4 and 11.9 respectively. In contrast, among adults blacks are more likely to report disability. This is particularly true of low income blacks. Except for urban blacks, the poor groups appear more likely to experience disability, given similar residence and race. However, age again plays an important part in this apparent relationship, according to the detailed tables. Relatively more nonpoor than poor children are actually reported to have experienced disability. Among adults, however, a higher proportion reporting disability among the low income group results in a higher overall rate for the poor.

The last column of Table 1-9 shows an important difference in the average number of disability days for persons with disability according to family income. Without exception, near poverty groups are disabled longer than the above near poverty groups. Overall, the mean number of disability days for the poverty group is one and one-half days longer.

Table 1-10 provides a picture of how people who reported disability in each population group used physicians. The first column shows some heterogeneity among the various groups with respect to the percentage of those with disability who saw a doctor. However, none of the major variables show consistent effects when controlling for the other major variables. It should be noted, however, that an income effect is particularly noticeable for children aged one to five when the detailed tables in the preliminary report (Andersen and Kravits, 1971) are examined. Above the poverty line, 56 percent of all children with disability days saw a doctor, compared with only 34 percent of those children below the poverty line.

The second data column of Table 1-10 shows the mean number of physician contacts for persons experiencing disability days. The main difference among the groups here appears to be a residential one. People living in urban areas tend to have more physician contacts than those living in rural areas.

The final data column in Table 1-10 presents the volume of physician care relative to the amount of disability people report. This column is the key data of this section from a policy standpoint, since its purpose is to look in some gross fashion at medical care relative to "need." The results are quite conclusive. The nonpoor population has considerably more physician contact per 100 disability days than does the poor population. Examination of the detailed tables (Andersen and Kravits, 1971) shows that these differences are found in every age group and are especially large for the very young and the elderly. Though not so strong as that of income, another apparent effect is that resulting from residence. The urban population consistently has more physician contacts per 100 disability days than does the rural population. There is no apparent difference in physician contacts per 100 disability days according to race. Thus, the poor and the rural population have fewer physician visits per 100 disability days but race per se does not appear related to this measure.

MEDICAL SEVERITY INDEX

The data from the previous sections on length of time since last examination and response to symptoms and disability show that some population subgroups delay longer than others in seeing a doctor. This suggests that when they do seek care it will be for more serious conditions.

The medical severity index permits this thesis to be tested more directly. The index is derived from physician evaluations of the medical urgency of the conditions of people who saw a physician in 1970.

The diagnoses for which people saw doctors were categorized by a panel of physicians with respect to whether (1) they were for preventive care, relief of symptoms or would not be affected by treatment, or whether (2) the person should or must see a doctor for such a condition. The first type of care was termed "elective" and the second "mandatory." Each respondent was classified according to whether all the diagnoses he reported were elective, some of the conditions were of one kind and some the other ("elective and mandatory care") or all were mandatory.

For the sample as a whole, approximately one-third of the respondents fell into each of the three medical severity categories (Table 1-11). Women, older adults, the poor, nonwhites, the less educated and the rural farm population had higher proportions of patients whose diagnoses were mandatory. On the other hand, those groups that had the highest proportions seeking elective care were males, children, nonpoor, the most highly educated and people who live in SMSAs outside the central city.

There was little or no difference in the proportion of whites and nonwhites seeking care for elective reasons only. These findings, then, generally support the proposition that those who are most likely to delay in seeing the doctor do, in fact, tend to be treated for more severe conditions when they do go to a physician.

SUMMARY

This chapter has examined where people get medical care and some of the reasons for that care. The summary will highlight some of the important trends discovered in comparing 1963 and 1970 findings, and major differences documented among subgroups in the population.

Trends from 1963 to 1970

In 1970 more people were reporting a clinic setting as their regular source of care and fewer were naming a particular physician. Physical examinations were reported as occurring more frequently. The main reason given for exams shifted from "symptom" to "preventive exam." The population was, generally, more likely to seek physician care in response to symptoms of illness in 1970 than in 1963.

Subgroup Differences

Females were more likely to have a regular source of care, have a recent examination, seek a physician in response to symptoms of illness and go to a physician for conditions classified as requiring physician care. Changes between 1963 and 1970 increased these differences between the sexes concerning regular source of care and examinations but reduced the difference in response to symptoms of illness.

Of all age groups, young children (infants to five years) are most likely to have a regular source of care, have had a recent examination, see a physician for particular symptoms and be given elective (rather than mandatory) care. Changes between 1963 and 1970 tended to accentuate these differences between young children and the rest of the population. Of all age groups, the elderly (65 and over) are most likely to receive care for "mandatory conditions." Their tendency to see a physician in response to symptoms of illness increased more between 1963 and 1970 than was true for the rest of the adult population.

According to income level, the low income population was least likely to have a regular source of care, have a recent examination and see a doctor in response to symptoms of illness or disability. When they did see the doctor, the conditions treated were judged most severe. Between 1963 and 1970 the position of the poor relative to the rest of the population worsened as far as having a regular source of care but improved with respect to frequency of exams and seeing a doctor in response to symptoms of illness.

The position of the nonwhite population relative to the rest of the population is generally similar to that of the low income population: they are less likely to have a regular source of care, they are more likely to report never having had a physical examination and they are treated for more severe conditions. Further, their relative position with respect to regular source of care worsened between 1963 and 1970 while their response to symptoms of illness became more like that of the rest of the population. However, nonwhites differed from the low income population in the following respects: they reported recent exams as frequently as the rest of the population and they seemed to have similar ratios of physician visits to disability days.

The findings for people in families with less educated heads were very similar to those for the low income population. One possible exception was that a reduction of differences in response to symptoms of illness between 1963 and 1970 was not as evident according to educational level as it was by income level.

According to residence, the rural farm and the central city people were least likely to have a regular source of care and, when treated, were most likely to be treated for severe conditions. They differed, however, in recency of exams and in seeing a physician for symptoms. While the rural farm population was also the residential group least likely to have recent exams or to see doctors for symptoms, the central city residents were among the most responsive in these respects. The rural population also had a lower ratio of physician visits to disability days than was true for the urban population.[2]

2. In this respect the central city residents did not differ from other urban residents and the farm population did not differ from other rural residents (Aday and Andersen, 1975:46).

Table 1-1. Regular source of medical care by selected characteristics: 1963 and 1970

Characteristic	Percent MD		Percent clinic		Percent osteopath, other		Percent no regular care		Total Percent 1963 and 1970
	1963	*1970*	*1963*	*1970*	*1963*	*1970*	*1963*	*1970*	
Sex (54)									
Male	71	65	11	18	5	4	14	13	100
Female	74	69	11	17	4	5	11	9	100
Age (1)									
1–5	78	69	11	21	3	4	8	6	100
6–17	72	67	13	20	5	5	10	8	100
18–34	69	65	10	18	4	4	17	13	100
35–54	72	69	9	14	5	4	14	13	100
55–64	75	67	9	16	4	5	12	12	100
65 and over	75	69	9	16	3	4	13	11	100
Family income (25)									
Low	63	56	17	24	4	4	16	16	100
Middle	75	68	10	17	4	5	11	10	100
High	75	74	7	14	6	4	12	8	100
Race (49)									
White	74	69	9	16	5	5	12	10	100
Nonwhite	62	51	20	30	3	3	15	16	100
Education of head (10)									
8 years or less	69	64	13	19	4	4	14	13	100
9–11 years	72	60	11	23	4	5	13	12	100
12 years	76	72	9	14	4	6	11	8	100
13 years or more	77	72	8	16	3	2	12	10	100
Residence (52)									
SMSA, central city	71 }	58 } 67	11 }	23 } 19	4 }	4 } 4	14 }	15 } 11	100
SMSA, other urban		73		13		4		10	100
Urban, non-SMSA		72		20		1		7	100
Rural, nonfarm	76	70	9	15	4	7	11	8	100
Rural, farm	77	65	9	20	3	3	11	12	100
Total	72	67	11	18	4	4	13	11	100

Regular Source of Care (51)[a]

[a] In this and subsequent tables, numbers in parentheses after variable names refer to variable definitions given in Appendix III.

Table 1-2.   Regular source of medical care by age, family income and residence: 1970[a]

Age (1)	Family Income (25)	Regular Source of Care (51)								
		Percent MD			Percent clinic			Percent no regular care		
		Residence (52)								
		SMSA, central city	Other urban	Rural	SMSA central city	Other urban	Rural	SMSA, central city	Other urban	Rural
0–17[b]	Low	26	57	64	56	27	22	18	16	14
	Middle	64	78	74	22	16	18	14	6	8
	High	77	82	81	20	17	17	3	1	2
18–64	Low	41	65	68	35	18	17	24	18	15
	Middle	62	75	72	19	15	19	18	10	9
	High	73	75	75	12	14	13	15	11	12
65 and over	Low	60	76	72	21	13	18	19	11	11
	Middle	77	80	80	18	17	14	5	4	6
	High	73	78	80	24	9	8	3	13	12
All ages	Low	41	67	68	39	18	18	21	15	14
	Middle	64	76	73	20	15	18	15	8	8
	High	74	78	78	15	15	15	10	7	8
All ages	Total	61	75	73	24	16	17	15	9	10

[a]In this table percentages are computed so that in any row the sum across a particular residence category equals 100, subject to rounding error. For example, in the first row for SMSA central city: 26 + 56 + 18 = 100.

[b]Includes infants under one year of age.

Table 1-3. Percent with clinic as regular source of care who usually see a particular doctor at the clinic by selected characteristics: 1970

	See Particular Doctor (51)		
Characteristic	*Percent yes*	*Percent no*	*Total percent*
Sex (54)			
Male	54	46	100	(1399)[b]
Female	61	39	100	(1543)
Age (1)			
1–5[a]	52	48	100	(327)
6–17	55	45	100	(952)
18–34	49	51	100	(588)
35–54	56	44	100	(508)
55–64	72	28	100	(197)
65 and over	78	22	100	(270)
Family income (25)			
Low	48	52	100	(1620)
Middle	60	40	100	(834)
High	64	36	100	(488)
Race (49)			
White	63	37	100	(1468)
Nonwhite	35	65	100	(1474)
Education of head (10)			
8 years or less	59	41	100	(1058)
9–11 years	61	39	100	(858)
12 years	57	43	100	(624)
13 years or more	51	49	100	(402)
Residence (52)			
SMSA, central city	46	54	100	(1896)
SMSA, other urban	50	50	100	(286)
Urban, non-SMSA	78	22	100	(156)
Rural, nonfarm	57	43	100	(375)
Rural, farm	84	16	100	(229)
Total	57	43	100	(2942)

[a]Excludes infants under one year of age.

[b]In parentheses are the unweighted numbers of observations which can be used in combination with the procedures described in Appendix I to calculate standard errors of the 1970 estimates. Since the 1970 sample is a weighted sample, these numbers should *not* be used for combining subcategories.

Table 1-4. Length of time since the last physical examination by selected characteristics: 1963 and 1970

					Time Since Last Examination				
	Percent one year or less		*Percent between one and five years*		*Percent over five years*		*Percent never*		*Total Percent*
Characteristic	*1963*	*1970*	*1963*	*1970*	*1963*	*1970*	*1963*	*1970*	
Sex (54)									
Male	52	52	30	32	8	10	10	6	100
Female	54	57	29	29	7	9	10	5	100
Age (1)									
1–5	65	72	20	18	—	—	15	9	100
6–17	49	53	27	31	6	7	18	10	100
18–34	56	57	32	32	6	8	6	3	100
35–54	50	48	33	35	11	15	6	2	100
55–64	50	54	32	28	11	14	7	4	100
65 and over	53	52	28	29	11	15	8	4	100
Family income (25)									
Low	45	51	26	29	10	12	19	8	100
Middle	51	54	32	32	7	9	10	5	100
High	59	57	29	31	6	9	6	4	100
Race (49)									
White	53	54	30	31	8	10	9	5	100
Nonwhite	55	57	25	26	4	7	16	10	100
Education of head (10)									
8 years or less	46	50	27	29	9	12	18	9	100
9–11 years	52	52	32	34	8	9	8	5	100
12 years	55	53	30	33	7	10	8	4	100
13 years or more	62	63	30	27	4	7	4	3	100
Residence (52)									
SMSA, central city ⎤	⎤	57 ⎤	⎤	30 ⎤	⎤	9 ⎤	⎤	4 ⎤	⎤
SMSA, other urban ⎬	56	56 ⎬56	29	31 ⎬30	7	9 ⎬9	8	4 ⎬5	100
Urban, non-SMSA ⎦	⎦	53	⎦	30	⎦	11	⎦	6	⎦
Rural, nonfarm	50	52	32	32	8	10	10	6	100
Rural, farm	38	49	26	26	8	13	28	12	100
Total	53	55	29	31	8	10	10	5	100

Table 1-5. Length of time since the last physical examination by person's regular source of medical care: 1963 and 1970

| | *Time Since Last Examination* | | | | | | | | |
| | *Percent one year or less* | | *Percent between one and five years* | | *Percent over five years* | | *Percent never* | | |
Regular Source of Medical Care (51)	*1963*	*1970*	*1963*	*1970*	*1963*	*1970*	*1963*	*1970*	*Total Percent*
Specialist	61	69	28	23	4	6	7	3	100 (2144)[a]
General Practitioner	52	54	29	33	8	9	11	5	100 (4427)
Clinic	52	54	27	31	7	9	14	7	100 (2842)
Osteopath, other	53	54	27	33	10	8	10	5	100 (403)
No regular care	39	28	36	35	18	25	12	12	100 (1547)

[a]In parentheses are the unweighted numbers of observations which can be used in combination with the procedures described in Appendix I to calculate standard errors of the 1970 estimates. Since the 1970 sample is a weighted sample, these numbers should *not* be used as weights for combining subcategories.

Table 1-6.   Reason for last physical examination by selected characteristics: 1963 and 1970

Characteristic	Reason for Examination (50)						
	Percent symptom 1963	Percent symptom 1970	Percent required 1963	Percent required 1970	Percent preventive 1963	Percent preventive 1970	Total percent
Age and Sex (1) (54)							
Male	35	30	40	38	25	32	100
1–5	34	26	14	14	52	60	100
6–17	26	28	43	39	31	34	100
18–34	23	22	61	59	16	20	100
35–54	42	34	39	38	19	29	100
55–64	51	37	27	31	22	31	100
65 and over	60	41	14	19	26	40	100
Female	43	34	24	23	33	43	100
1–5	32	27	14	17	54	56	100
6–17	31	29	38	32	31	39	100
18–34	37	26	33	33	30	41	100
35–54	49	41	17	14	34	45	100
55–64	57	44	15	16	28	40	100
65 and over	63	44	7	14	30	42	100
Family income (25)							
Low	51	39	24	28	25	33	100
Medium	38	31	35	33	27	35	100
High	34	28	34	29	32	42	100
Race (49)							
White	38	31	32	31	30	37	100
Nonwhite	44	32	31	26	25	40	100
Education of head (10)							
8 years or less	51	41	29	27	20	32	100
9–11 years	41	34	30	32	29	34	100
12 years	34	28	35	32	30	39	100
13 years or more	28	26	34	31	38	43	100
Residence (52)							
SMSA, central city ⎫		33		34		33	100
SMSA, other urban ⎬ 37		27 ⎱ 31	32	27 ⎱ 30	31	46 ⎱ 39	100
Urban, non-SMSA ⎭		36		28		37	100
Rural, nonfarm	41	32	32	32	27	36	100
Rural, farm	49	43	31	32	21	25	100
Total	39	32	32	31	29	37	100

Table 1-7. Length of time since seeing a physician for symptoms occurring during survey year: 1963 and 1970

Symptom[c]	Percent Seeing Physician Within Calendar Year 1963	1970	Percent Seeing Physician Earlier 1963	1970	Percent Never Seeing Physician[b] 1963	1970	Total Percent	
Unexpected bleeding	49	56	17	13	34	32	100	(891)[d]
Unexpected loss of ten pounds	56	58	14	6	30	36	100	(1363)
Shortness of breath	46	53	19	14	35	33	100	(1991)
Pains in the heart	55	62	20	16	25	23	100	(816)
Abdominal pains	55	61	14	17	31	22	100	(1514)
Pains in any joint	49	49	19	22	32	29	100	(879)
Cough for weeks	53	53	12	13	35	34	100	(497)
Sudden weakness or faintness	53	60	16	14	31	26	100	(1140)
Repeated vomiting	54	53	6	7	40	40	100	(1813)
Infections in eyes or ears	64	68	16	14	20	18	100	(1058)
Repeated indigestion	44	37	20	24	36	40	100	(1379)
Waking up with stiff joints	31	37	15	17	54	47	100	(267)
Frequent headaches	40	45	17	16	43	39	100	(755)
Feeling tired for weeks	42	50	16	12	42	38	100	(1110)
Diarrhea four or five days	50	46	12	11	38	43	100	(469)
Skin rash	53	53	25	24	22	23	100	(1586)
Frequent backaches	44	48	23	22	33	29	100	(792)
Getting up tired	31	37	10	11	59	52	100	(431)
Sore throat, fever	61	58	6	10	33	32	100	(790)
Nose stopped up	47	48	14	21	39	31	100	(992)

[a]Includes persons who saw physician in the year following the survey year up to time of interview. The majority of the interviewing was done in February of the year following the survey year.

[b]Includes cases where it was not known if doctor was seen.

[c]These symptoms are listed in order of increasing severity as judged by a panel of 40 physicians (Taylor, Aday and Andersen, 1975).

[d]In parentheses are the unweighted numbers of observations which can be used in combination with the procedures described in Appendix I to calculate standard errors of the 1970 estimates. Since the 1970 sample is a weighted sample, these numbers should *not* be used as weights for combining subcategories.

Table 1-8. Percent people with selected symptoms seeing a doctor within the year[a] by selected characteristics: 1963 and 1970

Characteristics	Percent getting up tired 1963	1970	Percent sore throat, fever 1963	1970	Percent waking up with stiff joints 1963	1970	Percent frequent headaches 1963	1970	Percent sudden weakness or faintness 1963	1970	Percent frequent backaches 1963	1970
Sex (54)												
Male	24	31	63	60	27	33	31	43	46	61	39	45
Female	35	40	60	56	35	39	44	46	57	59	47	50
Age (1)												
1–17	29	41	65	62	33	38	44	40	54	65	47	64
18–64	32	35	57	54	30	34	39	45	53	59	44	48
65 and over	32	43	45	49	36	45	41	47	54	61	45	48
Family income (25)												
Low	31	40	46	56	30	39	33	44	50	59	42	45
Middle	32	35	61	56	30	37	42	45	54	62	45	48
High	31	36	67	62	34	34	43	46	57	60	45	53
Race (49)												
White	31	38	62	59	32	36	40	46	55	60	45	48
Nonwhite	31	34	55	53	29	39	38	42	45	58	40	53
Education of head (10)												
8 years or less	30	39	57	55	30	37	38	39	54	59	42	47
9–11 years	30	37	61	51	33	40	37	50	58	56	45	46
12 years	33	36	62	57	34	34	38	40	51	60	47	46
13 years or more	34	37	68	68	33	38	52	55	51	65	51	57
Residence (52)												
SMSA, central city	31	38 } 37	61	53 } 58	32	36 } 35	42	52 } 48	54	61 } 62	44	50 } 48
SMSA, other urban		37		57		34		47		63		43
Urban, non-SMSA		32		74		34		40		61		53
Rural, nonfarm	36	40	64	59	34	43	39	43	54	59	47	51
Rural, farm	25	29	53	56	26	32	32	29	51	46	42	43
Total	31	37	61	58	32	37	40	45	53	60	45	48

[a]Includes persons who saw physician in the year following the survey year up to time of interview.

Table 1-9. Disability days during a two week period by income, residence and race: 1971[a,b]

Family Income (26)	Residence (52)	Race (49)	Percent with One or More Disability Days (8)		Mean Number of Disability Days for Those with Disability (8)	
Above near poverty	Urban	White	17	(2892)[c]	4.9	(491)[c]
Above near poverty	Urban	Black	17	(1188)	4.5	(132)
Above near poverty	Rural	White	16	(2356)	5.2	(353)
Above near poverty	Rural	Black	7	(81)	d	(6)
Below near poverty	Urban	White	22	(1444)	6.6	(273)
Below near poverty	Urban	Black	15	(1498)	6.8	(305)
Below near poverty	Rural	White	20	(1163)	6.5	(221)
Below near poverty	Rural	Black	18	(268)	6.4	(45)

[a]Revision of Table B in Andersen and Kravits (1971:11).

[b]Excludes infants under one year old.

[c]In parentheses are the unweighted numbers of observations which can be used in combination with the procedures described in Appendix I to calculate standard errors of the 1970 estimates. Since the 1970 sample is a weighted sample, these numbers should *not* be used as weights for combining subcategories.

[d]Based on fewer than 25 unweighted observations.

Table 1-10. Contacts with physicians by people with disability days during two week period by income, residence and race: 1971[a,b]

Family Income (26)	Residence (52)	Race (49)	Percent with Disability Contacting a Physician (8)	Mean Number of Physician Contacts for Persons with Disability	Physician Contacts per 100 Disability Days (41)
Above near poverty	Urban	White (491)[c]	44	0.8	17
Above near poverty	Urban	Black (132)	36	0.8	17
Above near poverty	Rural	White (353)	41	0.7	14
Above near poverty	Rural	Black (6)	d	d	d
Below near poverty	Urban	White (273)	33	0.8	12
Below near poverty	Urban	Black (305)	40	0.7	11
Below near poverty	Rural	White (221)	39	0.6	9
Below near poverty	Rural	Black (45)	37	0.6	9

[a]Revision of Table C in Andersen and Kravits (1971:14).

[b]Excludes infants under one year old.

[c]In parentheses are the unweighted numbers of observations which can be used in combination with the procedures described in Appendix I to calculate standard errors of the 1970 estimates. Since the 1970 sample is a weighted sample, these numbers should *not* be used as weights for combining subcategories.

[d]Based on fewer than 25 unweighted observations.

Table 1-11. Severity (53) of conditions treated by a physician during the year by selected characteristics: 1970

Characteristic	*Percent Treated for Conditions Requiring:*			
	Mandatory care only	*Both mandatory and elective care*	*Elective care only*	*Total*
Sex (54)				
Male	30	30	40	100
Female	33	33	35	101
Age (1)				
0–5	15	32	53	100
6–17	23	23	54	100
18–34	32	34	34	100
35–54	31	35	33	99
55–64	47	32	21	100
65 and over	50	34	15	99
Family income (26)				
Above near poverty	30	32	38	100
Below near poverty	39	29	33	101
Race (49)				
White	31	32	37	100
Nonwhite	38	23	39	101
Education of head (10)				
8 years or less	39	31	30	100
9–11 years	32	31	37	100
12 years	30	32	39	101
13 years or more	27	33	40	100
Residence (52)				
SMSA, central city	33	32	35	100
SMSA, other urban	27	32	40	99
Urban, non-SMSA	32	31	37	100
Rural, nonfarm	32	31	37	100
Rural, farm	38	29	33	100
Total	31	32	37	100

Chapter 2

Type and Volume
of Health Services
Received

The previous chapter dealt with use in a general fashion, in terms of people's usual source of care and conditions which lead them to seek services. This chapter deals with more direct and traditional measures of use of physicians, hospitals and dentists.

PHYSICIAN VISITS

An important measure of use of medical services is the percentage of the population who see a physician during the year. It is probably the clearest measure of gross exposure of the public to a physician's decisions. Obviously, the physician cannot prescribe care until he encounters a patient. Roughly two-thirds of the American population see a physician at least once each year.

Table 2-1 shows that in the period from 1958 through 1963 there was little or no change in the proportion of the population who saw a physician. Between 1963 and 1970, however, there was a small increase. The increase between 1963 and 1970 holds true for both sexes, though the proportion of females seeing a physician was higher than the proportion of males in each study. The increase was not consistent among age groups. Most of it was accounted for by people 55 and over.

A substantially greater proportion of the low income population was seeing a physician in 1970 than was true in 1963 (Table 2-1). The relative increase for middle income people was considerably less, while there was apparently no change in the proportion seeing a physician in the upper income group in 1970. Despite the relative gain by the poor, the proportion of the low income group seeing a physician in 1970 was still somewhat lower than the highest income group.

In 1970 the white population was clearly more likely to see a physician than was the nonwhite population (Table 2–1). Still, between 1963 and 1970 the gap closed considerably.

As education of the family head increases the probability that people in the family will see a doctor also increases (Table 2–1). However, as with income and race, the proportion of those least likely to see a physician (the less educated) increased between 1963 and 1970 while the percent seeing a doctor for those most likely to do so (the better educated) remained about the same over this interval.

People living in the central city of SMSAs and their rural counterparts on farms appeared less likely to see a doctor than other urban dwellers and rural nonfarm residents in 1970 (Table 2–1). Between 1963 and 1970 the percent seeing a doctor increased for all types of residents but the increase appeared greatest for the rural farm population.

The 1963 study showed that children from lower income families were considerably less likely to see a physician during the year than those from higher income families. These differences in use by income tended to disappear for older age groups. Table 2–2 suggests that in the interval since 1963 the gap has narrowed considerably. Among children one to five years of age the proportion seeing a doctor increased in the low income groups but actually appeared to decrease slightly in the middle and high income categories. The increase in proportions seeing a doctor for all children in the six to 17 age group was also primarily accounted for by the low income children. Thus, in 1970 the difference in the proportion of children seeing a doctor according to income, while still considerable, was nonetheless substantially smaller than had been the case in 1963.

Those 18 to 54 with low incomes were also more likely to see a doctor in 1970 than in 1963. The percentage increase among the poor was least for people 55 and over (Table 2–2). In contrast, among higher income people the only age groups where there were substantial increases were 55 to 64 and 65 and over.

These trends correspond to those which might be expected as a result of the implementation of Medicaid and Medicare in July 1966. Medicaid and most health center programs begun since 1963 were designed to serve the low income population of all ages. Consequently, decreases in the "health utilization deficit" of the poor might be expected. In contrast, the Medicare program was designed to benefit people of all incomes who were 65 and over. Some argue that features of the program, such as payment of the physicians on a fee for service basis, deductibles and coinsurance make it primarily a "middle class" program. The increased proportions of higher income elderly seeking care support such an argument.

Table 2-3 allows us to examine the joint influence of family income, age and residence on seeing a physician. Income is directly related to the proportion of children seeing a physician regardless of residence. On the other hand, residence, controlling for income, does not seem to be as important, although those urban children not living in central cities show a higher proportion seeing a doctor than children living elsewhere.

Adults aged 18 to 64 see the doctor in about the same proportions for all income-residence combinations (Table 2-3). For low and middle income groups 65 and over, the central city population is least likely to see a doctor. However, among the elderly with high family incomes, those living in the central city appear most likely to see a doctor.

The doctor's office is by far the most frequent place of visit. Eighty-five percent of all outpatient visits in 1970 were in a doctor's office (Table 2-4). Table 2-4 shows the shift in visit site between 1958 and 1970. Home visits decreased as a proportion of all visits from 11 percent to 2 percent in this time period. In contrast, office and clinic visits increased as a proportion of the total.

Traditionally, home visits have provided an important segment of care to those persons 65 and over. In 1970, old people were still more likely to be seen at home than younger patients (Table 2-4). Nevertheless, there was a major shift from home to office for the oldest group between 1958 and 1970. Home visits decreased by 18 percentage points, while office visits increased by about the same proportion of all visits.

Table 2-5 provides a more detailed picture of where various types of people were having physician visits in 1970. As mentioned previously, home visits are most likely for the aged. Visits in outpatient departments of hospitals are most common for low income, non-white and central city residents. Emergency room and "other visits," which include visits at child health clinics, are the most frequent types of visits for young children up to five years of age.

Table 2-6 shows that the mean number of physician visits per person per year has actually decreased over the last 12 years.[1] This

1. This downward trend is particularly noteworthy for people 65 and over. The enactment of Medicare in 1966, which largely removed financial barriers to physician visits once a deductible had been met, might have been expected to result in an increased rather than a decreased mean number of physician visits for this age group.

general decrease of about one-half of a physician visit per person was mainly the result of decreased visits by females. However, in each time period the average number of visits per person for females exceeded those for males. Prenatal visits account for a portion of the extra visits by females.

The trend between 1963 and 1970 of decreasing mean number of visits per person appeared for every group except for children under six and adults 55 to 64. Some consistent differences among age groups are found in each time period (Table 2-6). The mean number of visits for children from birth to age five is higher than that for children aged six to 17. The latter group has the lowest mean number of visits of any age group. The number of visits among adults increases in the older age groups. However, our data suggest that number of visits for those 55 to 64 became more similar to the number for those 65 and over between 1958 and 1970.

The low income group reports considerably more physician visits than the middle and high income groups in 1970 (Table 2-6). This finding for mean number of visits is exactly opposite to the relationship between family income and the fact of seeing a physician. In other words, the poor appear to be less likely to see a doctor, but once .they make a physician contact, the volume of services is on average considerably higher. In contrast, the average number of visits for whites exceeds that for nonwhites by one-half a visit (Table 2-6). Thus, whites are not only more likely to see a physician but also have a higher mean number of visits. Still, between 1963 and 1970 the gap in mean number of visits between the races narrowed as the mean number for whites decreased while it increased for nonwhites.

Visits according to educational level show relationships more similar to those for race than income level. That is, while the gap narrowed considerably between 1963 and 1970, the group with the largest number of visits in the former period (the best educated) still had more visits in the latter period as well.

People living in urban areas see a physician more often than those living in rural areas (Table 2-6). It might be recalled that the central city dwellers and the rural farm population were least likely to see a doctor during the year according to Table 2-1. While the rural farm population is also the group with the fewest physician visits, central city dwellers are above average for mean number of visits.

It should also be noted that while groups with the fewest visits in 1963 according to other social and demographic characteristics (low income, low education, nonwhite) increased their visits by 1970, the farm population experienced a decrease during the interval.

Table 2-7 shows the joint effects of income and age on physician visits for 1970. The pattern that emerges is very different for children and adults. For children from birth to age 17 the mean number of visits rises consistently with increasing income. For the group 18 to 64 the reverse is true; the mean number of visits actually decreases with increasing income. For the elderly the mean number of visits is fairly constant over income groups.

The second half of Table 2–7 gives the mean number of visits for those persons who actually saw a doctor. This measure allows us to look at mean number of visits controlling for the effect of the proportion of people in a given group who saw a physician. Visits per person seeing a doctor are relatively higher for the low income groups. Thus, for children who actually saw a doctor, there is less of a deficit for the low income groups than there appeared to be when looking at visits per person-year. For adults in every age group, the mean number of visits per person seeing the doctor is considerably higher for the low income group than for the upper income groups.

Table 2–8 shows age-income relationships to physician visits for both whites and nonwhites. Not controlling for age, mean number of visits per person-year is greater for whites than for nonwhites for every income group. However, within age groups this is not always the case. Low income nonwhite adults appear to see the doctor more often than do low income white adults. The mean number of visits per person-year, however, continues to be higher in the white population for all children and adults in the higher income groups.

The second half of Table 2–8 shows the volume of visits for those people seeing a doctor. The relative use of physicians by nonwhites compared to whites increases when contrasted with the findings for visits per person-year. For low income people of all ages the mean number of visits for the nonwhites tends to exceed that for whites. For the middle and high income groups, however, the mean number of visits per person seeing the doctor continues to be higher for the whites than for the nonwhites. The mean number of visits per person seeing a doctor not considering age and income is very similar for whites and nonwhites.

HOSPITAL USE

In some respects, the monitoring of general hospital services use by the population is more crucial than the monitoring of physicians' services. This is because of the serious nature of illnesses treated in the hospital and the extraordinary expense of hospital services.

Table 2–9 provides a view of trends for hospital admissions per 100 person-years over the entire span of years covered by the four national studies. These trend data show that there has been a rise in hospital admissions during this 17 year period. The increase has been experienced by both males and females. The female rate includes admissions for pregnancies and is in each time period considerably greater than that for males.

The change in admission rate for different age groups over the time spanned by these studies has not been uniform. The traditional pattern is relatively low rates of admission for children; relatively high rates in the 18 to 34 category, which includes most pregnancy admissions; a dropoff in the middle years; and an increase for the aged population. Although this general pattern exists in each time period, trend data suggest that most of the overall increase in admission rates has been accounted for by the older age groups, 55 to 64 and 65 and older. While Medicare might account for a portion of the increase for the 65 and over group between 1963 and 1970, it is obvious that this is a trend that began before the passage of Medicare and applies not only to those eligible for Medicare but also to those in the age group 55 to 64. A shorter term trend that should be pointed out between 1963 and 1970 is the increase in admission rates for children from birth to five years old.

Table 2–9 also suggests some rather definite changes in the relationship between income and admission over time. The 1953 study showed a relatively flat distribution over all income groups. In 1958 the lower income groups tended to have higher admission rates. The two later studies have accentuated this trend, so that by 1970 the lowest income groups had a hospital admission rate of about twice that of the highest income groups. Medicare and Medicaid may well account for some of these basic changes. However, again it should be pointed out that the changes we are observing were beginning to take place before the passage of these programs.

The admission rate for the white population exceeded that for the nonwhite in 1970 (Table 2–9). Despite the relatively high correlation between income and race, there are different relations between each characteristic and admissions: low income people had high admission rates, but nonwhites (who also tend to be low income) had relatively low admission rates. The younger mean age of the nonwhite population accounts for part of this discrepancy.

Over time the most consistent relationship between residence and hospital admissions has been the high rate for the rural nonfarm population and the relatively low rate for the population living in the large urban areas (Table 2–9). Between 1963 and 1970 the main increases appeared to be in the large urban and rural farm areas.

One possible reason for the high admission rates among the lowest income group is that older people who have higher admission rates tend to cluster in the low income groups. However, when we look at the rates for various age levels in 1963 and 1970 we see that this is not the entire answer (Table 2–10). Among people aged 18 to 54 the rates for the lowest income group still exceed the rates for other income groups. For children from birth to age 17 this is also the case in 1970. In 1963 the rates for low income children had been lower than for other children. For older persons 55 and over the relationship between income and use is not consistent. Between 1963 and 1970 the greatest gains in use were found among the higher income older people. Medicare might explain part of this trend if in fact it has been of particular benefit to the better-off elderly population.

Table 2–11 shows general trends in length of stay and total hospital days for the population from 1953 to 1970. Overall, length of stay remained relatively constant over the period. Because of increasing admission rates, total number of hospital days increased from 87 to 100 hospital days per 100 people per year.

Both length of stay and total hospital days tend to increase with increasing age (Table 2–11). Over time, these differences have grown larger. Between 1953 and 1970 length of stay decreased for people under 55 and increased slightly for those 55 and over. Total days of hospital care decreased for children, remained about the same for adults 18 to 54 and increased substantially for those 55 and over. Length of stay for females was about one day longer than it was for males throughout the period. Number of hospital days per 100 persons per year increased for both sexes but the increase appeared greater for females than males.

HOSPITALIZED SURGERY

Treatment by hospitalized surgery represents a substantial part of the health services delivered in this country. Surgical admissions account for over one-third of all admissions to short term general hospitals. Surgical rates have potential value for monitoring the population's use of services, given the concern in this country about the performance of "unnecessary" surgery. In addition, there is concern that some population groups are not getting "necessary" surgery.

Table 2–12 indicates that in-hospital surgical procedure rates increased in 1970 compared to the rates of 1958 or 1963. This was true for both sexes, with females continuing to have a higher rate than males. In each time period the surgical rates were generally higher in the older age groups than in the younger age groups (Table 2–12).

The findings from each of the three studies show relatively low rates for surgical procedures in the highest income groups (Table 2–12). Between 1963 and 1970 the increase seems to have been largely accounted for by increasing surgical procedure rates in the lower income groups. Thus, the overall pattern in 1970 is somewhat different from what it was in 1963. The lowest income groups in 1970 have the highest general hospital admission rates for surgery while in 1963 the lowest income groups had a rate very similar to that of the highest income groups.

White-nonwhite differences in surgical procedure rates appear negligible in Table 2–12. The differences according to residence also appear to be small. In earlier time periods the rural farm population appeared to have a considerably lower rate but this no longer appears to be the case.

In monitoring trends in surgery, indicators of surgeons' ability to keep abreast of new knowledge and to apply it effectively are of special concern. Heart surgery, transplanting of organs and similar procedures are dramatic examples of the intricacy of some modern-day procedures. Surgical effectiveness is directly related not only to new medical knowledge but also to the long and complicated training presently necessary before a physician becomes a surgical specialist. Therefore, some characteristics of the physicians performing surgery in each of the studies are considered below.

Involvement in surgery can be assessed by considering the physician's own classification of his or her practice. The distribution in Table 2–13 shows the type of practice reported by physicians performing surgery in 1963 and 1970. In 1963, 79 percent of the surgical procedures were performed by physicians reporting primary or secondary specialties involving surgery. By 1970 this proportion had increased to 87 percent.

Sixty percent of all hospitalized surgery in 1970 was performed by board-certified specialists—physicans who have had some seven years of training and practice beyond college and medical school (Table 2–14). Thirty-five percent were certified by a surgical examining board and an additional 25 percent were certified by boards for specialties that included surgery. With the passage of time, a greater proportion of surgical procedures is being performed by board-certified specialists. The proportion rose from 37 percent in 1953 to 46 percent in 1963 and to 60 percent in 1970. Thus, a large and growing proportion of all surgery is performed by physicians with considerable training and experience.

An issue of continuing interest is the characteristics of physicians performing more complicated and less complicated surgery. Table

2–15 shows that between 1963 and 1970 the percent of the common and usually less complicated procedures—tonsillectomies, adenoidectomies and appendectomies—performed by physicians with special interest in surgery increased from 42 percent to 57 percent. These physicians performed 84 percent of all other operations in 1963 and 90 percent of such operations in 1970. Apparently, most complicated surgery is performed by physicians who at least claim a special interest in a surgical specialty. A considerable proportion of the less complicated surgery was performed by physicians not claiming such an interest in 1970. However, this proportion appears to have been decreasing fairly rapidly between 1963 and 1970.

OBSTETRICAL CARE

A traditional measure of preventive medicine is the use of physicians' services by pregnant women. A commonly accepted norm is that a visit should be made to a physician during the first trimester of the pregnancy. Table 2–16 shows the proportion of mothers having live births during each of the survey years who saw a doctor in the first trimester. This proportion increased in each successive study, but rate of increase has not been consistent for all income and education categories.

With respect to income, Table 2–16 indicates that, over the 17 year period, increases in the proportion of pregnant women seeing a physician by the end of the first trimester have been restricted to the low and middle income groups. In contrast, the proportion among high income women has remained relatively stable over this time period. Similar trends are apparent with respect to education; that is, major increases have been made by the women with less education. The results of these two trends are that by 1970 we find much smaller differences by income and education categories. In fact, it is no longer clear that the highest income and education groups are most likely to see a physician by the end of the first trimester.

In 1970 differences still existed according to race and residence (Table 2–16). Expectant mothers in the central cities and those who are nonwhite are least likely to see a physician during the first trimester. In contrast, those women living in urban but non-SMSA areas and those living in rural areas but not on farms appear most likely to see a physician by the end of the third month of pregnancy.

Improved prenatal care is indicated by the increasing number of prenatal visits as well as by earlier initial exposure to a physician. With each succeeding study, the median number has increased starting with 8.4 in 1953 and reaching 10.9 in 1970 (Table 2–17). In 1953 there was a direct relationship between income and educational level and median number of visits. During the ensuing years the medians for the highest income and educational groups changed little. However, the number of visits of the middle and lower levels continued to increase, so that by 1970 the discrepancies according to income and education had largely been eliminated. Also, in 1970 differences in number of visits according to race and residence appeared minor.

The 1970 study showed an apparent cessation in the trend toward shorter length of hospital stay for delivery (Table 2–18). While the median decreased from 4.5 to 3.7 between 1953 and 1963, it remained at 3.7 in 1970. In 1953 median length of stay was over twice as long for the highest income group as for the lowest. These differences converged with each study, so that by 1970 the discrepancy had been reduced to seven-tenths of a day. In 1970 there was little apparent difference in median length of stay by race and no significant differences according to residence.

DENTAL CARE

For the purposes of monitoring the public's use of health services, dental care provides a marked contrast to most of the other services we have examined. It is generally viewed by the public as more "elective" and less "necessary" than physicians' services. However, by most objective standards, the level of unmet need for dental care is high, possibly even higher than for physicians' services. Dental care is also a service paid for largely out-of-pocket by the consumer with only very limited coverage by third party payers.

Table 2–19 shows a consistent increase in the proportion of the population seeing a dentist in each period from 1953 through 1970. While this proportion has been increasing for both males and females, the relative increase appears to have been greater for males. By 1970 the traditional discrepancy between the sexes—with females being more likely to see a dentist—had largely disappeared.

The unusual nature of dental care compared to other medical services is best pointed out by the established pattern among the age categories in percent seeing a dentist. The so-called "inverted U" pattern can be noted in each survey year, with the youngest and oldest age groups least likely to see a dentist. Over the 17 year time period there was an increase in the proportion seeing a dentist in each age category. However, the rate of increase, particularly in the period from 1963 to 1970, was greatest among those groups least likely to see a dentist. Consequently, over the 17 year period the percent seeing a dentist has doubled for the youngest age category and the oldest age category while the increase has been much more modest for the intervening age groups.

The traditional relationship between use of services and income which used to exist for hospital, physician and dental care exists today only for dental care. Looking at broad income categories, the percent using a dentist has increased for each income group. It is probably true that the relative increase has been greater for the lowest income groups than the higher income groups. Even in 1970, however, tremendous differences still existed. Thus, we find a person in the highest income group has a probability of seeing a dentist within a year about three times that of a low income person.

The major discrepancies with respect to income are also found according to race and education. Table 2–19 shows that the proportion of whites seeing a dentist is twice that for the nonwhite population, and the most educated group is more than twice as likely to see a dentist as the least educated. Differences exist with respect to residence, but these are not so large. Still, residents of SMSAs not living in the central cities are more likely to see a dentist than any other residential group.

Table 2–20 shows age and income effects simultaneously. For the youngest and oldest age groups, the proportion using a dentist tended to increase between 1963 and 1970 for all income groups. The actual percentage increase tended to be greatest for the low income groups. For the other age categories the increases in the seven year period were accounted for almost entirely by the low income groups. In fact, for the higher income categories, there appeared to be an actual decrease in the percentage of the group seeing a dentist in 1970 compared to 1963.

Table 2–21 provides mean number of visits per person per year for selected social and demographic characteristics. There is little in this part of the table which could not have been predicted, knowing the general magnitude of visits. However, when we look at mean number of visits per person seeing a dentist in the second column in the table, some new relationships are indicated. First, children aged one to five who do see the dentist have more visits than the visits per person-year might suggest. Further, people 65 and over seeing the dentist have about the same number of visits as people in the intermediate age categories.

For social characteristics, some of the changes in relative magnitude are even more pronounced (Table 2–21). For example, it appears that the mean number of visits for persons seeing a dentist might actually be higher for nonwhites than it is for whites. Also, the mean number of visits for low income and less well-educated people who see the dentist seems to be as high as for the rest of the population. In other words, once these groups get into the system, they appear to consume as much care as other groups. This was also found for physician care and was implied for hospital care. The finding for central city residents reinforces this general trend. The only major population groups not supporting this trend are the rural groups. People in rural areas were less likely to see a dentist than were urban people. Those who do see a dentist from rural areas also have a smaller mean number of visits.

SUMMARY

This chapter has considered the utilization rates for physician visits, hospital admissions, inpatient surgery, obstetrical care and dental visits. This summary presents major trends shown by the four studies and salient differences discovered among subgroups in the population.

Trends

In the period between 1958 and 1970 these studies show the proportion of people seeing a doctor increasing slightly, while the mean number of visits per person actually decreased. The hospital admission rate rose between 1953 and 1970, while the length of stay was similar in 1953 and 1970. The inpatient surgical rate appeared higher in 1970 than it had been in earlier studies. The proportion of surgical procedures performed by board-certified surgeons continually increased. Between 1953 and 1970 the proportion of women having live births who saw a doctor in the first trimester of pregnancy increased, as did the median number of physician visits per live birth. The percent of the population seeing a dentist increased over the period covered by the studies, but the rate of increase appears greater in recent periods than it was earlier.

Subgroup Differences

This chapter, as well as the previous one, presents a mixed picture of the nation's success in obtaining a more equitable distribution of health care among various social groups. Findings from this report that support the view that the United States is attaining equalization of health care opportunity include:

1. The gap between the percentage of low and high income people seeing a physician during the year narrowed considerably between

1963 and 1970. Most of the change was accounted for by an increase in the percentage of low income persons under age 55 seeing a doctor.

2. The increase in the proportion of the population seeing a doctor between 1963 and 1970 among all age groups appeared greatest for the elderly.
3. Once they see a physician, low income people average more visits than those of higher income.
4. For those people seeing the doctor, the mean number of visits by nonwhites is almost as great as the mean for whites.
5. The lowest income people were about twice as likely to be admitted to a hospital as those with the highest incomes in 1970, while in 1953 the admission rates were much the same for all income groups.
6. In 1953, the chances that pregnant women in the lowest income and education classes would see a doctor in the first trimester of pregnancy were less than one-half the chances for women with a college education and high family incomes. By 1970, most pregnant women, regardless of income or education, were seeing a doctor during the first trimester.
7. By 1970 the mean number of dental visits for persons seeing the dentist did not differ greatly according to income or race.

However, findings which contradict this picture of equalization of health care opportunities include:

1. A smaller proportion of the children living in central cities and rural areas see a doctor than is true for other children in the population.
2. The rural farm population is not only less likely to see a physician than the rest of the population, but also has on average fewer visits.
3. Although nonwhites and central city residents have longer lengths of stay once they are admitted to the hospital, their admission rates still were lower than those for the rest of the population in 1970.
4. Expectant mothers in the central cities are less likely to see a physician during the first trimester of pregnancy than are pregnant women living elsewhere.
5. Large differences still exist in the percent of the population seeing a dentist by income and race. The highest income group is three times more likely to see a dentist during a year's period than is the lowest income group. Whites are twice as likely as are nonwhites to see a dentist.

In conclusion, while great improvements in health care for disadvantaged groups have occurred over the last ten to 20 years, these groups are still not equal to the remainder of the population. In fact, in order to be "equal," they may well have to exceed higher income groups in their use of services to compensate for a greater rate of illness and disability.

A POSTSCRIPT:
CHANGES FROM 1970 TO 1974

Some significant changes in the utilization of health services have taken place in the United States since 1970. While it is not the general purpose of this report to provide "up to the minute" estimates using secondary sources, these recent changes extend and clarify trends documented by the earlier CHAS-NORC studies and provide additional information on progress toward equitable distribution of health services in the U.S. Consequently, published and unpublished data from the health interview survey of the National Center for Health Statistics (NCHS) for the years 1970 and 1974 are used here.

NCHS data, rather than CHAS data, are used for the 1970 estimates because the categories of socioeconomic variables used by NCHS do not always correspond to those used by CHAS. Further, there are some differences between the 1970 estimates of NCHS and those of CHAS. Since the main purpose of this section is to examine change between 1970 and 1974, it is appropriate to use NCHS estimates in both periods to limit the extent to which apparent changes over time actually reflect different study methodologies in the two periods. The major difference in operational definitions between NCHS and CHAS for the variables shown in Table 2–22 is that the NCHS estimates for percent of persons with physician visits and mean number of physician visits include telephone calls, while calls are excluded in the CHAS estimates. As a result, the estimated mean number of visits is about 0.6 visits higher using NCHS data than it is using CHAS data. Table 2–22 shows changes in various measures of utilization according to sex, age, race, family income, education of family head and place of residence.

Percent of the population seeing a physician increased from 72 percent to 75 percent between 1970 and 1974. Relative increases were greatest for the youngest and oldest, females, nonwhites, lower income groups and the least educated.

Mean number of visits per person per year also increased during the interval. The same groups that showed the greatest relative increase in proportion seeing a physician had the greatest relative increase in number of physician visits. In addition, the relative increase was greater for farm than for nonfarm residents.

Discharges from short term hospitals similarly increased from 1970 to 1974. Again, the increase tended to be greatest among those groups that showed the greatest relative increase in physician utilization.

Average length of stay decreased slightly in the four year period since 1970. The decrease tended to be concentrated in the groups that had increased their use of physicians and their hospital admission rate. The decrease in length of stay was particularly notable for the aged, nonwhite and lowest income groups, although the highest income group also experienced a significant reduction.

Percent of the population seeing a dentist increased slightly from 1970 to 1974. The pattern of increase paralleled that for physician use and hospital admissions. The relative increase appeared greatest for the nonwhite and low income population. The highest income groups actually registered a decrease in proportion seeing a dentist.

In sum, health service utilization rates generally appeared to increase beween 1970 and 1974 with the exception that length of stay decreased slightly. Generally, these changes were in the direction of more equitable distribution of service. That is, socioeconomic groups that were traditionally low utilizers increased their use rates relative to the rest of the population. The gains were particularly notable for the low income and nonwhite population.

Table 2-1. Percent seeing a physician during the survey year by selected characteristics: 1958, 1963 and 1970

	Percent Seeing a Physician (42)		
Characteristic	1958	1963	1970
Sex (54)			
Male	62	62	65
Female	70	68	71
Age (1)			
1–5	73	75	75
6–17	64	58	62
18–34	68	67	70
35–54	64	65	67
55–64	66	68	73
65 and over	68	68	76
Family income (25)			
Low	a	56	65
Middle	—	64	67
High	—	71	71
Race (49)			
White	—	68	70
Nonwhite	—	49	58
Education of head (10)	a		
8 years or less	—	56	62
9–11 years	—	63	66
12 years	—	69	69
13 years or more	—	76	76
Residence (52)			
SMSA, central city ⎫	a		65 ⎫
SMSA, other urban ⎬	—	66	72 ⎬ 69
Urban, non-SMSA ⎭	—		71 ⎭
Rural, nonfarm	—	66	68
Rural, farm	—	57	62
Total	66	65	68

[a]Not available for 1958.

Table 2-2. Percent seeing a physician (42) during the survey year by age and family income: 1963 and 1970

| | Family Income (25) | | | | | |
| | Percent low | | Percent middle | | Percent high | |
Age (1)	1963	1970	1963	1970	1963	1970
1–5	52	60	76	73	87	83
6–17	41	49	53	58	70	70
18–34	57	68	67	70	70	71
35–54	54	64	64	65	69	68
55–64	69	71	70	75	66	72
65 and over	68	73	66	85	71	82
Total	56	65	64	67	71	71

Table 2-3. Percent seeing a physician (42) during the survey year by age, family income and residence: 1970

| | | Residence (52) | | | |
Age (1)	Family income (25)	Percent SMSA, central city	Percent other urban	Percent rural	Percent total
1–17	Low	49	63	45	51
	Middle	58	67	60	62
	High	72	75	72	73
18–64	Low	71	69	63	68
	Middle	65	71	70	69
	High	66	72	69	70
65 and over	Low	69	74	75	73
	Middle	80	88	90	85
	High	93	78	73	82
All ages	Total	66	72	67	68

Table 2-4. Percent out-of-hospital physician visits by place of visit for all persons and for persons 65 and over: 1958, 1963 and 1970

	Place of Visit (45)										
	Home			Office			Clinic			Total	
Age (1)	1958	1963	1970	1958	1963	1970	1958	1963	1970		
All ages	11	5	2	80	83	85	9	12	13	100	
65 and over	26	12	8	67	81	84	7	7	8	100	

Characteristic	Place of Visit (45)					
	Home	Office	Outpatient department	Emergency room	Other	Total
Sex (54)						
Male	1	80	8	2	6	100 (3287)[a]
Female	3	88	6	1	2	100 (4018)
Age (1)						
0–5	1	75	8	6	10	100 (901)
6–17	1	84	9	3	3	100 (1561)
18–34	1	83	8	2	6	100 (1572)
35–54	1	85	8	2	4	100 (1438)
55–64	2	91	5	1	1	100 (706)
65 and over	8	84	6	1	1	100 (1127)
Family income (26)						
Above near poverty	2	88	5	2	3	100 (4529)
Below near poverty	3	77	14	2	4	100 (2776)
Race (49)						
White	2	87	6	2	3	100 (5301)
Nonwhite	2	70	19	2	6	100 (2004)
Education of head (10)						
8 years or less	2	85	9	1	3	100 (2259)
9–11 years	2	83	9	3	3	100 (1606)
12 years	2	88	5	2	2	100 (1912)
13 years or more	2	84	6	2	6	100 (1528)
Residence (52)						
SMSA, central city	2	76	13	3	6	100 (3146)
SMSA, other urban	1	89	5	2	3	100 (1058)
Urban, non-SMSA	5	89	3	1	2	100 (585)
Rural, nonfarm	3	89	4	2	2	100 (1854)
Rural, farm	1	91	4	3	1	100 (662)
Total	2	85	7	2	4	100 (7305)

[a]In parentheses are the unweighted numbers of observations which can be used in combination with the procedures described in Appendix I to calculate standard errors of the 1970 estimates. Since the 1970 sample is a weighted sample, these numbers should *not* be used as weights for combining subcategories.

Table 2-6. Mean number of physician visits per person-year (40) by selected characteristics: 1958, 1963 and 1970

Characteristic	Mean Number of Physician Visits (44)		
	1958	1963	1970
Sex (54)			
Male	3.5	3.8	3.6
Female	5.3	5.0	4.5
Age (1)			
0–5	4.6	3.9	4.2
6–17	2.7	2.5	2.2
18–34	4.1	5.0	4.2
35–54	4.7	4.9	4.0
55–64	5.1	5.7	6.3
65 and over	7.4	6.8	6.4
Family income (25)			
Low	_[a]	4.4	4.9
Middle	—	4.3	3.9
High	—	4.6	3.6
Race (49)			
White	_[a]	4.7	4.1
Nonwhite	—	3.2	3.6
Education of head (10)			
8 years or less	_[a]	3.9	4.2
9–11 years	—	4.7	3.6
12 years	—	4.7	3.6
13 years or more	—	5.3	4.5
Residence (52)			
SMSA, central city	_[a]		4.2 ⎫
SMSA, other urban	—	4.6	4.2 ⎬ 4.2
Urban, non-SMSA	—		4.4 ⎭
Rural, nonfarm	—	4.4	3.7
Rural, farm	—	3.6	3.4
Total	4.4	4.4	4.0

[a]Not available for 1958.

Table 2-7.   Mean number of physician visits by age and family income (25): 1970

Age (1)	Visits per Person-Year (44)			Visits per Person Seeing MD (44)		
	Low income	Middle income	High income	Low income	Middle income	High income
0–5	3.2	4.4	4.6	4.0	5.1	5.1
6–17	1.7	2.2	2.4	3.4	3.8	3.3
18–34	5.2	4.2	3.9	7.5	6.0	5.5
35–54	5.1	4.0	3.7	7.8	6.0	5.4
55–64	7.1	6.3	5.5	9.8	8.3	7.5
65 and over	6.3	6.4	6.7	8.6	7.4	7.9
Total	4.9	3.9	3.6	7.3	5.7	5.1

Table 2-8. Mean number of physician visits by age, family income and race (49): 1970

Age (1)	Family Income (25)	Visits per Person-Year (44)		Visits per Person Seeing MD (44)	
		White	Nonwhite	White	Nonwhite
0–17	Low	2.3	1.7	3.6	3.8
	Middle	3.0	1.9	4.4	3.3
	High	3.0	1.5	4.0	1.9
18–64	Low	5.6	6.1	8.1	9.3
	Middle	4.5	3.6	6.5	5.6
	High	4.0	2.9	5.7	5.2
65 and over	Low	6.0	8.8 —[a]	8.2	11.9 —[a]
	Middle	6.1	—	7.1	—
	High	6.8	—	8.0	—
All ages	Low	5.0	4.4	7.2	7.7
	Middle	4.0	3.1	5.7	5.0
	High	3.7	2.3	5.1	3.7
Total		4.1	3.6	5.8	6.0

[a]Based on fewer than 25 unweighted observations.

Table 2-9. Hospital admissions per 100 person-years by selected characteristics: 1953, 1958, 1963 and 1970

Characteristic	*Hospital Admissions per 100 Person-Years (30)*			
	1953	*1958*	*1963*	*1970*
Sex (54)				
Male	9	9	10	11
Female	15	15	15	16
Age (1)				
0-5	8	10	8	11
6-17	8	6	6	6
18-34	16	20	19	19
35-54	12	11	14	12
55-64	12	10	17	19
65 and over	13	18	18	21
Family income (25)				
Under $2,000	12	14	16	19
$ 2,000- 3,499	12	12	12	15
3,500- 4,999	12	14	12	17
5,000- 7,499	12	12	14	16
7,500- 9,999	⎫		14 ⎫	16 ⎫
10,000-12,499	11	10	11 ⎬ 12	12 ⎬ 12
12,500-14,999	⎬			11 ⎪
15,000 and over	⎭		10 ⎭	9 ⎭
Race (49)				
White	—a	—a	—a	15
Nonwhite	—	—	—	11
Residence (52)				
Large urban	10	11	10	12
Other urban	11	14	13	14
Rural, nonfarm	14	14	15	15
Rural, farm	12	13	11	13
Total	12	12	13	14

aNot available for three earlier studies.

Table 2-10. Hospital admissions per 100 person-years (30) by age and family income: 1963 and 1970

	Age (1)					
	0-17 years		18-54 years		55 and over	
Income (25)	1963	1970	1963	1970	1963	1970
Under $2,000	5	11	20	24	21	19
$ 2,000- 4,999	6	7	15	22	14	18
5,000- 9,999	7	9	19	18	19	23
10,000-14,999 ⎱	7	5	12	15	15	23
15,000 and over ⎰		7		9		18
Total	7	7	16	15	18	20

Table 2-11. Mean length of stay and hospital days per 100 person-years by age and sex: 1953, 1963 and 1970[a]

	Mean Number of Days per Admission (32)			Hospital Days per 100 Person-Years (31)		
Age and Sex (1) (54)	1953	1963	1970	1953	1963	1970
Age						
0-17	5.3	4.9	4.2	41	30	32
18-54	6.8	6.6	6.1	96	108	94
54 and over	11.9	11.9	12.3	148	208	242
Sex						
Male	8.3	8.0	8.1	71	83	83
Female	7.0	7.1	7.1	101	108	117
Total	7.4	7.4	7.5	87	96	100

[a]Selected observations excluded from this table for 1970. For exclusion criteria and estimates including all observations, see Appendix Table II-1.

Table 2-12. Mean in-hospital surgical procedures per 100 person-years by selected characteristics: 1958, 1963 and 1970

Characteristic	In-Hospital Surgical Procedures per 100 Person-Years (56)		
	1958	*1963*	*1970*
Sex (54)			
Male	4	4	5
Female	5	6	7
Age (1)			
0-5	3	3	6
6-17	4	4	3
18-34	5	5	7
35-54	5	6	6
55-64	5	6	9
65 and over	7	5	7
Family income (25)			
Under $2,000	5	3	7
$ 2,000- 3,499	4	4	6
3,500- 4,999	5	4	7
5,000- 7,499	5	6	8
7,500- 9,999 ⎫		7 ⎫	6
10,000-12,499 ⎪ 4		5 ⎬ 6	6 ⎫
12,500-14,999 ⎪		⎫	5 ⎬ 6
15,000 and over ⎭		⎭ 4 ⎭	5 ⎭
Race (49)			
White	_a	_a	7
Nonwhite	-	-	6
Residence (52)			
Large urban	5	5	6
Other urban	5	5	6
Rural, nonfarm	5	6	6
Rural, farm	3	4	5
Total	5	5	6

aNot available for 1958 and 1963.

Table 2-13. Percent distribution of specialty of physicians performing in-hospital surgery: 1963 and 1970

Specially Reported by Surgeon for Hospitalized Surgical Procedures: 1963 and 1970[a] (56) (57)	*1963*	*1970*
Surgical specialties only	72	83
Surgical specialties with "other" specialties[b]	7	4
Specialties not involving surgery[c]	5	4
No specialty reported	16	9
Total	100	100
N	(339)	(580)

[a]Surgical specialties include general surgery, opthalmology, otolaryngology, anesthesiology, colon and rectal surgery, neurological surgery, orthopedic surgery, plastic surgery, thoracic surgery, urology, and obstetrics and gynecology. "Other" specialties include all specialties recognized by the American Medical Association not included under surgical specialties above. Source: AMA (1969).

[b]Surgeon reports both a primary and secondary specialty, one being a surgical specialty as defined in footnote a and the other being an "other" specialty.

[c]Includes internists and pediatricians performing cardiac catherizations and exchange transfusions. These procedures are classified as surgery because of the extensive use of the operating room and blood but are properly done by non-surgical specialists. Almost half of the surgery (47%) done in 1970 by specialists without a surgery specialty fell into this category.

Table 2–14. Percent distribution of hospitalized surgical procedures by American Board certification of physicians who performed the operations: 1953, 1958, 1963 and 1970

	Percent Hospitalized Surgical Procedures[a]			
Certification (57)	1953	1958	1963	1970
Certified by a surgical examining board	21[b]	25[b]	28	35
Orthopedic surgery	5	4	6	7
General surgery	13	18	15	21
Plastic surgery	1	1	3	1
Neurological surgery	1	1	1	2
Thoracic surgery	1	1	2	3
Colon and rectal surgery[c]	1	1	1	1
Certified by other specialty boards which include surgery in the specialty	16[b]	17[b]	18	25
Urology	2	2	1	7
Obstetrics and gynecology	4	4	8	8
Ophthalmology and otolaryngology	10	12	10	10
Not certified for surgery	63	58	54	40
Total	100	100	100	100
N	(338)	(552)	(339)	(580)

	1953	1958	1963	1970
Table N	338	552	339	580
Physician not identified				
Dentist	36	43	36	68
Osteopath	7	8	4	14
Chiropodist	8	7	3	13
	—	—	—	1
Sample N	389	610	382	676

[a] Caesarean deliveries included in 1963 and 1970 but excluded in 1953 and 1958.

[b] The sum of the components does not equal the total because a few operations were performed by physicians certified by more than one board.

[c] Classified as "proctology" in the 1953 and 1958 surveys.

Table 2-15. Specialty interest of physician performing tonsillectomies, adenoid-ectomies, appendectomies and other hospitalized surgical procedures: 1963 and 1970

	Percent Surgical Procedures (56)					
Surgical Specialty Reported[a] (57)	*Tonsillectomy, adenoidectomy, appendectomy*		*Others*		*All procedures*	
	1963	*1970*	*1963*	*1970*	*1963*	*1970*
Yes	42	57	84	90	79	87
No	58	43	16	10	21	13
Total	100	100	100	100	100	100
N	(66)	(60)	(273)	(520)	(339)	(580)

[a]If the physician reports more than one specialty, he is considered to have a surgical specialty if *either* primary or secondary specialty involves surgery.

	1963	*1970*
Table N	339	580
Physician not identified	36	68
Dentist	4	14
Osteopath	3	13
Chiropodist	–	1
Sample N	382	676

Table 2-16. Percent women having live births who saw a doctor in the first trimester of pregnancy by family characteristics of mother: 1953, 1958, 1963 and 1970

Characteristic	Percent Seeing Physician by End of First Trimester (47)			
	1953	*1958*	*1963*	*1970*
Family income (25)				
Low	42	67	58	66 (136)[c]
Middle	66	77	86	92 (112)
High	89	86	88	85 (42)
Education (10)				
8 years or less	42	57	68	71 (34)
9–11 years	58	75	88	81 (96)
12 years	72	79	80	88 (107)
13 years or more	90	88	88	81 (53)
Race (49)				
White	_[a]	_[a]	_[a]	86 (172)
Nonwhite	–	–	–	65 (118)
Residence (52)				
SMSA, central city	_[a]	_[a]	_[a]	72. (154)
SMSA, other urban	–	–	–	84 (44)
Urban, non-SMSA	–	–	–	96 (26)
Rural, nonfarm	–	–	–	90 (46)
Rural, farm	–	–	–	b (20)
Total	65	77	80	83 (290)

[a]Not available for earlier studies.

[b]Based on fewer than 25 unweighted observations

[c]In parentheses are the unweighted numbers of observations which can be used in combination with the procedures described in Appendix I to calculate standard errors of the 1970 estimates. Since the 1970 sample is a weighted sample, these numbers should *not* be used as weights for combining subcategories.

Table 2-17. Median[a] number of prenatal physician visits by family characteristics of mother: 1953, 1958, 1963 and 1970

	Median Number of Prenatal Visits (46)			
Characteristic	1953	1958	1963	1970
Family income (25)				
Low	4.8	6.3	6 5	9.6 (136)[d]
Middle	9.6	9.5	10.9	12.2 (112)
High	10.5	11.7	11.1	11.0 (42)
Race (49)				
White	_b	_b	_b	11.0 (172)
Nonwhite	–	–	–	10.5 (118)
Education (10)				
8 years or less	5.1	5.4	8.0	10.1 (34)
9–11 years	7.3	8.8	10.0	9.7 (96)
12 years	8.9	10.5	10.8	11.3 (107)
13 years or more	12.2	12.0	10.6	11.2 (53)
Residence (52)				
SMSA, central city	_b	_b	_b	10.5 (154)
SMSA, other urban	–	–	–	11.6 (44)
Urban, non-SMSA	–	–	–	9.8 (26)
Rural, nonfarm	–	–	–	12.0 (46)
Rural, farm	–	–	–	c (20)
Total	8.4	9.8	10.5	10.9 (290)

[a]The median is that number of visits that exceeds the number of visits made by one-half of the mothers and is less than the number made by the other half.

[b]Not available for 1953, 1958 or 1963.

[c]Based on fewer than 25 unweighted observations.

[d]In parentheses are the unweighted numbers of observations which can be used in combination with the procedures described in Appendix I to calculate standard errors of the 1970 estimates. Since the 1970 sample is a weighted sample, these numbers should *not* be used as weights for combining subcategories.

Table 2-18. Median[a] number of days for delivery admission for live births by family characteristics of mother: 1953, 1958, 1963 and 1970

| Characteristic | *Median Length of Stay (32)* | | | |
	1953	*1958*	*1963*	*1970*
Family income (25)				
Low	2.2	3.6	3.1	3.2
Middle	4.8	4.5	4.0	4.0
High	5.0	4.8	4.2	3.9
Race (49)				
White	_b	_b	_b	3.8
Nonwhite	–	–	–	3.6
Residence (52)				
SMSA, central city	_b	_b	_b	3.5
SMSA, other urban	–	–	–	4.2
Urban, non-SMSA	–	–	–	3.4
Rural, nonfarm	–	–	–	3.7
Rural, farm	–	–	–	c
Total	4.5	4.4	3.7	3.7

[a]This median calculation is based only on hospital days of the admission during which the delivery took place and excludes days during any prior admissions for prenatal complications or false labor. Nonhospitalized deliveries were coded 0 days and included in the calculation.

[b]Not available for 1953, 1958 or 1963.

[c]Based on fewer than 25 unweighted observations.

Table 2-19. Percent seeing a dentist during the survey year by selected characteristics: 1953, 1963 and 1970

	Percent Seeing a Dentist (6)		
Characteristic	*1953*	*1963*	*1970*
Sex (54)			
Male	31	36	44
Female	36	40	46
Age (1)			
1–5	10	12	21
6–17	44	47	56
18–34	44	46	52
35–54	39	43	46
55–64	25	32	34
65 and over	13	19	26
Family income (24)			
Under $2000	17	16	23
$ 2,000– 3,499	23	25	23 } 28
3,500– 4,999	33		33
5,000– 7,499	44	40	35 } 40
7,500– 9,999			44
10,000–12,499			51
12,500–14,999	56	58	50 } 55
15,000–17,499			53
17,500 and over			67
Race (49)			
White	–[a]	43	47
Nonwhite	–	20	24
Education of head (10)			
8 years or less	–[a]	25	27
9–11 years	–	35	39
12 years	–	48	49
13 years or more	–	55	61
Residence (52)			
SMSA, central city	–[a]		41
SMSA, other urban	–	42	54 } 47
Urban, non-SMSA	–		45
Rural, nonfarm	–	37	41
Rural, farm	–	27	40
Total	34	38	45

[a]Not available for 1953.

Table 2-20. Percent seeing a dentist during the survey year by age and family income: 1963 and 1970

Age (1)	Income (24)	Percent Seeing a Dentist (6)	
		1963	*1970*
1–5	Under $2,000	0	4
	$ 2,000– 4,999	4	9
	5,000– 9,999	13	14
	10,000–14,000 }	23	30 } 30
	15,000 and over }		29 }
6–17	Under $2,000	11	24
	$ 2,000– 4,999	30	35
	5,000– 9,999	48	53
	10,000–14,999 }	71	57 } 65
	15,000 and over }		74 }
18–34	Under $2,000	31	47
	$ 2,000– 4,999	33	41
	5,000– 9,999	49	43
	10,000–14,999 }	57	57 } 60
	15,000 and over }		65 }
35–54	Under $2,000	23	31
	$ 2,000– 4,999	28	30
	5,000– 9,999	42	38
	10,000–14,999 }	58	46 } 53
	15,000 and over }		60 }
55–64	Under $2,000	16	20
	$ 2,000– 4,999	25	27
	5,000– 9,999	32	29
	10,000–14,000 }	52	44 } 44
	15,000 and over }		44 }
65 and over	Under $2,000	12	16
	$ 2,000– 4,999	18	18
	5,000– 9,999	24	35
	10,000–14,999 }	39	48 } 49
	15,000 and over }		50 }

Table 2-21. Mean number of dentist visits by selected characteristics: 1970

Characteristic	Visits per Person-Year (7)	Visits per Person seeing a Dentist (7)
Sex (54)		
Male	1.3	3.0
Female	1.5	3.4
Age (1)		
1–5	0.5	2.2
6–17	1.7	3.1
18–34	1.6	3.2
35–54	1.6	3.5
55–64	1.1	3.4
65 and over	0.8	3.3
Race (49)		
White	1.5	3.2
Nonwhite	0.8	3.5
Family income (25)		
Low	0.9	3.2
Middle	1.2	3.0
High	1.9	3.3
Education of head (10)		
8 years or less	0.5	3.3
9–11 years	1.0	3.3
12 years	1.2	3.0
13 years or more	1.7	3.3
Residence (52)		
SMSA, central city	1.4	3.4
SMSA, other urban	1.8	3.5
Urban, non-SMSA	1.3	3.0
Rural, nonfarm	1.1	2.8
Rural, farm	1.1	2.7
Total	1.4	3.2

Table 2-22. Utilization of health services by selected characteristics according to NCHS data[a]: 1970 and 1974

	Type of Utilization									
Characteristic	*Percent seeing a physician*		*Mean number of physician visits*		*Hospital discharges per 100 persons per year*		*Average length of hospital stay*		*Percent seeing a dentist*	
	1970	*1974*	*1970*	*1974*	*1970*	*1974*	*1970*	*1974*	*1970*	*1974*
Age										
0–5	83	88	5.9	6.3	8.9	10.4	7.3	6.4	17	21
6–16	64	68	2.9	3.2	6.0	5.5	5.1	5.1	61	63
17–24	76	77	4.6	4.5	16.9	14.0	5.9	5.6	56	57
25–44	73	76	4.6	5.0	15.0	15.6	6.9	7.4	52	55
45–64	70	74	5.2	5.0	14.7	17.5	11.1	10.2	44	47
65 and over	73	77	6.3	6.7	23.4	25.4	13.1	11.7	26	29
Sex										
Male	69	71	4.1	4.3	10.9	12.1	10.0	9.8	46	48
Female	75	79	5.1	5.6	15.5	16.0	7.6	7.4	48	51
Family income										
Under $2,000	71	76	5.3	5.9	19.0	20.8	11.5	9.7	29	36
$ 2,000– 3,999	69	76	5.1	5.3	17.1	21.6	10.1	10.9	29	32
4,000– 6,999	69	74	4.4	5.0	14.5	17.0	9.0	8.8	37	36
7,000– 9,999	72	75	4.3	5.1	12.4	15.2	7.4	7.7	46	42
10,000–14,999	74	75	4.6	4.6	11.7	12.8	7.4	8.0	56	51
15,000 and over	77	78	4.9	4.9	10.8	10.7	8.0	6.8	68	64
Race										
White	73	76	4.8	5.0	13.5	14.2	8.3	8.2	49	51
Nonwhite	65	71	3.8	4.4	11.4	13.7	10.7	9.8	30	35

(Continued)

Table 2-22 continued

Characteristic	Type of Utilization									
	Percent seeing a physician		Mean number of physician visits		Hospital discharges per 100 persons per year		Average length of hospital stay		Percent seeing a dentist	
	1970	1974	1970	1974	1970	1974	1970	1974	1970	1974
Education of head										
8 years or less	65	70	4.4	4.8	14.7	17.7	10.0	10.1	29	31
9-11 years	68	72	4.4	4.6	14.3	15.0	8.7	9.0	39	41
12 years	74	76	4.6	4.8	12.8	13.6	7.8	7.2	52	52
13 years or more	79	81	5.1	5.4	11.7	11.5	7.6	7.2	65	65
Residence										
SMSA	73	76	4.8	5.2	12.6	13.0	9.2	8.9	49	52
Non-SMSA, nonfarm	71	74	4.5	4.5	14.8	17.0	7.7	7.6	42	44
Non-SMSA, farm	65	68	3.3	4.1	11.5	13.8	7.5	6.7	43	46
Total	72	75	4.6	4.9	13.3	14.1	8.6	8.4	47	49

[a]The sources for 1970 and 1974 data by age and sex are NCHS (1972a) and NCHS (1975), respectively. The remainder are unpublished data provided by Ronald Wilson, Division of Analysis, National Center for Health Statistics.

Chapter 3

Expenditures for Personal Health Services

This chapter considers the expenditures for the health service use described in Chapter Two. These expenditures will be assessed at both the family and individual level. The four surveys permit rather detailed documentation of increasing expenditures—a trend that has been of major concern to the public and to those who provide health services.[1] Because a question of continuing interest from a policy perspective is the extent to which these health expenditure increases represent increased delivery of services rather than rising prices, a final section will be devoted to this issue.[2]

Since one of the main purposes of this chapter is to discuss trends in health service expenditures, the 1970 data are presented so that they can be compared to the three earlier studies. Thus, where possible, comparable definitions and categories of data were used. However, new categories have been created solely for the 1970 data

1. The trend analyses are based largely on mean estimates. Some of the mean estimates of expenditures from the 1970 data are subject to considerable sampling variability due to the large expenditures and high weights of certain cases in the sample. Consequently, to reduce this variability, the text tables exclude all observations that account for 10 percent or more of the weighted expenditures for any table cell. Estimates *including* these observations are provided in Appendix II. In addition, this chapter provides a fair number of median and distributional estimates that are less influenced by extreme cases.

2. Of course, medical care expenditures have continued to rise rapidly since the most recent data reported here were collected. Rather than stressing absolute magnitudes of expenditures that are continuously increasing, emphasis is given to relationships and trends that have relevance for longer periods of time. For recent expenditure and price data for medical care, the reader is referred to current issues of the *Social Security Bulletin* and the *Consumer Price Index*.

where special expenditure analyses appear appropriate. Most important is the distinction made between "free" and "nonfree" sources of payment for care. Nonfree sources are all those for which expenditures were reported in the earlier studies. This categorization allows trend analysis over time using comparable categories. Although there was no Medicare program in 1963, when the last study was done, Medicare has been included in the nonfree category since it is in large part a substitute for voluntary health insurance and no requirements regarding income level are involved in its use. CHAMPUS (Armed Forces dependents' coverage) was considered nonfree in both the 1963 and the 1970 studies.

The "free" categories are those for which no expenditure estimates were made in previous studies. Because of the increasing importance of these sources in financing health care in the United States, the decision was made to include estimates of expenditures in the 1970 study. Medicaid is included in the "free" group since it is designed to serve public aid recipients and, in some states, those just above the public aid income level. Thus, it has fairly stringent income eligibility requirements. Also included is care given by tax-supported hospitals and clinics when there was no other source of reimbursement. Certain other categories accounting for small amounts of care, including vocational rehabilitation, care for members of the Armed Forces and care provided by the Office of Economic Opportunity, are included in the free care totals.

This division into "free" and "nonfree" care allows an estimation of total expenditures for personal health services, including public expenditures, and provides fairly complete details on the financing of medical care for the poor. At the same time it produces data that can be compared with the earlier studies.

FAMILY EXPENDITURES

An analysis of family expenditures[3] is crucial for policymaking purposes because the family is the unit that has major impact on the medical care utilization and expenditures of its members. For example, the earnings and health insurance coverage of the head of the

---

3. "Family expenditures" as used in this study refer to charges incurred by families for the medical goods and services used by family members during the survey year. These goods and services include physicians services, general hospital care, prescribed and nonprescribed drugs and medications, dental care and "other" goods and services for health such as use of nonphysician health personnel, eyeglasses, and orthopedic appliances. These expenditures include amounts paid by health insurance but exclude health insurance premiums. They also include charges incurred by the family during the survey year which had not been paid at the time of interview. For detailed definitions of the components of total expenditures see Appendix III.

family are significant determinants of the medical care received by the rest of the family. In this section family expenditures for all health services as well as expenditures for various types of services will be examined. Further, family outlay which represents what the family actually spends out-of-pocket for medical care and health insurance will be explored. For legislative and planning purposes, families who experience excessive financial burden because of illness are of special interest. Consequently, families with "catastrophic" expenditures for medical care will also be studied.

Expenditures for All Services

Table 3–1 shows that mean family nonfree expenditures have increased continuously since 1953, with the greatest increase occurring between 1963 and 1970 (an average of 8.0 percent per year, compared with an average of 5.7 percent per year between 1953 and 1963). The amount of expenditures for medical care was directly related to a family's income, varying from $318 for low income families (those with family income of less than $2,000) to $979 for high income families (with earnings of $15,000 and over).[4]

As noted in the introduction, a more inclusive measure of expenditures, which estimates the cost of "free" care, was used in the 1970 study. When this measure combining both free and nonfree expenditures is used, differences in total expenditures among income groups are reduced, although those families in the highest income category have over twice the mean expenditures of those in the lowest income group (Table 3–2). If, however, the above/below near poverty measure, which adjusts income for family size, is used, the discrepancy is further reduced.[5]

4. It should be noted that with rising incomes the proportion of families represented by the lower income categories declined in each time period. The percentages of families in each income group in each survey year is as follows:

	Percent of All Families			
Income	*1953*	*1958*	*1963*	*1970*
Under $2,000	21	17	13	10
2,000–3,499	22	17	14	11
3,500–4,999	25	20	14	9
5,000–7,499	20	26	25	16
7,500 and over	12	20	34	54
Total	100	100	100	100

5. A measure that reflects family size has advantages for estimating the relationship of income and family health services use and expenditures over measures that do not take the family size variable into account. The latter tend to concentrate elderly poor living alone in the low income group while large families with very modest incomes appear in the "middle income" categories.

Table 3-2 also shows median family expenditures for 1970. The median for all families is less than one-half of the mean, illustrating the skewed nature of the expenditure distribution. As with the mean, expenditures increase with increasing income level. However, for the lower income levels the median is generally a smaller proportion of the mean. This suggests an especially skewed distribution among low income families: a large proportion have low expenditures, but a few have relatively high expenditures. It should be pointed out that serious illness in the family, particularly of wage earners, can reduce family income at the same time it increases medical expenditures. The elderly are also proportionately overrepresented in both the low income and high medical care use categories.

Table 3-3 documents the increasing proportion of families having large nonfree expenditures for personal health services. Between 1963 and 1970 the percent of families with expenditures of $1,000 or more increased from 8.1 percent to 18.1 percent. By 1970, 6.1 percent of all families were spending $2,000 or more, compared to 1.6 percent in 1963.

The proportion of families with low nonfree expenditures has not decreased as rapidly as one might expect, given the rapidly increasing numbers of families with high expenditures. Between 1963 and 1970 the proportion of families with nonfree expenditures of $1 to $49 per year decreased only slightly—from 16 percent to 13.2 percent— and the proportion reporting no expenses actually increased. Probably, two factors can largely account for this finding. One is that a greater proportion of families are now receiving "free" services than in the past. Including families receiving "free" care in the total, as is done in the last column in Table 3-3, serves to reduce the proportion of families with less than $50 of expenses in 1970 from 16 percent to 11.5 percent. The second is simply that a significant number of families actually continue to get no or few medical services in a given year, so that increasing prices have little effect on the magnitude of their expenditures.

Expenditures by Type of Service

Table 3-4 shows family expenditures for various types of services. Family expenditures for hospital services rose much more rapidly over the years covered by these studies than they did for other services so that by 1970 hospital expenditures had replaced physician expenditures as the largest type of expenditure. Further, the last column of Table 3-4 shows that the free component is primarily for hospital services. Thus, including the free component further increases the proportion of 1970 family expenditures accounted for by hospital services.

Family Outlay for Personal Health Services

A more direct measure of the financial impact of medical care on families than expenditures is the percentage of income spent on medical care. The measure "aggregate outlay for personal health services" is calculated as a percentage of family income. It includes direct out-of-pocket family health expenditures during 1970, including the employee's share of premiums and Medicare Part B premiums, but excludes expenditures for services met by any third party, including insurance companies, Medicare and Medicaid.

In 1970 the average family devoted 4.2 percent of its income to purchasing health services (Table 3–5). In 1958 the average family spent 5.5 percent of its income on health services, but since then the proportion spent on the same services has been dropping. This has taken place in spite of an overall increase in the utilization of health services and rapidly increasing prices in medical care. There are several explanations for this trend. They include growing public expenditures for medical care and increasing employee fringe bene-. fits in the form of employer payment of health insurance premiums, neither of which represents direct outlays from a family's income.[6]

Table 3–5 illustrates the relatively large burden of medical care costs on low income families throughout the 17 year period. In each study year the proportion of income devoted to health services has been inversely related to income, with the poorest families devoting a proportion of their income to health services that was three or four times greater than that of the highest income groups. Adjusting for family size reduces this disparity somewhat. Still, in 1970, families below the near poverty line were spending about twice as high a percentage of their income for medical care as those above the near poverty level.

The Medicare and Medicaid programs, which began to operate in 1966, midway between the 1963 and 1970 studies, had as one of their prime functions reducing the financial hardship of medical care costs on low income people, both aged and nonaged. Results show that in 1970 as in the earlier studies the poor continued to spend much more of their income on medical care than the rest of the population (Table 3–5). There has actually been a slight increase between 1963 and 1970 in outlay as a percent of family income for those families earning less than $10,000[7] with the exception of those with family income below $2,000. Several factors, however, should

6. An employee's earned income is reduced by some proportion of his employer's contributions to Medicare and voluntary health insurance. Inclusion of these costs in the outlay variable would increase outlay as a proportion of income, particularly as the level of employer contribution rises.

7. Including the cost of employer contributions in the outlay variable might conceivably alter the apparent relative expenditures of the poor and nonpoor.

be kept in mind in examining these findings: (1) Fewer families are represented by the lowest income categories in the later studies. (2) Families in the lowest income groups are more likely to have had serious illnesses which tend to reduce family income at the same time that they increase medical care expenses. (3) In addition, as pointed out in previous chapters, there has been an overall increase in the utilization of health services, particularly among the poor, and a rapid increase in medical care prices. Medicare, Medicaid and other public programs may have helped contain the earlier upward trend in the proportion of income spent on medical care by low income families.

Table 3-6 separates from all other families those families in which at least one member is 65 or over. These are, of course, families for whom Medicare is a potential third party payer. Among the lowest income families (yearly income less than $2,000), aggregate outlay as a percent of income is 12-13 percent for both younger and older families. At higher income levels the aggregate outlay percent tends to be greater for older families than for younger ones. The differences appear greatest among families with incomes between $2,000 and $7,500. For example, older families with yearly income from $2,000 to $3,499 spend 11.3 percent for health purposes compared to 6.4 percent for younger families in the same income bracket. The special financial problems for low income families with older members are illustrated when family size is considered along with income. Older families with incomes below the near poverty level spent 12.3 percent of that income for health purposes compared to 6.0 percent for younger families with incomes below the near poverty level.

Catastrophic Expenditures

This section addresses issues relating to the financial impact of catastrophic illness on families. As our data will show, different definitions of "catastrophic" result in very different target populations. Before programs to aid those burdened by catastrophic expenditures are developed, the implications of alternative definitions of "catastrophic" need to be explored. Three definitions or categories of catastrophic expenditures are used here. Excessive expenditures are measured by the absolute amount of a family's outlay for medical care ($1,000 or more), its outlay as a percentage of family income (15 percent or more) and as a gross expenditure ($5,000 or more).

In 1970, 8.5 percent, or over five and one-half million families, had outlays of $1,000 or more for medical care. Ten percent, or almost seven million families, spent at least 15 percent or more of their family incomes. And the group of families with gross expenditures for medical care of $5,000 or more comprised about 1 percent of all families. These are the portions of the population defined by the three measures of catastrophic illness used here.

Tables 3-7 and 3-8 provide a profile of the three types of families that incur gross expenditures greater than $5,000, outlays of $1,000 or more, or costs greater than 15 percent of their family incomes. The largest group (38 percent) in the gross expenditure column has incomes of at least $15,000 (Table 3-7). Families with outlays of $1,000 or more are also heavily weighted toward the higher income brackets, with 65 percent of these families having incomes of $10,000 or more. In contrast, families who spent at least 15 percent of their family income for medical care are predominantly low income—38 percent have incomes under $2,000 and 76 percent have incomes below $5,000. Further, as indicated in Table 3-5, outlay as a proportion of income actually started to decline for the population as a whole after 1958, but not for low income families. Even the advent of Medicare and Medicaid in July 1966 did not prevent a rise between 1963 and 1970 in outlay as a percent of income for families with incomes under $7,500, except for the very lowest income group.

Table 3-8 describes the characteristics of families with gross expenditures of $5,000 and "excessive" outlays for medical care. Those families in the gross expenditure category are more likely to have younger family heads who are highly educated and employed full time. The same characteristics fit families with outlays of $1,000 or more. Both groups are more likely to be white and above the near poverty level than families with outlays which equal 15 percent or more of their family incomes. Fifty-three percent of the latter families have family heads who are 65 or older, 61 percent of the family heads have fewer than 12 years of education and one-third of them are retired. The family size variable suggests the presence of large numbers of older people in these families with large percentage outlays; 87 percent of such families have three members or less. The residential distribution shows that a large percentage of the first two types of families are urban dwellers who do not live in the inner city (46 and 47 percent respectively). The distribution of central city residents is about equal for all three groups of families. More of the families with 15 percent or greater outlays are rural (37 percent, compared to 24 percent for families with $5,000 and over expenditures, and 21 percent for those with outlays of $1,000 or more).

Tables 3-7 and 3-8 suggest differences in policy implications depending on the definition of catastrophic illness expenditures emphasized. A national health insurance plan designed to reduce excessive family outlays for medical care (or aimed at those with gross expenditures above a certain level) without direct consideration of family income level would benefit a considerably different group of families than would a plan that seeks primarily to reduce outlay as a proportion of family income. A different group of services would also undoubtedly be paid for. Outlay at low income levels can exceed 15 percent paying for fairly common services. A plan addressed to outlay as a percent of income might well be paying for such items as eyeglasses and drugs while one addressed to large expenditures would probably be paying for hospital and physician services.

INDIVIDUAL EXPENDITURES

In order to understand patterns of health care expenditures for age and sex and the interaction between these demographic variables and other characteristics such as income, race and residence, it is necessary to go beyond the family and examine individual expenditures. The individual is also a logical unit of analysis for looking at expenditures for various kinds of services, including hospital, physician, drug, dental and obstetrical, which are examined in this section. In addition, using the individual as the unit of analysis eliminates any effects of changes in family size on expenditure comparisons over the period covered by the studies.

Expenditures for All Services

Mean nonfree expenditure per individual for all personal health services increased from $65 in 1953 to $112 in 1963 and $209 in 1970 (Table 3-9). The average annual increase was considerably greater in the latter period (8.9 percent) than it had been in the former (5.2 percent).

Table 3-9 shows that in each study expenditures for females exceed those for males. However, the rate of increase appeared greater for males than females.

Each study showed expenditures generally increasing with increasing age (Table 3-9). The average annual increase during the first ten year period tended to be greater for adults than for children. Between 1963 and 1970 the rate of increase was greater for adults 55 and over, but children from birth to five years also had a relatively high rate of expenditure increase.

In 1963 expenditures still tended to be directly related to income level (Table 3-9). Between 1963 and 1970 the rate of expenditure increase was considerably greater for the lowest income group so that by 1970 the total spent per year by the low income group was greater than the middle income group.

Table 3-10 shows per capita expenditures for various kinds of services in 1953, 1963 and 1970. It also shows the rate of expenditure increase for each in the intervals between the studies.[8] In the 1953 study, expenditures for physician services were highest, followed by hospital, drugs, dental and "other" services. Between 1953 and 1963 the rate of expenditure increase was greatest for drugs and hospital services, but physician expenditures continued to rank first. Between 1963 and 1970 expenditure increases for hospital services far exceeded those for other types of health services. Consequently, hospital services had replaced physician services as the service with the largest expenditures by 1970. During this latter period expenditures for physician care in the hospital and those for nonmedical practitioners such as optometrists and chiropractors also rose at a relatively rapid rate.

The distribution of medical expenditures by level of expenditures and how that distribution is changing over time is useful for assessing the impact of new health legislation. For example, one concern is the effect of universal catastrophic type health insurance coverage on total expenditures and particularly on expenditures for patients receiving intensive and costly medical treatment. A picture of trends in expenditures for people with expensive illness episodes is necessary background information for considering the impact of catastrophic coverage.

Table 3-11 indicates that in 1963 the top 1 percent of users in terms of expenditures were responsible for 17 percent of the total amount spent for nonfree health services. By 1970, they accounted for 23 percent of the expenditures for nonfree care excluding Medicare (24 percent including Medicare) and 26 percent of total expenditures. The proportion of total expenditures accounted for by the top 5 and 10 percent of users also increased between 1963 and 1970, but the most dramatic increase was for the top 1 percent. The percentages for the four quartiles show little variation in the proportion of the total each accounted for from 1963 to 1970.

Table 3-12 shows that the average annual increase in mean health expenditures for the top 1 percent of users by magnitude of expenditures has been 17.2 percent per year between 1963 and 1970. The increase has been less for nonfree care excluding Medicare (11.4 percent) and nonfree care including Medicare (13.3 percent). The highest average annual increases have been among the top percentage

8. Detailed definitions of the various services and expenditures for them in 1963 and 1970 are found in Appendix III.

groups, although the bottom quartile shows a 13.2 percent annual increase for total health care expenditures. It is clear from these tables that people with catastrophic type illnesses are taking a large, and apparently growing, proportion of the medical care dollar. What requires further study is the extent to which extending catastrophic insurance benefits might give added impetus to a current trend.

Expenditures by Type of Service: 1970

While the previous section emphasized trends in individual expenditure patterns over time, this section examines expenditures in 1970 according to selected demographic and socioeconomic characteristics. Also, while the previous section emphasized nonfree expenditures so that comparisons could be made over all studies, the tables in this section report on nonfree plus free expenditures, thus giving a more complete picture of total expenditures in 1970. Each table in the section shows the mean expenditure for all people in each population group. In addition, it shows the mean and median for only those people who actually had expenditures for the service.

Table 3–13 shows the sum of free plus nonfree expenditures for all services for 1970. For all the measures shown, expenditures for females exceed those for males. Expenditures also tend to increase with increasing age. Total expenditures for people above the near poverty level are, on average, somewhat higher than those for people below the near poverty level. The median differences by poverty level are relatively greater than the mean differences for the total population. This suggests that while the majority of low income persons have relatively low expenditures, there are some with high expenditures, thus bringing the mean average close to the rest of the population. People with the most education have the highest mean expenditures and those with the least education have the second highest mean expenditures. The median figures do not show this pattern. This suggests a distribution for the low education group similar to that for the low income group: a large proportion with low expenditures but also a sizable group with very high expenditures. Suburbanites living in SMSAs but not in the central cities have the highest expenditures among all types of residents. The central city dwellers have the second highest expenditures but are still considerably lower than the suburbanites.

Table 3–14 shows hospital expenses divided into inpatient and outpatient categories. The former includes expenses for stays in long term care institutions; the latter includes emergency room and hospital outpatient department expenses. Females had a higher mean expense for inpatient services for the total population but males had a higher mean among people with expenses. This indicates that fewer males are hospitalized but that those who are hospitalized tend to have higher expenses.

Inpatient expenditure rates tend to increase with increasing age by all of the measures used in Table 3-14. An exception is that children aged six to 17 are less likely to have expenses than those zero to five, but when older children are hospitalized their expenditures are similar to expenses for the younger ones. The relatively high expenditures for persons aged 18 to 34 reflect hospital costs for obstetrical services, which are concentrated in this age group. There is not the same relationship between age and hospital outpatient expenses as was observed for inpatient expenditures. The variance is much less and, indeed, middle-aged persons 35 to 54 appeared to have the highest average expenditures.

For both inpatient and outpatient services the low income and least educated groups had the highest expenditures (Table 3-13). The poor and the least educated were more likely to use these hospital services and also had the highest average expenditures among people using services.

Urban residents living in SMSAs had higher hospital expenses than people living elsewhere (Table 3-13). Central city residents had much higher outpatient expenses than any other residential group.

Table 3-15 divides physician expenses into those incurred while patients were hospitalized and those resulting from ambulatory care. Inpatient care includes charges for inpatient surgery and for visits physicians make to hospital inpatients. It excludes the charges for care provided by salaried physicians to hospitalized patients that are included in hospital expenses. Outpatient expenses include charges for care in doctors' offices and clinics, charges for physician home visits and physician charges for all obstetrical care.

The average expense for males and females for inpatient physician care is similar. Outpatient expenses for physician care were higher for females than for males.

Physician expenses generally increase with increasing age, but there are some exceptions (Table 3-15). Children under six years of age have relatively high expenditures for outpatient physician services, reflecting the preventive examinations received by the young. Also, expenses for persons 55 to 64 rival those of the elderly for being the highest among all age groups.

In 1970, the above near poverty group was still spending more for physician services than were the poor (Table 3-15). Only among people having expenditures for outpatient care were the expenses for the poor as high as those for the rest of the population.

The highest average physician expenditures according to education of the family head was for the group with the most education (Table 3–15). This was particularly true for outpatient services. Those with the least education had mean inpatient expenses similar to those with most education when all persons are considered. However, among people with physician expenditures, those with the least education ranked second behind the best educated.

People living in SMSAs but not in the central city (suburbanites) had higher physician expenditures than any other residential group. The mean and median expenses for people with expenses for the central city residents was second highest to the suburbanites. Further, the outpatient average charges for people with charges were higher for the central city residents than for any other group.

Prescribed drug expenses are higher for females than for males according to Table 3–16. However, for nonprescribed drugs the expenses are similar for the sexes. As with physician and hospital expenses, drug expenses tend to grow larger with increasing age (Table 3–16). Exceptions are that expenses for the youngest children tend to be higher than for those six to 17 and that nonprescribed expenses are high for persons 55 to 64.

Drug expenses appear similar according to poverty level (Table 3–16). Among people with prescribed drug expenses, the poor tended to spend more per person. The group with the lowest education had the highest prescribed drug charges (Table 3–16). There did not seem to be important differences in expenditures for nonprescribed drugs according to education level.

Central city residents had the highest average expenditures for prescribed drugs among all residential groups (Table 3–16). As was the case for education and income groupings, no major differences appeared in expenditures for nonprescribed drugs according to residential groupings.

Table 3–17 shows that females had somewhat higher expenditures for dental services than males. Expenditures for dental care reach a peak among middle-aged persons according to Table 3–17. However, if we consider only people with expenditures, the mean and median expenditures tended to be similar for persons 35 and older.

Higher income persons show larger expenditures for dental care than do the poor regardless of the expenditure measure examined (Table 3–17). Dental expenditure is also directly related to level of education, as indicated by mean expenditure for the total population. But, for people with expenditures, the least educated probably had the highest mean expenditures, and median expenditures similar to those for other educational groups.

SMSA residents who do not live in central cities have considerably higher dental expenditures than any other residential group (Table 3–18). At the other extreme, rural farm residents have considerably lower dental expenditures than the rest of the population.

Table 3–18 shows expenditures for non-MD health practitioners, including optometrists, physical therapists and chiropractors, and for other medical expenditures, including laboratory tests and medical appliances such as glasses, hearing aids and wheelchairs. Females tended to have higher total "other" expenditures than did males. Expenditures for non-MD practitioners tended to increase with age both for the total population and for people with services. However, the median expenditure for those with services is more similar for the various age groups. Expenditures for medical tests and appliances also increase with age, with the exception that expenditures peak in the 55 to 64 age group.

The above poverty and best educated groups have higher "other" medical expenditures than do the poor and those with the least education (Table 3–18). These differences tend to disappear if we look only at the mean and median expenditures for people with expenditures. People in families headed by a person with nine to 12 years of education had lower expenditures than either the better or less well educated groups.

SMSA residents tended to have higher "other" expenditures than other urban and rural residents (Table 3–18). The median expenditures for people with expenditures were similar for all residential groups.

EXPENDITURES FOR LIVE BIRTHS

This section examines changes in health service expenditures associated with live births from 1953 to 1970. Both free and nonfree expenditures are available for 1970 so that expenditures by all major sources of payment for obstetrical services according to income level of the mother can be analyzed.

Table 3–19 shows that nonfree expenditures per live birth rose from $193 in 1953 to $532 in 1970. The rate of increase, as with other health services, was greater in the period between 1963 and 1970 than between 1953 and 1963. Of total expenditures in 1970, 61 percent were for hospital services, while about one-third were for physician services. Over the 17 year period covered by the studies, hospital services have accounted for more and more of the total bill, while the proportion spent for physician services, drugs and other medical services has declined. This has occurred despite a drop in the average number of days spent in the hospital for a delivery.

Table 3–20 shows that in each time period the nonfree expenditures for women in the upper income groups were considerably higher than the nonfree expenditures for women in the lowest income groups. Further, the rate of increase has been greater for the higher income groups so that the disparity appeared to be increasing between 1953 and 1970.

One reason for the increasing disparity might be that an increasing proportion of the expenses for live births by low income mothers is in the "free care" category. Table 3-21 allows us to compare free plus nonfree mean and median expenditures for the different income groups. This table shows that, at least for 1970, the discrepancy in expenditures by income is greatly reduced when the free component is included. Considering only the nonfree component, mean expenditures for the low income group were only 38 percent of the high income mean. Including the nonfree component increased this percentage to 80.

PRICE AND USE INCREASES[9]

A question of continuing interest from a policy perspective is the extent to which health expenditure increases represent increased delivery of services or rising prices. This section examines the contributions of price and use to health expenditure increases over the 1953 to 1970 time period using data from the series of household interview surveys. In addition to confirming some of the general findings of studies based on other data sources (Klarman et al., 1970b), data from household interviews permit separate analyses to be done for different population groups. This section examines the contributions of price and use to expenditure increases by different age, sex, income, race and residence groups and by source of payment.

Throughout the section, increases will be analyzed separately for the 1953-1963 period and the 1963-1970 period. The first period, 1953-1963, can be characterized as one in which a primary shift in financing patterns occurred: from consumer out-of-pocket payments for medical care to payments by voluntary health insurance. The coverage was mainly for hospital and inpatient physician services. The groups that benefited most from the growth in voluntary health insurance were the working population and their dependents. The second period, 1963-1970, witnessed the passage of the Medicare and Medicaid legislation. Both programs went into effect in mid-1966 although the time of implementation and range of benefits for

9. This section is a condensed and edited version of Andersen, Foster and Weil (1976). It is presented here with the permission of *Inquiry*.

Medicaid varied from state to state. In this latter period, the proportion of the personal health care dollar accounted for by voluntary insurance remained relatively constant. The main trend here was a decrease in the percentage paid for by government. Given the target populations of Medicare and Medicaid, it seems fair to say that, in a relative sense, the changes in financing mechanisms were greatest for the elderly and the medically indigent during this period.[10]

The total expenditures analyzed in this section include both a nonfree and free component. For this analysis, the free component of total per capita expenditures for the earlier studies was estimated using aggregate data published by the Social Security Administration (SSA, 1973). Since SSA estimates are based on the total population, while the CHAS studies include only the noninstitutionalized population, these aggregate estimates were adjusted to exclude expenditures for the institutionalized population.[11]

Allocation to Price and Use

Any effort to discuss "price" and "use" increases in the health field is inevitably complicated by quality considerations. Conceptually, a price increase means that more money is spent to purchase *the same service*. All other expenditure increases are properly considered use increases.[12] If a "completely new" product or service is purchased, the entire expenditure represents a use increase. If a "higher quality" product is purchased at greater expense than the lower quality product purchased previously, the difference between the cost of the new product and the cost of the old one represents purchase of additional services. It is for this reason that Klarman et al., (1970a) refer to our "use" category as "all other." While a further division of our "use increase" category into "increased use of

10. See Chapter Four for data concerning insurance coverage and third party payments.

11. The following procedure was used to obtain estimates for free care in fiscal 1953: Using Tables 8 and 9 of the Social Security estimates (SSA), an estimate for 1953 fiscal year was arrived at by adding to the free estimate for 1950 one-half of the difference between the 1950 and 1955 free estimate. The CHAS value was determined for the noninstitutionalized population by the following ratio:

$$\frac{\text{CHAS free 1970 X SSA free 1953}}{\text{SSA free 1970}} = \text{CHAS free estimate 1953}$$

The identical procedure was employed in obtaining CHAS estimates for free care in 1963 using SSA free estimates for 1960 and 1965 with the exception that the difference was multiplied by 0.6 to obtain and estimate for calendar year 1963.

12. When price and use are both increasing, some of the increase in expenditure results from the interaction of the two. That is, higher prices are paid on the additional services purchased originally. Use of annual average percentage increases drastically reduces this interaction effect, however.

the same services" and "use of new and better services" categories would be desirable, it would require a more detailed specification of the services purchased than the specification for which we have data.

While the concept of price employed here is the conventional one in economics and is the one that guides the U.S. Department of Labor in the construction of its Consumer Price Index (CPI), another concept lies at the base of some of the "price" indexes familiar in the health field. Hospital expense per patient day, for example, is better suited to answering the question, How rapidly is the amount which a patient should expect to pay for a day in the hospital increasing? than is the hospital component of the Consumer Price Index. However, hospital expense per patient day includes tests and other ancillary services which have been increasing over time. Consequently, we feel the CPI which is based only on room and board charges, is conceptually better suited to measure "price" as used in this study.

In practice, an index that captures only "pure price" increases is difficult to construct. The hospital component of the Consumer Price Index, for example, is unable to make any adjustment for the increases in intensity of services that presumably have accompanied increased nurse staffing levels which are included in room and board charges. The effects of such changes in the nature of the product will be attributed therefore to price increases. It is for such reasons that we are unwilling to assert generally that the effects of technology and changing quality are included in the use term, although that is clearly the intent of the method. The success with which pure price increases are measured varies by type of expenditure, and these differences will be discussed as results are presented.

Components of Expenditure Increases

Price increases are computed using various components of the Consumer Price Index (U.S. Department of Labor, 1973), although alternative price measures are available. Table 3-22 indicates that price increases account for more of the increase in per capita expenditures that do use increases, over both the 1953-1963 and the 1963-1970 periods. Although prices increased much more rapidly during the 1963-1970 period than previously, use also increased more rapidly, with the relative contributions of price and use not greatly changed. If adjustments are made for changes in the general purchasing power of the dollar by subtracting the rate of increase of the CPI for all items (1.4 percent for the 1953-1963 period and 3.4 percent for the 1963-1970 period) from the rates of price increase in Table 3-22, the rate of increase in medical prices in real terms is seen to have increased from 1.9 percent per year in the 1953–1963 period to 2.7 percent per year in the 1963–1970 period.

During both periods, the component showing by far the highest rate of price increase is hospital care. Since the hospital price index is based on daily service charges, and the quality of room, board and nursing services is presumed to have increased over time, there is some concern that the figures in Table 3–22 may overstate hospital price increases (and, correspondingly, understate use increases by excluding "use of higher quality services" from use increases).

One means of assessing this possibility is to compare the results in Table 3–22 with results obtained using different price indexes. Hospital expense per inpatient day and per adjusted patient day both have the characteristic that expenditure increases resulting from greater use of ancillary services per day in the hospital will be allocated to the price effect. Since increased use of ancillary services is known to have occurred, we would expect the per diem expense indexes to show greater price increases than an index based on changes in the price of a uniform product. In fact, expense per inpatient day and expense per adjusted patient day give results virtually identical to those in Table 3–22.[13] We conclude that much of the effect of increasing quality of hospital care has been attributed to price in Table 3–22.[14]

Still another method of determining price and use increases is to determine use increases from direct measures of use and attribute the remainder of per capita expenditure increases to price. As long as the price index measures the price of the same "unit of service" as measured by the use index, this method should give the same results as the one used in constructing Table 3–22. Price and use increases were computed using short term hospital days per capita as the use measure. The results are virtually identical to those in Table 3–22 for the 1953–1963 period (a 6.2 percent rate of price increase and a 0.9 percent rate of use increase) but gave a much smaller rate of use increase (1.5 percent) over the 1963–1970 period. This discrepancy is probably attributable in part to the inclusion of care provided in long term hospitals, nursing homes and extended care facilities in the expenditure data but not in the patient days data. We thus conclude

13. Using expense per inpatient day as the price index gives price increases of 6.5 percent in the 1953–1963 period and 10.5 percent in the 1963–1970 period. Using expense per adjusted patient day gives a rate of price increase of 10.6 percent over the 1963–1970 period (adjusted patient days have not been published for years prior to 1963).

14. Unfortunately, we still have no measures of the amount by which "pure price" increases are overstated.

that much of the hospital use increase reported in Table 3–22 actually represents increased use of these institutions.[15]

Price increases also exceeded use increases for physician services. Although some increases in quality of physician services may be attributed to price in Table 3–22, the physician fee component of the CPI probably comes much closer to pricing a uniform product than does the hospital component.[16] There is no physician index comparable to hospital expense per patient day, however. The only direct measure of physician use available from survey data is the number of office visits, and even this is only available since 1963. Physician office visits per capita actually declined at the rate of 1.4 percent per year over the 1963–1970 period, in contrast to the 2.3 percent rate of use increase indicated in Table 3–22. If a crude direct measure of physician use is constructed by adding to the number of office visits the number of hospital patient days (our expenditure data include payments to physicians for services provided to inpatients, as long as the physician is paid separately from the hospital), the result is still a slight reduction (–0.8 percent per year) in physician use over the 1963–1970 period. We conclude that virtually all of the 2.3 percent per year use increase reported in Table 3–22 represents changes in the nature of services rendered per physician contact. Such changes would include more surgery, greater tendency to be seen by a specialist and provision of more separately billed services per physician contact.[17] While Table 3–22 indicates virtually no change in physician use over the 1953–1963 period, this may understate the rate of increase in use by as much as 1 percent per year due to the increased rate at which the customary fees priced by the CPI were actually collected over this time period (Klarman et al.,

15. It seems reasonable to expect that utilization of these institutions increased more rapidly during the 1963–1970 period than during the earlier period due to extended care facility coverage under Medicare and the general aging of the population. Use of long term hospitals and nursing homes is still not as great a factor as the reader might initially suspect, even for 1970, since our data cover only the noninstitutionalized population.

16. Although the nature of a family physician's office visit (an important element of the CPI physician fee component) may have changed somewhat over time, changes in the nature of medical practice are believed to be more related to use of procedures for which physicians price separately. It is not at all clear that the nature of the surgeon's input to such procedures as tonsillectomies and herniorrhaphies (other important components of CPI) has changed appreciably over time.

17. If physicians do not provide additional services, but merely begin to price separately for items that used to be included in the price of an office visit, the result will be an overstatement of use increases and corresponding understatement of price increases. The magnitude of such a fractionation effect is unknown, however.

1970b). The rate of increase in physician use over this period would still be less than the rate of increase from 1963–1970, however.

Dental care also showed a greater rate of use increase from 1963–1970 than during the earlier period. Although survey data on dental visits are available only for 1970, data from the National Center for Health Statistics (NCHS, 1965b and 1972a) indicate that dental visits per capita declined at the rate of 1 percent per year from 1963–1970. All of the increase in dental use, then, represents changes in the nature of a dental contact. Such changes can include greater number of restorations per visit, greater incidence of orthodontal work and greater incidence of cleaning by hygienists.

Drugs were the only component of health expenditures to show a slower rate of use increase over the 1963–1970 period than earlier. Drugs also showed by far the lowest rate of price increase of any of the expenditure components. Both the expenditure data and the CPI component used in Table 3–22 include both prescription and non-prescription drugs. The CPI drug component has been the object of substantial criticism because of the limited number of prescription items priced, and also because the items that are priced do not include "new" drugs even though new drugs account for a substantial share of the market. Firestone (1970), however, constructed a much more broadly based index with the priced items changed frequently and found that, except over short time periods, it gave virtually the same results as the prescription component of the CPI. Firestone also showed that indexes such as average price per prescription have over-estimated price increases due to increases over time in the average dosage per prescription. We conclude that virtually all of the increase in drug expenditures is attributable to use when use is defined more broadly than the number of prescriptions.

Relative Impact of Type of Service and Payer

Table 3–23 indicates the contribution of each service to the total expenditure increase per person and also to the expenditure increase attributable to increased use.

Increases in hospital expenditures accounted for 37 percent of the total per capita expenditure increase in 1953–1963 and over one-half of the total increase in the later period. In contrast, they accounted for a much smaller proportion of the increase in expenditures attributable to use in each period. Still, hospitals accounted for a third of the total use increase between 1963 and 1970. Physician services accounted for almost one-fifth of the expenditure increase in each period but were a factor in the use increase only in the second period. Table 3–23 suggests that dental services contributed between

10 and 15 percent to both total expenditure and use increase in both periods. Drugs appeared to be a much bigger factor in both expenditures and use increases in the earlier period than in the later one.

Table 3–23 also allows us to assess the relative impact of the free and nonfree sources. An assumption is made that price increases are the same in the free and nonfree sector. Table 3–23 shows that increasing expenditures by the free sources accounted for only 5 percent of the expenditure increase in the early period and apparently did not contribute at all to use increase. In the latter period, however, the free sources accounted for 16 percent of the increase in expenditures and about one-quarter of the total use increase. Contributions to the increase in expenditures and use by the free component were primarily for hospital and physician services. In general, Table 3–23 permits the conclusion that the free component in expenditure increases trebled in the period 1963–1970 and that actual use of health care services which were paid for on behalf of the needy accounted for one-fourth of the overall use increase.

Price and Use Increases by Population Characteristics

Table 3–24 provides an opportunity to examine the impact of price and use increases for various subgroups of the population. Since separate price indexes are not available by population group, this requires the assumption that the rate of price increase for each service is the same for all population groups. Differences in rates of price increases in Table 3–24, therefore, reflect differences in the distribution of medical expenditures among services with varying rates of price increases. While it is often argued that prices paid by different population groups vary (especially between white and non-white and between urban and rural), reasons for expecting different *rates of increases* are unclear.[18]

Table 3–24 suggests that price increases as defined here are relatively constant over the various population groups examined. In both periods, the rates of price increase tend to be somewhat higher for

18. The major concern with possible differences in rates of increase appears to be with respect to the urban-rural differential. Direct evidence on this point is available from the Consumer Price Index only since 1967. Annual rates of increase in the CPI for all items between 1967 and 1973 ranged from 5.1 percent for cities with populations of 3.5 million or more to 4.5 percent in cities with populations of 2,500 to 50,000. Evidence that is less direct with respect to the urban-rural distinction but more direct with respect to the items considered in this study can be obtained by examining rates of increase in hospital expense per patient day in the ten most rural versus the ten most urban states. Annual rates of increase were 5.9 percent in the rural states versus 6.6 percent in the urban states over the 1953–1963 period and 10.1 percent versus 10.8 percent over the 1963–1970 period. Both sets of evidence are consistent with the belief that prices in urban areas have risen only slightly more rapidly than in rural areas.

groups who are high users of hospital services (the service with the highest price increases)—for example, women at childbearing ages 18 to 34. Also, price increases for nonwhites in the latter period are slightly over the norm.

Use increases showed considerable variability for the population groups considered. In the pre–Medicare-Medicaid period, those groups with the greatest use increases were the middle-aged population, males and the low income population. The smallest use increases were found among children aged six to 17. In the latter period, which experienced the advent of Medicare and Medicaid, the rate of use increase for the low income population accelerated and the male rate of increase continued to exceed the female. Also, as might be expected, the rate of increase was greater for those 65 and over than for the population as a whole. However, similar high rates of use increase were seen for the zero to five and 55 to 64 age groups. One group, those aged 35 to 54, apparently had a decrease in annual rate of use.

Rates of use increase appeared similar for the white and nonwhite population. Even though the nonwhite population is disproportionately low income, its rate of use increase was considerably lower than for the low income population as a whole.

SUMMARY

The main purposes of this chapter have been to (1) document expenditures for providing medical care to various groups defined according to age, income and residential characteristics and changes that have taken place in these expenditures over the period from 1953 through 1970; (2) provide an indication of the direct financial burden on these various population groups by indicating their outlay for medical care; (3) show the relative influence of "price" and "use" on expenditure increase over time.

Some main findings concerning expenditures for medical care include:

1. Expenditures for medical care have been increasing at an accelerating rate over the 17 year period documented by these studies, reaching an average increase of 9 percent per year in the period from 1963 through 1970.
2. Among the various health services, the expenditures for hospital care have been increasing most rapidly, averaging over 14 percent per year in the period from 1963 to 1970.
3. Expenditures for medical care are greatest for the oldest age

groups, for whites and for people living in suburban areas. The population groups with consistently low expenditures from all sources for most types of services include nonwhites and low income children living in rural areas.

4. Overall expenditures tend to be highest for individuals in the lowest income groups, but when adjustment is made for family size, differences between individuals above and below the near poverty income level are small.

5. In the period between 1963 and 1970, increases in total expenditures were greatest for people in the youngest and oldest age groups.

Concerning the financial burden of medical care, highlights include:

1. The poor spend a greater proportion of their income on health care than the nonpoor. The lowest income families spent 13 percent of their income for medical care in 1970 compared to 3 percent for the highest income families.

2. The proportion of aggregate family income spent for health services dropped from a high of 5.5 percent in the 1958 study to 4.2 percent in 1970, reflecting, among other factors, increased public expenditures and increased payments of insurance premiums by employers.

3. While families overall are spending less of their incomes on medical care, the percent of income generally spent by low income families has continued to rise between 1963 and 1970 despite the enactment of the Medicare and Medicaid programs during this interval.

4. Between 1963 and 1970 the proportion of all medical expenditures accounting for people with the highest (catastrophic) expenditures rose substantially.

5. The typical family with large outlays for medical care might be described as suburban, white, in the middle or upper income bracket and headed by a full time worker. In contrast, the family spending 15 percent or more of its income for medical care is more likely to be rural, older, in the lower income bracket and with a head who is not a full time worker. These contrasts suggest that a national health insurance plan designed to reduce excessive family outlays for medical care without direct consideration of family income level would benefit a considerably different group of families than would a plan which primarily seeks to reduce outlay as a proportion of family income.

The investigation of price and use contributions to the increases in expenditures for medical care of the U.S. noninstitutionalized population in two recent periods suggests the following:

1. Price increases contributed substantially more to overall expenditure increases in both periods than did use increases.
2. Hospital price increases contributed most to overall price increases in both periods. Drug use in the first period and hospital use in the second period contributed most to overall use increases.
3. The so-called "free" services made a substantial contribution to increases in use between 1963 and 1970 while apparently making no contribution in the earlier period.
4. In the pre-Medicare-Medicaid period, use increases were greatest among the working age male population and among the low income group.
5. In the more recent period, use increases shifted not only to the elderly and the very young, but also to the group 55 to 64. The relatively high rate of use increase for males and the low income group continued.

These findings, then, suggest that institution of the Medicare and Medicaid programs were accompanied by:

1. Acceleration of some trends which were already taking place, i.e., relatively high rates of increase for the low income population and the aged;
2. A reduction in rates of increase for some groups not considered to be a target population for the program, such as those 35 to 54, but an increase for others, such as the 55 to 64 group;
3. Rates of increase for the nonwhite population which appear no greater than for the white population, even though the former presumably would be considered a target population.

Table 3-1. Mean expenditures for nonfree personal health services per family by family income: 1953, 1963 and 1970

Family Income (24)	Mean Nonfree Expenditures (13)			Average annual Percent Increase[a]	
	1953	1963	1970	1953-63	1963-70
Under $2,000	$130	$228	$318	5.4	4.8
$ 2,000- 3,499	156	245	394	4.3	6.8
3,500- 4,999	207	289	502	3.1	7.9
5,000- 7,499	259	409	620	4.4	5.9
7,500- 9,999			604 ⎫		
10,000-14,999	353	480	676 ⎬ 752	3.0	6.4
15,000 and over			979 ⎭		
Total	$207	$370	$624	5.7	8.0

[a]Average annual percent increases in this report are computed according to the technique outlined by G. Barclay (1958:28-33) using logarithms to the base 10. The shifts in proportion of the population represented by each income category make it possible for the average annual increase for all families to equal or exceed the computed increase for any income category.

Table 3-2. Mean and median expenditures for free and nonfree health services per family by family income and poverty level: 1970

Income and Poverty Level (24) (26)	Free and Nonfree Expenditures (1)		
	Mean		Median
Under $2,000	$ 469	(595)[a]	$149
$ 2,000- 3,499	551	(609)	186
3,500- 4,999	600	(450)	295
5,000- 7,499	723	(676)	306
7,500- 9,999	668	(499)	365
10,000-14,999	719	(600)	432
15,000 and over	1,013	(336)	475
Above near poverty	746	(2187)	368
Below near poverty	593	(1578)	219
Total	$ 707	(3765)[b]	$326

[a]In parentheses are the unweighted numbers of observations which can be used in combination with the procedures described in Appendix I to calculate standard errors of the 1970 estimates. Since the 1970 sample is a weighted sample, these numbers should *not* be used as weights for combining subcategories.

[b]Excludes 115 families where survey information was collected only for selected family members.

Table 3-3. Percent distribution of families by level of nonfree expenditures for personal health services: 1953, 1958, 1963 and 1970

Level of Family Expenditures	Percent Distribution of Families				
	Nonfree expenditures (13)				Free and nonfree expenditures (14)
	1953	1958	1963	1970	1970
None	29.8	2.9 ⎫	1.8 ⎫	2.8 ⎫	2.0 ⎫
Under $50	15.8 ⎫	17.3 ⎬ 20.2	16.0 ⎬ 17.8	13.2 ⎬ 16.0	9.5 ⎬ 11.5
$ 50- 99	20.1	14.0	11.7	11.2	10.5
100- 199	11.8	20.7	18.7	14.0	13.9
200- 299	7.0	13.5	12.8	11.3	11.4
300- 399	4.9	9.2	9.5	7.9	8.1
400- 499	6.3	5.7	6.3	4.8	5.7
500- 749	2.3	8.3	10.0	10.2	11.0
750- 999	1.6	3.8	5.1	6.5	7.2
1,000-1,999	0.4 ⎫	3.9	6.5	12.1	13.7
2,000-2,999	⎬	0.7	1.6	3.5 ⎫	3.9 ⎫
3,000-4,999	⎬ 0.4			1.4 ⎬ .5.9	1.9 ⎬ 7.0
$5,000 and over	⎭			1.0 ⎭	1.2 ⎭
Total	100	100	100	100	100

Table 3-4. Mean expenditures per family by type of service: 1953, 1958, 1963 and 1970

Service	Mean Nonfree Expenditures (13)				Mean Expenditures, 1970, Free and Nonfree (14)
	1953	1958	1963	1970	
Hospital (17)	$ 39	$ 68	$ 97	$235	$284
Physician (19)	77	98	115	167	184
Drugs (16)	31	60	75	88	94
Dental (15)	33	44	48	79	86
Other (18)	27	24	35	54	59
Total	$207	$294	$370	$624	$707

Table 3-5. Aggregate family outlay for personal health services as a percent of family income, by income group: 1953, 1958, 1963 and 1970

Family Income and Poverty Level (24) (26)	Aggregate Outlay as Percent of Family Income (39)			
	1953	1958	1963	1970
Under $2,000	11.8	13.0	15.7	12.6
$ 2,000– 3,499	6.1	8.4	8.5	9.0
3,500– 4,999	5.4	6.4	6.8	7.3
5,000– 7,499	4.7	5.4	5.6	5.7
7,500– 9,999 ⎫				4.5 ⎫
10,000–14,999 ⎬	3.0	3.9	3.8	3.7 ⎬ 3.5
15,000 and over ⎭				3.1 ⎭
Above near poverty	_a	_a	_a	3.0
Below near poverty	–	–	–	8.2
Total	4.8	5.5	5.0	4.2

[a] Not available.

Table 3-6. Aggregate family outlay for personal health services as a percent of family income, by income group and by age of oldest member: 1970

Family Income and Poverty Level (24) (26)	Aggregate Outlay as a Percent of Family Income (39) (24)			
	Families whose oldest member is 65 or over		Families whose oldest member is under 65	
Under $2,000	13.1	(325)[a]	11.9	(295)[a]
$ 2,000– 3,499	11.3	(290)	6.4	(295)
3,500– 4,999	8.8	(152)	6.7	(313)
5,000– 7,499	8.9	(163)	5.1	(541)
7,500– 9,999	5.7	(107)	4.3	(420)
10,000–14,999	5.0	(79)	3.6	(544)
15,000 and over	3.8	(66)	3.0	(290)
Above near poverty	5.9	(566)	3.7	(1735)
Below near poverty	12.3	(616)	6.0	(963)
Total	7.4	(1182)	3.8	(2698)

[a]In parentheses are the unweighted numbers of observations which can be used in combination with the procedures described in Appendix I to calculate standard errors of the 1970 estimates. Since the 1970 sample is a weighted sample, these numbers should *not* be used as weights for combining subcategories.

Table 3-7. Percent distribution of family expenditures for medical care by family income: 1970

Family Income (24)	Expenditures			Income distribution of all families
	Gross expenditure greater than $5,000 (14)	Outlay is $1,000 or more (39)	Outlay is 15 percent or more of family income (39)	
Under $2,000	5	1	38	10
$ 2,000– 3,499	8	4	25	11
3,500– 4,999	3	6	13	9
5,000– 7,499	20	13	14	16
7,500– 9,999	8	12	4	15
10,000–14,999	18	28	3	22
15,000 and over	38	37	4	17
Total	100 (47)[a]	100 (209)[a]	100 (451)[a]	100 (3765)[a]

[a]In parentheses are the unweighted numbers of observations which can be used in combination with the procedures described in Appendix I to calculate standard errors of the 1970 estimates. Since the 1970 sample is a weighted sample, these numbers should *not* be used as weights for combining subcategories.

Table 3-8. Percent distribution of families by expenditures for medical care and family characteristics: 1970

	Percent			
Characteristic	*Gross expenditure (14) greater than $5,000*	*Outlay is $1,000 or more (39)*	*Outlay is 15 Percent or more of family income (39) (24)*	*Distribution of all families*
Age of Head (1)				
21–35	11	17	11	27
36–50	42	40	12	28
51–64	33	33	25	25
65 and over	13	10	53	20
Major activity of[b] main earner (37)				
Employed full time	57	77	26	65
Retired	12	8	34	14
Other	30	15	40	21
Race (49)				
White	94**	96	90	89
Nonwhite	6	4*	10	11
Near poverty level (26)				
Above	81**	93	34	74
Below	18	7	66	26
Education of head[b] (10)				
8 years or less	15	18	43	27
9–11 years	10	15	18	18
12 years	17	27	22	28
13 years or more	57	40	17	27
Family size (23)				
Small	45**	48	87	67
Medium	37	39	9	22
Large	19	14	4*	12

Residence (52)				
SMSA, central city	27	23	27	32
SMSA, other	46	47	26	26
Urban, non-SMSA	4	10*	10	13
Rural, nonfarm	23	16	26	23
Rural, farm	1	5*	11	6
Total	100[a] (47)[c]	100[a] (209)[c]	100[a] (451)[c]	100[a] (3765)[c]

[a]Columns do not add to 100 percent due to rounding error.

[b]Excludes cases with no answer and don't know.

[c]In parentheses are the unweighted numbers of observations which can be used in combination with the procedures described in Appendix I to calculate standard errors of the 1970 estimates. Since the 1970 sample is a weighted sample, these numbers should *not* be used as weights for combining subcategories.

*Fewer than 25 unweighted cases in cell.

**Every cell in the expenditures greater than $5,000 column has fewer than 25 cases with the exception of these cells.

Table 3-9. Mean nonfree expenditures per person by age, sex and income: 1953, 1963 and 1970*

Characteristic	Mean Nonfree Expenditures (13)			Annual Percent Increase	
	1953	*1963*	*1970*	*1953-1963*	*1963-1970*
Sex (54)					
Male	$ 51	$ 92	$187	5.6	10.1
Female	80	131	231	4.7	8.1
Age (1)					
0-5	28	47	94	4.9	9.9
6-17	38	56	85	3.7	6.0
18-34	70	124	212	5.4	7.7
35-54	80	151	209	6.0	4.6
55-64	96	165	346	5.2	10.6
65 and over	102	184	387	5.6	10.6
Family income (25)					
Low	-[a]	95	205	-[a]	11.0
Middle	-	105	191	-	8.5
High	-	128	228	-	8.2
Total	$ 65	$112	$209	5.2	8.9

[a]Not available for 1953.

*Selected observations are excluded from this table. For exclusion criteria and estimates including all observations, see Appendix Table II-2.

Table 3-10. Mean nonfree expenditures by type of service: 1953, 1963 and 1970

Type of Service	Mean Nonfree Expenditure (13)			Percent Annual Increase	
	1953	*1963*	*1970*	*1953-1963*	*1963-1970*
Hospital (17)	$ 13	$ 29	$ 70	7.6	14.3
Inpatient	—[a]	28	77	—[a]	14.4
Outpatient	—	1	2	—	9.9
Physician	25	35	56	3.2	6.7
Inpatient (20)	—[a]	11	21	—[a]	9.2
Outpatient (21)	—	24	35	—	5.4
Drugs (16)	10	23	29	7.9	3.3
Prescribed	—[a]	16	20	—[a]	3.2
Nonprescribed	—	7	9	—	3.6
Dental (15)	10	15	26	3.9	7.9
Other (18)	8	10	19	2.1	9.2
Practitioners	—[a]	3	6	—[a]	9.9
Goods and services	—	7	13	—	8.8
Total	$ 65	$112	$209	5.2	8.9

[a]Not available for 1953.

Table 3-11. Total expenditures for health services for population groups ordered by magnitude of expenditures: 1963 to 1970

Percent of Population Ordered by Magnitude of Expenditures	1963 Nonfree (13)	1970 Nonfree excluding Medicare (13)	1970 Nonfree including Medicare (13)	1970 Total (14)
		Percent of total expenditures		
Top 1 percent	17	23	24	26
Top 5 percent	43	48	49	50
Top 10 percent	59	63	65	66
Top quartile	81	84	85	85
Third quartile	14	12	11	11
Second quartile	5	4	3	4
Bottom quartile	1	*	*	1
Total	100[a]	100	100[a]	100[a]
		Mean expenditures per person		
Top 1 percent	$1,942.61	$4,322.83	$4,919.78	$6,469.44
Top 5 percent	956.86	1,776.10	2,051.41	2,484.04
Top 10 percent	659.00	1,183.52	1,355.99	1,613.73
Top quartile	363.25	625.22	705.38	836.03
Third quartile	62.24	90.40	92.08	106.27
Second quartile	20.53	28.56	28.87	36.11
Bottom quartile	2.38	3.38	3.70	5.98
Total	$ 112.10	$ 186.89	$ 207.51	$ 246.10

[a]Columns do not add to 100 percent due to rounding error.

*Less than 0.5 percent.

Table 3-12. Average annual increase in mean expenditures for population groups ordered by magnitude of expenditures: 1963 and 1970

Percent of Population Ordered by Magnitude of Expenditures	Nonfree Excluding Medicare (13)	Nonfree Including Medicare (13)	Total Health Care Expenditures (14)
Top 1 percent	11.4	13.3	17.2
Top 5 percent	8.8	10.9	13.6
Top 10 percent	8.4	10.3	12.8
Top quartile	7.8	9.5	11.9
Third quartile	5.3	5.6	7.6
Second quartile	4.7	4.9	8.1
Bottom quartile	5.0	6.3	13.2
Total	7.3	8.9	11.2

Table 3-13. Mean and median total (14) expenditures per person by selected characteristics: 1970*

Characteristic	Total Population Mean	People with Expenditures Mean	People with Expenditures Median
Sex (54)			
Male	$213	$232	$ 62
Female	260	275	79
Age (1)			
0-5 years	106	114	47
6-17 years	96	105	41
18-34 years	246	260	80
35-54 years	244	259	89
55-64 years	379	415	135
65 years and over	429	456	135
Poverty level (26)			
Above near poverty	243	256	75
Below near poverty	217	246	50
Education of head (10)			
8 years or less	238	265	63
9-11 years	197	213	64
12 years	209	223	67
13 years or more	298	307	86
Residence (52)			
SMSA, central city	236	256	71
SMSA, other	301	318	88
Urban, non-SMSA	195	207	69
Rural, nonfarm	202	216	60
Rural, farm	184	203	55
Total	$238	$254	$ 70

*Selected observations are excluded from this table. For exclusion criteria and estimates including all observations, see Appendix II-3.

Table 3–14. Mean and median total (14) hospital expenditures per person by selected characteristics: 1970*

Characteristic	Inpatient Hospital (17)			Outpatient Hospital (17)		
	Total population Mean	People with expenditures Mean	Median	Total population Mean	People with expenditures Mean	Median
Sex (54)						
Male	$ 71	$ 832	$461	$4	$48	$26
Female	101	764	451	3	60	28
Age (1)						
0–5 years	32	378	279	3	41	30
6–17 years	18	368	308	2	38	24
18–34 years	94	602	396	3	44	23
35–54 years	75	741	507	4	70	34
55–64 years	153	1141	839	3	45	25
65 years and over	199	1209	796	3	61	32
Poverty level (26)						
Above near poverty	89	816	451	3	44	25
Below near poverty	101	906	478	6	75	35
Education of head (10)						
8 years or less	98	904	558	5	65	30
9–11 years	74	701	482	5	49	27
12 years	78	722	397	2	38	27
13 years or more	79	719	442	4	53	25
Residence (52)						
SMSA, central city	86	874	537	6	66	32
SMSA, other	94	852	526	3	40	24
Urban, non-SMSA	65	503	320	1	b	b
Rural, nonfarm	67	611	397	2	39	21
Rural, farm	75	736	385	a	22	15
Total	$ 92	$ 837	$455	$4	$57	$27

aLess than 50¢.

bFewer than 25 unweighted cases in cell.

*Selected observations are excluded from this table. For exclusion criteria and estimates including all observations, see Appendix

Table 3-15. Mean and median total (14) physician expenditures per person by selected characteristics: 1970*

Characteristic	Inpatient, Including Surgery (20)			Outpatient[a] (21)		
	Total Population	People with expenditures		Total population	People with expenditures	
	Mean	Mean	Median	Mean	Mean	Median
Sex (54)						
Male	$22	$294	$140	$33	$55	$26
Female	21	261	178	46	70	30
Age (1)						
0–5 years	10	153	85	36	50	32
6–17 years	6	165	125	18	33	16
18–34 years	19	246	123	48	76	31
35–54 years	22	277	253	43	70	31
55–64 years	39	317	287	58	87	41
65 years and over	41	291	162	55	79	45
Poverty level (26)						
Above near poverty	23	284	167	42	63	30
Below near poverty	17	248	112	33	64	28
Education of head (10)						
8 years or less	23	253	161	34	61	29
9–11 years	16	228	157	35	59	29
12 years	20	259	140	36	56	25
13 years or more	23	312	190	53	75	33
Residence (52)						
SMSA, central city	17	269	189	43	75	33
SMSA, other	28	359	240	46	69	30
Urban, non-SMSA	20	201	99	36	55	28
Rural, nonfarm	18	209	135	32	52	25
Rural, farm	17	214	129	28	48	23
Total	$21	$277	$156	$40	$63	$30

[a]Includes all obstetrical care including delivery.
*Selected observations are excluded from this table. For exclusion criteria and estimates including all observations, see Appendix Table II-5.

Table 3-16. Mean and median total (14) drug expenditures per person by selected characteristics: 1970*

Characteristic	Prescribed Drugs (16)			Nonprescribed Drugs (16)		
	Total population	People with expenditures		Total population	People with expenditures	
	Mean	Mean	Median	Mean	Mean	Median
Sex (54)						
Male	$19	$49	$17	$ 9	$12	$ 5
Female	26	56	24	9	13	6
Age (1)						
0–5 years	9	19	10	6	9	5
6–17 years	6	20	10	6	8	5
18–34 years	17	40	16	9	12	5
35–54 years	28	62	27	10	14	7
55–64 years	42	86	50	14	21	10
65 years and over	56	92	52	12	18	10
Poverty level (26)						
Above near poverty	23	51	20	9	13	6
Below near poverty	23	60	22	7	12	5
Education of head (10)						
8 years or less	28	69	29	8	13	5
9–11 years	19	47	19	8	11	5
12 years	21	47	20	9	13	6
13 years or more	23	50	17	9	13	6
Residence (52)						
SMSA, central city	25	60	20	9	13	5
SMSA, other	22	47	20	8	12	7
Urban, non-SMSA	23	51	20	9	13	5
Rural, nonfarm	21	51	20	9	12	5
Rural, farm	21	54	29	8	12	5
Total	$23	$53	$20	$ 9	$13	$ 5

*Selected observations are excluded from this table. For exclusion criteria and estimates including all observations, see Appendix Table II–6.

Table 3-17. Mean and median total (14) dental expenditures per person by selected characteristics: 1970*

| | Dental (15) | | |
| | Total population | People with expenditures | |
Characteristic	Mean	Mean	Median
Sex (54)			
Male	$27	$65	$25
Female	30	70	26
Age (1)			
0–5 years	3	26	17
6–17 years	29	54	22
18–34 years	33	66	27
35–54 years	38	83	29
55–64 years	27	84	31
65 years and over	20	80	28
Poverty level (26)			
Above near poverty	33	70	25
Below near poverty	14	54	20
Education of head (10)			
8 years or less	20	74	25
9–11 years	24	66	25
12 years	28	61	24
13 years or more	38	69	26
Residence (52)			
SMSA, central city	26	68	25
SMSA, other	43	86	30
Urban, non-SMSA	22	53	20
Rural, nonfarm	21	54	22
Rural, farm	16	43	18
Total	$28	$67	$25

*Selected observations are excluded from this table. For exclusion criteria and estimates including all observations, see Appendix Table II-7.

Table 3-18.   Mean and median total (14) other expenditures per person by selected characteristics: 1970*

Characteristic	Non-MD Practitioners (18)			Tests, Glasses, Other Goods and Services (18)		
	Total population	People with expenditures		Total population	People with expenditures	
	Mean	Mean	Median	Mean	Mean	Median
Sex (54)						
Male	$ 5	$33	$14	$13	$47	$33
Female	6	40	14	17	51	32
Age (1)						
0–5 years	a	b	b	4	35	20
6–17 years	2	15	12	7	35	28
18–34 years	4	29	13	16	44	30
35–54 years	5	30	14	20	55	36
55–64 years	9	35	16	27	62	40
65 years and over	11	55	14	22	57	35
Poverty level (26)						
Above near poverty	6	40	14	16	50	33
Below near poverty	3	26	14	11	48	32
Education of head (10)						
8 years or less	6	35	14	16	55	34
9–11 years	3	19	13	13	46	32
12 years	4	28	14	12	41	30
13 years or more	8	51	14	20	55	35
Residence (52)						
SMSA, central city	6	33	14	17	52	33
SMSA, other	5	42	15	16	51	31
Urban, non-SMSA	4	28	15	13	46	33
Rural, nonfarm	3	21	12	14	48	32
Rural, farm	4	24	13	12	41	32
Total	$ 6	$39	$14	$15	$50	$32

a Less than 50¢.

b Fewer than 25 unweighted cases in cell.

* Selected observations are excluded from this table. For exclusion criteria and estimates including all observations, see Appendix Table II–8.

Table 3-19. Mean nonfree expenditures per live birth (22) by type of service: 1953, 1958, 1963 and 1970

Type of Service	*Mean Nonfree Expenditures (13)*			
	1953	*1958*	*1963*	*1970*
Hospital (17)	$ 82	$128	$162	$327
Physician (19)	91	118	133	184
Drugs (16)	10	17	16	15
Other (18)	10	8	5	6
Total	$ 193	$272	$316	$532

Table 3-20. Mean nonfree expenditures per live birth (22) by family income level: 1953, 1958, 1963 and 1970

Family Income (25)	*Mean Nonfree Expenditures (13)*				
	1953	*1958*	*1963*	*1970*	
Low	$112	$172	$194	$270	(136)[a]
Middle	208	283	327	598	(112)
High	276	348	393	712	(42)
Total	$193	$272	$316	$532	(290)

[a]In parentheses are the unweighted numbers of observations which can be used in combination with the procedures described in Appendix I to calculate standard errors of the 1970 estimates. Since the 1970 sample is a weighted sample, these numbers should *not* be used as weights for combining subcategories.

Table 3-21. Mean and median total expenditures per live birth (22) by type of service and family income level: 1970

Type of Service	Family Income (25)							
	Low		Middle		High		Total	
	Mean	*Median*	*Mean*	*Median*	*Mean*	*Median*	*Mean*	*Median*
Hospital (17)	$402	$345	$423	$410	$439	$400	$421	$393
Physician (19)	144	141	204	225	255	244	199	208
Drugs (16)	20	2	18	10	11	—[a]	17	6
Other (18)	6	—[a]	6	—[a]	9	—[a]	7	—[a]
Total	$572	$489	$651	$637	$714	$709	$644	$627

[a]The median expenditure is zero for any distribution in which more than half of the observations fall into the category "none."

Table 3-22. Average annual percent increase in expenditures (14) per person in price and use by type of health service: 1953-1963 and 1963-1970

	Annual Percent Increase			
	1953-1963		*1963-1970*	
Service	*Price[a]*	*Use[b]*	*Price[a]*	*Use[b]*
Hospital (17)	6.1	1.0	10.5	3.9
Physician (19)	3.0	0.1	5.4	2.3
Dental (15)	2.3	1.6	4.5	4.2
Drugs (16)	0.8	7.4	0.4	3.7
Other[c] (18)	1.4	0.7	3.4	6.3
Total[d]	3.3	1.5	6.1	3.6

[a]Price increases are estimated on the basis of the medical care component of the United States Department of Labor's Consumer Price Index (U.S. Department of Labor, 1973).

[b]The residual increase in expenditure not accounted for by price increase was defined as increase due to "use."

[c]Uses the CPI component for optometrists' fees and glasses.

[d]Computed using as weights the expenditure by service in the initial time period.

Table 3-23. Percent increase in expenditures (14) per individual accounted for by type of service and source of payment in current and constant dollars: 1953–1963 and 1963–1970

Service	Source of Payment	Percent Increase			
		1953–1963		1963–1970	
		Total expenditures[a]	Use[b]	Total expenditures[a]	Use[b]
Hospital (17)		37	13	52	32
	(Nonfree) (13)	(33)	(14)	(43)	(26)
	(Free) (12)	(4)	(–1)	(9)	(6)
Physician (19)		19	–1	22	18
	(Nonfree) (13)	(20)	(3)	(18)	(10)
	(Free) (12)	(–1)	(–5)	(4)	(8)
Dental (15)		11	13	11	15
	(Nonfree) (13)	(10)	(12)	(10)	(11)
	(Free) (12)	(*)	(1)	(1)	(3)
Drugs (16)		27	72	7	21
	(Nonfree) (13)	(26)	(69)	(6)	(17)
	(Free) (12)	(1)	(2)	(1)	(4)
Other (18)		5	4	8	15
	(Nonfree) (13)	(5)	(4)	(7)	(13)
	(Free) (12)	(*)	(*)	(1)	(2)
All services		100	100	100	100
	(Nonfree) (13)	(95)	(102)	(84)	(76)
	(Free) (12)	(5)	(–2)	(16)	(24)

*Less than 0.5 percent.

[a]Proportional expenditure increase with no consideration of price changes.

[b]Expenditures in the latter period are deflated (by appropriate components of the Consumer Price Index) to price levels in the earlier period before percentage increases are computed.

Table 3-24. Average annual percent increase in expenditures (14) per person in price and use for all personal health services by selected characteristics of the population: 1953-1963 and 1963-1970

| | *Annual Percent Increase* | | | | |
| | *1953-1963* | | *1963-1970* | | |
Characteristic	*Price[a]*	*Use*	*Price[a]*	*Use*	*Mean 1970 Expenditures (14)*
Age (1)					
0-5	3.3	1.5	5.5	5.2	$106
6-17	3.1	0.5	5.3	1.0	96
18-34	3.4	1.4	6.6	2.1	246
35-54	3.3	2.7	6.2	-0.4	244
55-64	3.2	1.7	6.0	5.0	379
65 and over	3.3	2.1	5.9	5.1	429
Sex (54)					
Male	3.2	2.3	5.9	4.7	213
Female	3.3	1.2	6.2	2.6	260
Family income (25)					
Low	3.2	3.1	6.4	6.2	280
Middle	3.2	1.1	6.2	3.3	216
High	3.2	0.6	5.8	2.8	239
Race (49)					
White	_b	_b	6.0	3.5	245
Nonwhite	—	—	6.6	3.7	166
Residence (52)					
Urban	3.3	1.2	6.0	3.9	259
Rural, nonfarm	3.3	0.9	6.2	3.0	202
Rural, farm	3.3	1.0	6.1	4.7	184
Total	3.3	1.5	6.1	3.6	238

[a]Price increases are adjusted according to the mix of services purchased by each group.

[b]Information not available in 1953.

Chapter 4

How Personal Health Services
are Financed

Methods of financing personal health services are important because these services account for over 8 percent of the gross national product. Further, as the previous chapter has documented, health services expenditures have special characteristics that make financing of particular concern at both the individual and the family level. Medical expenditures are often unexpected. They are distributed unequally among the population. They are incurred by families regardless of income. Therefore, they are difficult to plan and budget for. In addition, some families experience extraordinary medical expenses that can cause severe economic hardship. For example, in 1970, 7 percent of the families interviewed had total expenditures of $2,000 or more, and over 1 percent, or some three-quarters of a million families, had expenses of $5,000 or more.

Major methods of financing health services in the U.S. include Medicare for the aged and voluntary health insurance for the rest of the population. The first section of this chapter considers the extent and type of coverage various groups in the population have and how this coverage has changed over the two decades covered by this series of national studies. Subsequent sections consider trends in employer contributions to health insurance premiums and sources of payment for various types of health services. The sources considered include out-of-pocket payments, voluntary insurance, Medicare, Medicaid and welfare, other "nonfree" sources, and other "free" sources. A following section looks directly at the proportion of the public's expenditures for health services covered by health insurance benefits.

A final section deals with debt incurred by the population in meeting the costs of medical care.

HEALTH INSURANCE COVERAGE

This section examines health insurance coverage of the noninstitutionalized population of the United States as it existed at the conclusion of calendar year 1970. Since the most recent study paralleled earlier studies conducted in 1953, 1958 and 1963, it is possible to look at trends in coverage over a 17 year period. The situation in 1970 and trends over time will be considered (1) for families, (2) for individuals, (3) according to type of insurer and method of enrollment, and (4) according to employer contribution for group policies.

Family Coverage

Table 4-1 shows that 83 percent of all families had some health insurance coverage in 1970 — up 20 percentage points from 1953 and 9 percentage points from 1963. In 1970, families headed by women and those with other characteristics associated with "minority" or "disadvantaged status" were less likely to have health insurance than other families in the population. However, Table 4-1 suggests that differences in coverage according to sex and education of the head of the family, as well as main activity of the main earner, family income and residence, were considerably less in 1970 than they had been in earlier studies.

Table 4-2 indicates that two out of every five families had some major medical insurance coverage in 1970. There has been rapid growth in this type of insurance since the late 1950s. In contrast to general health insurance coverage, large differences continue to exist in the proportion covered by major medical insurance according to family income and work activity of the main earner. Low income families and those headed by a person not working full time are much less likely to be covered by a major medical policy.

Individual Coverage

Table 4-3 shows the proportion of individuals with health insurance covering various types of medical care. This table shows that about three-quarters of the population had hospital and surgical-medical coverage in 1970. Further, physician visit coverage has expanded over the past few years, so that it covered over half the population by 1970. Much of the expansion of physician visit coverage is due to the increasing prevalence of major medical coverage which had covered one-fifth of the population in 1963 but was up to two-fifths by 1970. The expansion of outpatient drug coverage in recent years is also largely through major medical type coverage. Thus, most people shown to have doctor visit and drug coverage are not covered for the first dollar cost but only after a deductible (of $50 or $100, for example) has been paid. Coverage of the costs of regular dental care is a relatively recent phenomenon which covered 11 percent of the population in 1970 and has increased considerably since then.

Table 4–4 shows trends in coverage of persons for hospital care according to age. In the period from 1953 through 1963 the elderly and young persons 18 to 24 were the groups least likely to have coverage. In the interim between 1963 and 1970 Medicare was signed into law so that in the latter year virtually all old people had hospital coverage. In 1970 the 18 to 24 age group continues to be the age group with the least coverage (about one-third had no hospital insurance). Many of those younger people are no longer covered by their parents' insurance but are not yet employees covered through their own places of work.

Table 4–5 indicates the proportion of people with various social and demographic characteristics who were covered by hospital, doctor visit and major medical insurance in 1970. Older people 55 to 64 who are not yet eligible for Medicare appear somewhat less likely to have doctor visit and major medical insurance than younger people. Only 5 percent of the elderly had major medical insurance to supplement their Medicare coverage. Coverage in 1970 did not differ according to sex, but persons with family incomes below the near poverty level were much less likely to have any of the coverages than were those with incomes above the near poverty level. The lower the educational level of the family head, the less likely it was that family members would be covered by insurance. The difference in proportion covered according to education was much greater for doctor visit and major medical coverage than for hospital insurance. Central city and rural farm residents were less likely to have insurance than other urban and rural nonfarm residents. This discrepancy was found for all types of coverage reported in Table 4–5.

Twenty-three percent of the population were not covered by hospital insurance in 1970. Table 4–6 attempts to shed some light on two questions: Who are these people? and How do they differ from persons with insurance? The uninsured are a relatively young population, with 44 percent of them being 17 or under. Of course, few of the uninsured are over 65, but a smaller proportion of them are 35 to 64 than is true for the insured population.

Half of the uninsured are males and half are females, indicating no difference from the insured population in sex composition. Also, approximately one-half of the uninsured are below the near poverty income level, but in this respect they differ greatly from the insured population. Only 14 percent of the latter have incomes below the near poverty level.

Over one-third of the uninsured live in families headed by a person with eight or fewer years of formal education. About three-fifths were in families where the head had not completed high school. Two-fifths of the insured persons were from families with heads who had not completed high school.

Thirty-seven percent of the uninsured live in the central city of an SMSA, compared to 28 percent of the insured. While they are largely an urban group, the uninsured also include a disproportionate number of rural farm residents. In sum, then, the uninsured population can be described as relatively young, low income, poorly educated and living in urban areas.

Type of Insurer and Method of Enrollment

Table 4-7 shows that Blue Cross and the private insurance companies each insured about one-third of the population against the cost of hospital and inpatient surgery care in 1970. Prepaid groups and other independent insurers accounted for another 6 percent of the population. Medicare's share was about one-tenth, representing the population 65 and over. The CHAMPUS group are the dependents of armed forces personnel who receive care at government institutions or have their care paid for by the government.

Table 4-8 distinguishes those people and their dependents who are insured through place of work or through some other group they belong to from those who purchase health insurance directly. There has been a decline in the proportion of the population covered by nongroup insurance from 1963 to 1970. In 1970, 15 percent of the population were covered by health insurance purchased directly. The decrease between 1963 and 1970 can, in part, be explained by the advent of Medicare. Before Medicare, many of the elderly who were not covered by employer insurance purchased policies directly. The incentive to buy insurance was greatly reduced after Medicare, although supplementary policies for the elderly are not uncommon.

Since nongroup policies tend to be less comprehensive than group coverage, and because they return less on the premium dollar, it is of interest to look at the methods of enrollment of different social and demographic groups in the population. Table 4-9 illustrates that persons 55 to 64 and the elderly were the groups most likely to have nongroup coverage in 1970. People 55 to 64 were less likely to have group coverage than other ages and appear to compensate by purchasing nongroup insurance, resulting in 27 percent having nongroup coverage. Thirty-six percent of those 65 and over had some nongroup coverage. This proportion indicates the extent to which the elderly are supplementing their Medicare coverage.

There is little difference in the type of enrollment according to sex. While similar portions of the poor and nonpoor have nongroup coverage, 76 percent of the people above the near poverty level have group coverage compared to about one-half that percentage below the near poverty level. Thus, the low income group is not only less likely to have insurance than the rest of the population, but those who have insurance are more likely than higher income families to have nongroup coverage that is less comprehensive and more expensive to buy.

The proportion of people with group coverage increases as the education of the family head increases, while the proportion with nongroup coverage shows no discernible pattern according to education. Fifty-five percent of individuals in families headed by a person with an eighth grade education or less have group coverage, compared with 79 percent of individuals in families with a family head who attended college. Thus, in a fashion similar to that for low income families, those with little education who have insurance are less likely to have group coverage. However, the differences according to education are considerably smaller than according to income.

Central city and rural farm residents are less likely than other residents to have group coverage. Actually, less than one-half of all rural farm residents had group coverage in 1970. In contrast, 24 percent of the rural farm residents had nongroup coverage compared to 15 percent for the population as a whole.

EMPLOYER CONTRIBUTION TO
HEALTH INSURANCE PREMIUMS

Employer participation in the payment for work group health insurance increased steadily over the period from 1953 to 1970 according to Table 4-10. By 1970 employers were paying all of the group health insurance premiums for 39 percent of the families with group insurance. In addition, 53 percent of the families with group health insurance had some of the premiums paid for by employers. Thus, only 8 percent of the families with health insurance through a work group were paying all of the premium in 1970, compared to 21 percent in 1963 and 41 percent in 1953.

SOURCES OF PAYMENT
FOR HEALTH SERVICES

This section is devoted to an examination of the proportion of health services expenditures paid for by various sources. The sources are divided into "free" and "nonfree." "Free" refers to expenditures for medical goods and services provided to the family at no direct cost or at substantially reduced rates and without benefits being provided by any type of health insurance plan. Free care is further divided into that provided by Medicaid, welfare and free institutions versus "other free" expenditures. The latter includes care provided by the Veterans Administration, by workmen's compensation and by certain governmental agencies such as federally funded crippled children's programs.

"Nonfree" expenditures are generally considered to be expenditures for care that the consumer pays for himself, either directly or through some third party to which he pays premiums or has premiums paid on his behalf. Nonfree subcategories include payments by voluntary insurance, Medicare payments, out-of-pocket expenditures and a residual "other nonfree" category that includes payments by CHAMPUS and those made by accident and liability insurance carried by some member of the patient's family.

All tables in this section with the exception of the first (Table 4–11) are based on our "best estimate" data. The best estimate data incorporates cost information provided by physicians, hospitals and third party payers. Table 4–11 shows trends between 1963 and 1970 and, for comparability, uses best estimate data for hospital inpatient expenditures only, since verification of ambulatory care was not carried out in 1963.

In the following section, the contribution of each source of payment is examined for various subgroups in the population defined by the standard demographic and socioeconomic variables that have been used throughout the volume. Subsections are devoted to total expenses and to expenses for hospital, physician, drugs, dental and other services.

Total Expenses

Table 4-11 shows that for people with expenditures, nonfree expenditures more than doubled between 1963 and 1970. However, out-of-pocket expenditures as a proportion of total expenditures decreased due to the greater share covered by insurance benefits.

In each period, inpatient hospital services were most expensive and were also most likely to be covered by health insurance benefits

(Table 4-11). Inpatient physician services were next most expensive but were also reduced considerably by insurance benefits. Despite the fact that insurance picked up a greater proportion of the costs of these expensive services, people with expenses were still left on average with sizable bills to pay out of their own pocket in 1970. Thus, those who were hospitalized had out-of-pocket expenditures that averaged over $200 and those with hospitalized surgery had personal physician bills that averaged $141.

While insurance benefits for services other than inpatient hospital and inpatient physician services also increased between 1963 and 1970, most people with nonfree expenditures for other health services in 1970 were meeting these expenditures with out-of-pocket payments (Table 4-11). Only expenditures for physician office and home visits were reduced appreciably by insurance benefits in 1970, and even here the reduction was only 17 percent (from $52 to $43) for the major expense category of office visits. In both 1963 and 1970, nonfree expenditures for ophthalmologists, drugs, dental care and for other medical goods and services were mostly out-of-pocket payments by the consumer.

Table 4-12 shows sources of payment for free and nonfree expenditures for various social and demographic groups in 1970. Out-of-pocket payments account for 44 percent of all expenditures, making it the most important source of payment. Ranked as the second major source of payment is voluntary health insurance, accounting for 31 percent of the total. Medicaid and welfare rank third (13 percent), followed by Medicare (8 percent). Other free and nonfree sources account for a relatively small proportion of the total expenditures.

Table 4-12 shows that Medicaid and welfare pay relatively more of the expenditures for children than for adults. Medicare paid about one-half of the total expenditures for people 65 and over. Voluntary insurance paid the greatest proportion for older adults 55 to 64 and the smallest (apart from the elderly) for children six to 17. These same children have a greater proportion of their expenditures paid for out-of-pocket than any other age group.

People with family incomes below the near poverty level had a quarter of their total expenditures paid for by Medicaid and welfare. As would be expected, the proportion paid for by Medicaid and welfare decreased with increasing income (Table 4-12). Because persons 65 and over tend to have low incomes, Medicare also pays proportionately more of the expenditures for low income persons than is true for higher income persons. Contrarily, voluntary insurance pays a greater proportion for higher income persons, covering 50 percent or more of the expenditures for persons with family incomes of $10,000 or more in 1970.

Whites and nonwhites pay a greater proportion of their total expenditures out-of-pocket than is paid by any other source (Table 4-12). However, this proportion is considerably greater for whites (45 percent) than for nonwhites (32 percent). The second most important source for nonwhites is Medicaid (28 percent), while for whites it is voluntary insurance (31 percent).

The patterns for educational level are similar to those for income (Table 4-12). The persons from families headed by someone with little education rely more on Medicaid and Medicare, while those with more education have greater proportions of their expenditures covered by voluntary insurance and pay for more out of their own pocket. The biggest differences according to residence are that Medicaid and welfare pays a greater proportion of the expenditures of persons living in central cities of SMSAs, and Medicare pays more of the total for rural farm residents than for people living elsewhere.

Hospital Expenses

In 1970 over one-half of the total expenses for inpatient hospital services were paid for by voluntary insurance (Table 4-13). No other source of payment accounted for as much as 20 percent. Out-of-pocket payments, which were the main source of payment for all health services combined, accounted for only 12 percent of the inpatient hospital bill.

Voluntary insurance paid the majority of the bill for all age groups except the elderly, who had four-fifths of their total hospital expenses covered by Medicare (Table 4-13). The low income and nonwhite populations had substantial proportions of their inpatient expenses paid for by Medicaid. The rural farm population had relatively less paid for by voluntary insurance and more paid for by Medicare than the rest of the population. Central city residents paid less out-of-pocket and had more paid for by Medicaid than other residents.

Expenditures for outpatient services in hositals are financed to a lesser extent by voluntary insurance and to a greater extent by Medicaid than are inpatient services (Table 4-14). This reflects the greater use of outpatient departments and emergency rooms by groups who are more likely to have services paid for by Medicaid. These groups include the low income, nonwhite, low education and central city residents.

Physician Expenses

Like hospital services, physician inpatient services are financed primarily by voluntary insurance (Table 4–15). In contrast to inpatient hospital expenses, out-of-pocket payments make up a quarter of the total for inpatient physician services and Medicaid accounts for only a small proportion. The latter apparently results because much of the Medicaid and welfare care is provided in institutions with salaried doctors. The services these physicians provide are taken into account in the inpatient hospital billing.

Physician outpatient expenditures reported in Table 4–16 refer to all care provided in ambulatory settings including visits in doctors' private offices. Two-thirds of the costs of these services were paid for out-of-pocket in 1970. Most groups shown in Table 4–16 paid 50 percent or more of the costs for these services themselves. Medicaid paid about one-quarter of the physician ambulatory cost for the low income and nonwhite groups and Medicare paid 29 percent for the elderly.

Drug Expenses

Table 4–17 shows that prescription drug expenditures are mostly paid for on an out-of-pocket basis. Medicaid pays about one-quarter of the cost of drugs for the lowest income and nonwhite populations. The highest income group has 18 percent of its drug bills paid by insurance. It includes the people most likely to have major medical insurance, which usually picks up some portion of drug costs after an initial deductible is met.

Dental Expenses

Dental services are also financed primarily by direct payments by users (Table 4–18). However, persons below the near poverty level and nonwhites have about one-third of their dental costs paid by Medicaid and welfare.

Other Expenses

"Other" expenses reported in Table 4–19 include expenses for the services of other health practitioners such as optometrists and chiropractors, the cost of appliances such as glasses and hearing aids, and the cost of tests done in private laboratories. Some three-fourths of these services are paid out-of-pocket. The below poverty group had about one-sixth of the total paid by Medicaid and welfare. However, voluntary insurance pays a larger proportion (14 percent) of the total than was true for dental care and drugs.

Expenses for Live Births

Table 4–20 shows that the average expenditures for live births, including hospital expenses, physician expenses, drugs and other medical services, was $648 in 1970. For the lowest group Medicaid and welfare paid about one-half of the total with voluntary insurance and out-of-pocket payments making up the rest. These low income families were to pay on average $168 themselves per live birth. The live births in middle and high income families were apparently financed about equally by voluntary insurance and out-of-pocket payments.

HEALTH INSURANCE BENEFITS
AS A PROPORTION OF
HEALTH SERVICES EXPENDITURES

This section examines changes in the proportion of expenditures for health services covered by voluntary health insurance from 1953 through 1970. The expenditures for 1970 in this section are the best estimate expenditures for hospital services and social survey expenditures for the other services. Expenditures for 1970 are limited to the nonfree component. This combination makes the 1970 estimates most comparable to those from the earlier studies. In examining these trends it should be remembered that benefits for 1970 generally include payments by Medicare, a program which did not exist at the time of the earlier studies. Further, the "free" component of care was considerably increased for the lower income groups in the 1970 study by the Medicaid program. Consequently, the "nonfree" component examined in this section represents a smaller proportion of the total expenses for the low income segment in 1970 than it did in earlier studies.

Table 4–21 indicates that insurance paid a greater proportion of expenditures in each succeeding study, increasing from 15 percent in 1953 to 37 percent in 1970. In addition, Medicare accounted for 9 percent of the total in 1970 so that together, Medicare and private insurance accounted for 46 percent of all nonfree expenditures.

Hospital services were most likely to be covered by insurance in each period (Table 4–21). While one-half of the hospital expenses were covered in 1953, the proportion rose to 84 percent in 1970. Of this total in 1970, 19 percent was accounted for by Medicare. The proportion covered by voluntary insurance actually appeared to decrease slightly between 1963 and 1970. This resulted from the shift of coverage of the elderly, who are heavy consumers of hospital services, from voluntary health insurance to the rolls of Medicare.

The proportion of physician services covered by insurance also increased with each study, reaching 43 percent in 1970 (Table 4-21). In each period, in-hospital surgery was the service most likely to be covered, followed by obstetrical care and other physician services (mostly ambulatory care visits) in that order.

Other types of health services were unlikely to be insured prior to 1970 (Table 4-21). By 1970 drugs, dental services, and other medical services and appliances were being covered to a greater extent by insurance. Even in 1970, however, the vast majority of expenditures for these health services was still being paid for directly by consumers.

The benefits received by insured families according to their level of expenditures is shown in Table 4-22. For insured families with expenditures of $500 or less the mean benefits paid did not change very much over the period covered by the studies. For families with expenditures over $500, however, benefits increased with each study.

One explanation for the lack of increases in benefits for the lower expenditure families is based on inflation. Lower cost services such as ambulatory physician visits, drugs and dental care are less likely to be covered by insurance, while the higher cost hospital and inpatient physician services are more likely to be covered. In the earlier years, expenditures of from $100 to $500 were more likely to include insured services. In the later periods it is unlikely that families with expenses of less than $500 have used the expensive services most likely to be insured. In contrast, the increasing benefits for families with large expenditures reflect the trend toward major medical type coverage. It offers additional protection against the large "catastrophic type" expenses of $1,000 to $2,000 or more that are becoming more and more common due to inflation and the use of more sophisticated and expensive medical techniques. The sum effect of these trends has been to raise the total mean benefits per insured family from $45 in 1953 to $346 in 1970.

The trends shown in Table 4-22 are elaborated further in Table 4-23, which indicates changes in the proportion of expenses paid for according to level of expenses. In each study, benefits as a proportion of expenditures increased as expenditures increased. The change over time shows that families with large expenditures are having a greater proportion of their expenditures paid by insurance. In 1953 families with expenditures of $1,000 or more had 23 percent of their expenditures covered. This proportion had increased to 45 percent in 1963 and 63 percent in 1970. In 1970 insured families as a whole were having about one-half of their medical care expenses paid for by insurance.

Table 4-24 allows the examination of change in the proportion of families with various levels of coverage. Among all insured families the proportion with at least 20 percent, 50 percent or 80 percent of their bills paid by insurance has tended to increase over time. The comprehensiveness of the coverage has also increased between 1963 and 1970.

For low expenditure families there was an actual decrease in the proportion with various types of coverage between 1953 and 1963 (Table 4-24). However, this trend was reversed in the 1970 study.

A consistent trend over the 17 year period was the increase in the proportion of families with expenditures of $500 or more who had various levels of coverage. Particularly significant is the proportion with 80 percent or more of their expenses covered, which rose from 2 percent in 1953 to 12 percent in 1963 and 17 percent in 1970.

Generally, 80 percent coverage of health service expenses might be considered a reasonably comprehensive level. While the level of family income and expense would obviously enter into judgments about the "adequacy" of coverage in individual situations, the 80 percent level is a useful norm against which to compare actual levels of coverage. Table 4-25 shows trends in the proportion of families having 80 percent or more of their expenses for various types of services paid by insurance. These proportions have not changed greatly in the period covered by the studies. The proportion of families with 80 percent coverage of hospital expenses increased from 59 percent to 70 percent between 1953 and 1970. The comprehensiveness of surgical coverage increased from 45 percent in 1953 to 54 percent in 1970. The proportion of physician obstetrical services covered by insurance does not appear to have increased over the 17 year period, being in the vicinity of one-third of the expenses throughout the period. Relatively few families have comprehensive benefits if total expenses are considered. Further, the proportion has not changed much: in 1953, 7 percent of all families had 80 percent or more of their health expenses covered by insurance and the proportion was 8 percent in 1970.

Table 4-26 shows the comprehensiveness of insurance coverage according to family income level. In 1953 the lowest income families appeared to have the greatest proportions of their expenses covered by insurance. By 1963 the middle income families ($5,000-$9,999) seemed to have the highest level of coverage. There appeared to be less relationship between family income and benefits as a percent of expenditures in 1970. In considering this table it should be remembered that total expenditures increase with family income, so that the percentages shown are of smaller amounts for the low income groups.

Table 4-27 allows the simultaneous consideration of the comprehensiveness of coverage by income level and type of service. In 1963 it appeared that low income families were less likely to have 80 percent or more of their hospital bill paid by insurance than were the rest of the population. However, by 1970 they were as likely as the rest of the population to have such comprehensive coverage. In 1963 low income families seemed to be more likely to have 80 percent or more of their surgical charges covered by insurance than higher income families. By 1970 no such pattern was evident.

The proportion of medical expenditures for live births paid for by insurance has increased consistently according to Table 4-28. Between 1953 and 1970 the proportion of expenditures covered for live births for which some benefits were received increased from 53 percent to 73 percent. If all live births are considered (including those for which insurance paid nothing), the percent of expenditures covered was 30 in 1953 and 54 in 1970.

In sum, this section has indicated that health insurance paid an increasing proportion of expenses for all health services between 1953 and 1970. The rate of increase was greatest for families with high levels of expenditure. Still, only 8 percent of families receiving health insurance benefits had 80 percent or more of their total expenses paid for by insurance in 1970. The comprehensiveness of coverage for insured families as measured by percent of nonfree expenses covered by insurance did not appear to be associated to any great extent with income in 1970. Coverage of expenditures associated with live births increased consistently from 1953 to 1970. While there is little question that voluntary health insurance is becoming more comprehensive in terms of people covered and benefits paid, the debate over its performance concerns its rate of growth, groups excluded, services covered and cost of administration.

FAMILY DEBT FOR PERSONAL HEALTH SERVICES

One measure of the financial hardship caused by the costs of health services is the proportion of families who must borrow or go into debt to meet the financial obligations resulting from medical treatment. Medical debt is generally considered an "unsatisfactory" method of financing health services because of their unique characteristics. If they could be purchased like other goods and services— when desired and of the quantity and quality the family could afford—perhaps the problem of medical debt would be of little more concern than the balance owed by a family on its automobile or television set. The cost of these items is known in advance and the consumer determines the time of purchase. The costs of many health services cannot be so predetermined and the consumer usually has no choice but to purchase these services when necessary. Systematic saving is only a partial solution, since families do not know how much should be saved annually.

Table 4–29 shows that the portion of families with medical debt decreased slightly from 20 to 17 percent between 1963 and 1970. However, the mean debt for families with debt increased from $157 to $286 and the median also increased. Further, the proportion with a debt of $300 or more increased from 15 to 23 percent.

Table 4–30 indicates the proportion of various kinds of families with debt. Younger families are more likely to have debts than older ones. Thus, one-quarter of the families headed by a person under 45 had a medical care debt in both 1963 and 1970. In contrast, only about one in 15 families headed by a person 65 or over had a medical care debt.

In 1963 families headed by someone working full time and those headed by other than a full time worker, including the retired, disabled, unemployed, housewives or students, were about equally likely to have debt. The reduction in percent with debt by 1970 seemed to be greater for families without a full time worker as head. In 1963 the insured were as likely as the uninsured to have a medical care debt. By 1970, however, the uninsured were more likely to have a medical care debt than the insured. Differences by race were inconsequential in both 1963 and 1970.

As might be expected, the percentage of families with debt increased as family medical expenditures increased. In both 1963 and 1970 there appeared to be a curvilinear relationship between income level and percent with debt. The middle income group was most likely to have a medical care debt, and this difference was more pronounced in 1970 than it had been in 1963. Differences in debt by residence were not great in 1970, although urban families not living in SMSAs and rural nonfarm families appeared somewhat more likely to have a medical care debt.

This analysis of family debt for medical care suggests that the situation improved somewhat between 1963 and 1970 with respect to the percent of families having a medical care debt. The increased amount of the debt in 1970 for those with a medical care debt is probably attributable to inflation. In 1970 the families most likely to have a medical care debt are young, lack insurance, have high medical expenditures and are of middle income.

SUMMARY

This chapter presents a picture of expanding coverage for hospital, surgical and major medical expenses in the U.S. Further, coverage for doctor visits, prescribed drugs and dental care is becoming more common. However, health insurance coverage is not so comprehensive that all covered persons are protected from financial catastrophe when confronted by serious illness. Also, about one person in four had no private insurance or Medicare coverage at all in 1970. While Medicaid and welfare pays for some of the medical care this group receives, the financial burden of medical care is still a substantial one for these people.

Table 4-1. Percent families with health insurance (28) by selected characteristics: 1953, 1958, 1963 and 1970

Family Characteristic	Percent Insured (35)			
	1953	1958[a]	1963[a]	1970[b]
Sex of head (54)				
Male	66	71	76	85
Female	48	60	65	78
Income level (25)				
Low	41	42	51	71
Middle	71	79	78	86
High	80	86	89	93
Residence (52)				
Urban	70	73	77	83
Rural, nonfarm	57	73	74	86
Rural, farm	45	44	54	75
Main activity of main earner (37)				
Working full time	69	78	82	87
Not working full time	25	39	56	75
Education of head (10)				
6 years or less	44	47	47	74
7-8 years	61	64	70	81
9-12 years	69	75	79	84
13 years or more	75	82	85	88
Total	63	69	74	83

[a]Includes CHAMPUS (Armed Forces dependent's coverage)
[b]Includes CHAMPUS and Medicare, Part A.

Table 4-2. Percent families with major medical insurance (34) by selected family characteristics: 1958, 1963 and 1970

Family Characteristic	*Percent with Major Medical Insurance[b] (33)*		
	1958	*1963*	*1970*
Income level (25)			
Low	1	6	15
Middle	7	22	49
High	11	38	61
Residence (52)			
Urban	7	26	41
Rural, nonfarm	7	19	44
Rural, farm	1	10	30
Main activity of main earner (37)			
Working full time	8	30	55
Not working full time	a	8	14
Total	7	24	41

[a]Less than 0.5 percent.
[b]Excludes CHAMPUS and Medicare.

Table 4-3. Percent individuals with health insurance by type of coverage: 1953, 1958, 1963 and 1970

Type of Coverage	Percent Covered (35)			
	1953	1958	1963	1970
Hospital (33)	57	65	68	77
Surgical-medical (55)	48	61	66	74
Outpatient doctor visit[a] (43)	b	b	35	57
Major medical (38)	b	b	22	41
Outpatient drug[c] (9)	b	b	26	42
Dental (5)	b	b	2[d]	11

[a]Includes first dollar doctor visit coverage as written by prepaid group practice plans, unions and certain other insurers; all major medical policies whether or not connected with a base plan; and Medicare, Part B. First dollar doctor visit coverage, excluding major medical policies and Medicare, Part B, both of which have a deductible, is estimated at 11 percent of the population for 1970.

[b]Not available.

[c]Includes first dollar drug coverage as written by some prepaid group practices, unions and certain other insurers and by major medical policies. First dollar drug coverage excluding major medical policies is estimated at 5 percent of the population for 1970.

[d]Source: Table 706, U.S. Bureau of the Census (1971b).

Table 4-4. Percent of persons insured against costs of hospital care by age: 1953, 1958, 1963 and 1970

Age (1)	Percent Insured (35) (33)			
	1953	1958[a]	1963[a]	1970[b]
0-5	57	67	68	69
6-17	58	57	68	73
18-24	49	57	58	64
25-34	64	70	72	80
35-44	65	73	75	77
45-54	63	70	71	82
55-64	54	63	72	75
65 and over	31	43	56	97

[a]Includes CHAMPUS.

[b]Includes CHAMPUS and Medicare.

Table 4-5. Percent individuals with selected types of health insurance coverage by selected characteristics: 1970

Characteristic	*Percent of Individuals With: (35)*		
	Hospital insurance (33)	*Doctor visit insurance (43)*	*Major medical (38)*
Age (1)			
0–5	69	51	44
6–17	73	53	44
18–34	72	53	45
35–44	80	60	51
55–64	75	48	35
65 and over	97	85	5
Sex (54)			
Male	76	57	42
Female	77	56	40
Poverty level (26)			
Above near poverty	85	64	49
Below near poverty	47	33	14
Education of head (10)			
8 years or less	65	43	21
9–11 years	73	51	37
12 years	80	60	45
13 years or more	87	70	58
Residence (52)			
SMSA, central city	71	49	34
SMSA, other	82	64	45
Urban, non-SMSA	76	56	40
Rural, nonfarm	80	60	47
Rural, farm	66	48	33
Total	77	57	41

Table 4-6. Selected characteristics of the population uninsured for hospital coverage: 1970

Characteristic	*Percent Distribution by Demographic Characteristics*		
	Of the uninsured population	*Of the insured[a] population (35)*	*Of the total population*
Age (1)			
0-5	14	9	10
6-17	30	24	26
18-34	26	22	23
35-54	19	23	22
55-64	10	9	9
65 and over	1	13	10
Sex (54)			
Male	50	49	49
Female	50	51	51
Poverty level (26)			
Above near poverty	47	86	77
Below near poverty	53	14	23
Education of head (10)			
8 years or less	36	20	24
9-11 years	23	19	20
12 years	25	30	29
13 years or more	14	30	26
Residence			
SMSA, central city	37	28	30
SMSA, other	21	29	27
Urban, non-SMSA	12	12	12
Rural, nonfarm	20	26	24
Rural, farm	10	6	7
Total	100 (5185)[b]	100 (6434)[b]	100 (11619)[b]

[a]Includes Medicare and CHAMPUS.

[b]In parentheses are the unweighted numbers of observations which can be used in combination with the procedures described in Appendix I to calculate standard errors of the 1970 estimates. Since the 1970 sample is a weighted sample, these numbers should *not* be used as weights for combining subcategories.

Table 4-7. Percent individuals insured against the costs of hospital and surgical care by type of insurer: 1953, 1958, 1963 and 1970

	Type of Coverage (35)							
	Hospital insurance (33)				*Surgical insurance (55)*			
Type of insurer[a] *(36)*	*1953*	*1958*	*1963*	*1970*	*1953*	*1958*	*1963*	*1970*
Blue Cross or Blue Shield	27	31	31	37	19	28	29	34
Private insurance	29	32	36	34	27	33	36	33
Prepaid group practices, other independents	6	7	5	6	7	5	6	6
CHAMPUS	_b	1	1	1	_b	1	1	1
Medicare	—	_b	_b	10	—	_b	_b	8

[a] Individuals covered by two or more policies underwritten by different types of insurers are double counted in this table.
[b] Program not yet in existence

Table 4-8. Percent total population covered (35) by hospital insurance (33), by type of enrollment and type of insurer: 1953, 1958, 1963 and 1970

Type of Enrollment (11) and Insurer^a (36)	*Percent with Hospital Insurance Coverage*			
	1953	*1958*	*1963*	*1970*
Group				
Blue Cross	21	23	24	30
Private insurance	17	23	27	27
Prepaid group practices, other independents	5	6	5	6
CHAMPUS	$-^c$	1	1	1
Medicare	–	$-^c$	$-^c$	10
Nongroup				
Blue Cross	6	8	7	7
Private insurance	12	9	10	8
Prepaid group practices, other independents	b	1	1	b
Total	57	65	68	77

[a]Individuals covered by two or more policies carried through different types of enrollment or underwritten by different types of insurers are double counted in this table.

[b]Less than 0.5 percent.

[c]Program not yet in existence.

Table 4-9. Percent total population (35) covered by hospital insurance (33), by method of enrollment and selected characteristics: 1970

Characteristic	Method of Enrollment[a] (11)	
	Group	*Nongroup*
Age (1)		
0–5	63	7
6–17	64	11
18–34	64	11
35–54	69	13
55–64	55	27
65 and over	96	36
Sex (54)		
Male	67	13
Female	67	17
Poverty level (26)		
Above near poverty	76	15
Below near poverty	38	16
Education of head (10)		
8 years or less	55	17
9–11 years	67	11
12 years	69	17
13 years or more	79	14
Residence (52)		
SMSA, central city	63	14
SMSA, other	73	14
Urban, non-SMSA	68	17
Rural, nonfarm	71	15
Rural, farm	47	24
Total	67	15

[a]Individuals with both a group and nongroup policy are double counted in this table.

Table 4-10. Employer contribution toward family's premiums for health insurance policies carried through a work group or union: 1953, 1963 and 1970

Extent of Contribution	*Percent of Families Carrying One or More Health Insurance Policies Through Work Group or Union (28) (34)*		
	1953	*1963*	*1970*
Employer pays some of family's work group health insurance premiums	59	79	92
Employer pays all[a]	10	27	39
Employer pays part	49	52	53
Employer pays none of family's work group health insurance premiums	41	21	8
Total	100	100	100

[a]Includes premiums for any dependents covered under policy. If family has more than one policy through a work group, the employer must pay the entire premium for each policy for the family to be included in this category.

Table 4-11. Mean nonfree expenditures per person with expenditures[a] by type of service including and excluding health insurance benefits: 1963 and 1970

	Mean Nonfree Expenditures (13)					
	Per person with expenditures			Per person with expenditures excluding health insurance benefits[b] (29)		
Type of Service	1963	1970		1963	1970	
Hospital (17)						
Nonobstetrical hospital inpatient	$325	$882	(857)c	$84	$208	(491)c
Obstetrical hospital inpatient	175	388	(169)	77	207	(127)
Hospital outpatient	23	43	(523)	17	38	(369)
Physician (19)						
Hospital surgery	200	340	(407)	75	141	(245)
Out of hospital surgery	48	62	(157)	33	33	(135)
Obstetrics	142	157	(242)	96	103	(199)
Ophthalmologist	14	17	(507)	14	16	(477)
Other physician, in hospital	71	129	(580)	44	69	(362)
Other physician, house call	35	35	(190)	31	22	(173)
Other physician, office	20	52	(5005)	19	43	(4674)
Drugs (16)						
Prescribed	36	51	(3918)	35	47	(3793)
Nonprescribed	11	13	(7764)	11	13	(7757)
Dental care (15)	41	67	(3290)	41	65	(3225)
Other medical goods and services (18)						
Nonmedical practitioners	23	41	(1233)	22	38	(1190)
Other medical care	32	48	(2738)	30	40	(2463)
Total	$119	$254	(9993)	$86	$123	(9897)

[a]Includes observations where third party payments exceeded expenditures.

[b]Excludes payments by private insurance and CHAMPUS in 1963; excludes payments by private insurance, CHAMPUS, Medicare and person's liability insurance in 1970.

[c]In parentheses are the unweighted numbers of observations which can be used in combination with the procedures described in Appendix I to calculate standard errors of the 1970 estimates. Since the 1970 sample is a weighted sample, these numbers should *not* be used as weights for combining subcategories.

Table 4-12. Distribution of best estimate (3) expenditures (14) for all personal health services by selected characteristics and source of payment: 1970*

Characteristic	Medicaid, welfare, free institutions	Other free care	Medicare	Voluntary insurance	Out-of-pocket	Other nonfree care	Total Mean Expenditures (14) per Person
			Percent Distribution by Source of Payment				
Sex (54)							
Male	6	6	9	32	47	a	$211
Female	10	1	9	33	46	1	258
Age (1)							
0-5	11	a	—b	37	51	1	105
6-17	11	1	—	26	61	1	96
18-34	9	4	—	36	48	3	246
35-54	8	6		35	51	a	236
55-64	6	2	a	45	46	1	376
65 and over	6	3	48	7	36	a	428
Poverty Level (26)							
Above near poverty	9	3	6	34	47	1	256
Below near poverty	26	4	20	16	33	1	213
Family Income (24)							
Under $2,000	29	3	28	8	32	a	302
$ 2,000- 3,499	24	5	24	11	35	1	259
3,500- 4,999	12	4	11	29	43	1	256
5,000- 7,499	9	5	12	33	41	a	255
7,500- 9,999	5	4	3	39	48	1	186
10,000-14,999	3	3	5	36	50	3	208
15,000 and over	2	2	2	37	56	1	231

Race (49)							
White	11	3	9	31	45	1	$258
Nonwhite	28	5	9	25	32	1	162
Education of Head (10)							
8 years or less	14	5	18	22	41	1	234
9–11 years	12	2	10	29	46	1	193
12 years	7	2	7	36	47	1	208
13 years or more	3	4	3	39	49	2	295
Residence (52)							
SMSA, central city	13	4	9	31	42	1	235
SMSA, other	6	3	7	34	48	2	299
Urban, non-SMSA	8	3	9	30	49	1	190
Rural, nonfarm	6	3	9	35	46	1	199
Rural, farm	6	5	16	24	48	1	181
Total	13	3	8	31	44	1	$248

*Selected observations are excluded from this table. For exclusion criteria and estimates including all observations, see Appendix Table II-9.

a Less than 0.5 percent.

b Not applicable.

Table 4-13. Distribution of best estimate (3) hospital inpatient (17) expenditures by selected characteristics and source of payment: 1970*

Characteristic	Percent Distribution by Source of Payment						Total Mean Expenditures (17) per Person
	Medicaid, welfare, free institutions	Other free care	Medicare	Voluntary insurance	Out-of-pocket	Other nonfree care	
Sex (54)							
Male	9	10	20	50	10	1	$ 71
Female	14	1	17	55	11	2	101
Age (1)							
0-5	18	a	– b	72	10	a	32
6-17	23	1	–	67	6	3	18
18-34	15	4	–	61	15	5	94
35-54	17	9	–	63	10	1	75
55-64	8	3	–	77	11	1	154
65 and over	3	5	81	7	4	a	199
Poverty level (26)							
Above near poverty	5	4	12	63	14	2	89
Below near poverty	30	5	33	23	8	1	101
Family income (24)							
Under $2,000	33	4	45	9	9	a	148
$ 2,000- 3,499	26	9	42	16	7	a	119
3,500- 4,999	18	6	23	37	15	1	83
5,000- 7,499	13	5	25	45	12	a	96
7,500- 9,999	6	6	5	70	12	1	73
10,000-14,999	6	4	14	62	10	4	68
15,000 and over	a	2	9	78	8	3	45

Race (49)							
White	9	4	18	54	13	2	$ 94
Nonwhite	37	9	19	31	4	a	62
Education of head (10)							
8 years or less	15	7	34	36	8	a	98
9–11 years	16	3	21	46	12	2	75
12 years	14	2	14	60	9	1	78
13 years or more	3	5	8	70	10	4	80
Residence (52)							
SMSA, central city	19	6	19	50	5	a	86
SMSA, other	8	3	18	55	13	3	94
Urban, non-SMSA	10	5	21	51	11	2	65
Rural, nonfarm	10	4	22	52	11	1	67
Rural, farm	8	8	32	38	12	2	75
Total	12	4	18	53	12	1	$ 92

* Selected observations are excluded from this table. For exclusion criteria and estimates including all observations, see Appendix Table II-10.

a Less than 0.5 percent.

b Not applicable.

Table 4-14. Distribution of best estimate (3) hospital outpatient (17) expenditures by selected characteristics and source of payment: 1970*

Characteristic	Percent Distribution by Source of Payment						Total Mean Expenditures (17) per Person
	Medicaid, welfare, free institutions	Other free care	Medicare	Voluntary insurance	Out-of-pocket	Other nonfree care	
Sex (54)							
Male	35	10	4	28	19	4	$5
Female	29	4	3	32	29	3	4
Age (1)							
0-5	47	—	—b	21	28	4	4
6-17	26	2	—	38	26	8	3
18-34	38	14	—	21	24	3	5
35-54	27	9	—	40	18	6	3
55-64	36	10	—	39	15	—a	4
65 and over	34	3	33	12	18	a	3
Poverty level (26)							
Above near poverty	12	7	3	44	28	6	4
Below near poverty	60	7	5	6	21	1	6
Family income (24)							
Under $2,000	67	6	10	5	12	a	6
$ 2,000- 3,499	58	4	8	5	25	a	6
3,500- 4,999	56	11	2	12	19	—a	6
5,000- 7,499	33	8	1	29	25	4	4
7,500- 9,999	13	12	—a	33	35	7	3
10,000-14,999	6	7	3	59	23	2	3
15,000 and over	—a	7	1	53	28	11	4

Race (49)							
White	26	8	4	34	24	4	$4
Nonwhite	53	4	4	13	25	1	7
Education of head (10)							
8 years or less	45	6	11	20	18	$-^a$	5
9–11 years	41	7	2	25	24	1	4
12 years	15	7	1	44	26	7	3
13 years or more	12	9	1	40	29	9	4
Residence (52)							
SMSA, central city	37	6	5	21	30	1	8
SMSA, other	21	9	1	45	21	3	4
Urban, non-SMSA	21	7	2	54	16	$-^a$	1
Rural, nonfarm	5	10	3	41	21	20	3
Rural, farm	20	3	5	40	31	1	1
Total	31	7	4	30	24	4	$4

*Selected observations are excluded from this table. For exclusion criteria and estimates including all observations, see Appendix Table II-11.

[a]Less than 0.5 percent.

[b]Not applicable.

Table 4-15. Distribution of best estimate (3) physician inpatient (20) expenditures by selected characteristics and source of payment: 1970*

Characteristic	Percent Distribution by Source of Payment						Total Mean Expenditures (20) per Person
	Medicaid, welfare, free institutions	Other free care	Medicare	Voluntary insurance	Out-of-pocket	Other nonfree care	
Sex (54)							
Male	2	a	11	58	28	1	$22
Female	6	a	11	56	23	4	22
Age (1)							
0-5	3	a	_b	69	27	1	11
6-17	8	1	–	60	29	2	7
18-34	5	1	–	61	23	10	17
35-54	6	1	–	71	22	a	22
55-64	3	a	–	60	36	1	38
65 and over	2	a	56	19	22	1	42
Poverty level (26)							
Above near poverty	1	a	7	63	26	3	24
Below near poverty	17	a	27	30	25	1	17
Family income (24)							
Under $2,000	14	1	36	22	26	1	21
$ 2,000– 3,499	20	a	30	19	29	2	22
3,500– 4,999	8	2	19	43	28	a	17
5,000– 7,499	4	a	18	54	24	a	24
7,500– 9,999	4	a	5	60	29	1	15
10,000–14,999	a	1	4	64	25	6	21
15,000 and over	a	-	6	68	24	2	15
Race (49)							
White	4	a	11	57	26	2	24

Nonwhite (13)	13	2	12	51	22	a	$ 8
Education of head (10)							
8 years or less	8	1	22	37	30	2	23
9–11 years	4	1	14	60	21	a	15
12 years	3	a	6	62	26	3	20
13 years or more	2	a	7	61	27	3	22
Residence (52)							
SMSA, central city	5	1	9	68	17	a	19
SMSA, other	1	a	12	48	33	6	24
Urban, non-SMSA	10	1	13	54	22	a	20
Rural, nonfarm	3	a	14	50	31	2	18
Rural, farm	8	a	17	46	27	2	18
Total	4	1	11	57	25	2	$22

*Selected observations are excluded from this table. For exclusion criteria and estimates including all observations, see Appendix Table II-12.

aLess than 0.5 percent

bNot applicable.

Table 4-16. Distribution of best estimate (3) physician outpatient[b] (21) expenditures by selected characteristics and source of payment: 1970

Characteristic	Percent Distribution by Source of Payment						Total Mean Expenditures (21) per Person
	Medicaid, welfare, free institutions	Other free care	Medicare	Voluntary insurance	Out-of-pocket	Other nonfree care	
Sex (54)							
Male	5	10	4	17	63	1	$29
Female	6	3	5	18	67	1	42
Age (1)							
0–5	10	1	—c	12	76	1	32
6–17	8	4	—	18	69	1	15
18–34	4	8	—	20	66	2	46
35–54	5	9	—	21	65	a	35
55–64	5	6	—	23	64	2	53
65 and over	8	a	29	8	55	a	54
Poverty level (26)							
Above near poverty	2	6	3	20	68	1	38
Below near poverty	23	3	11	7	54	2	29
Family income (24)							
Under $2,000	18	3	16	6	56	1	42
$ 2,000– 3,499	26	2	15	8	47	2	35
3,500– 4,999	11	4	14	11	59	1	39
5,000– 7,499	5	12	4	20	57	2	36
7,500– 9,999	4	3	2	17	72	2	33
10,000–14,999	2	7	1	24	66	0	36
15,000 and over	1	4	1	20	74	0	35
Race (49)							
White	4	6	4	19	66	1	37

	23	6	6	11	50	4	$29
Nonwhite	23	6	6	11	50	4	$29
Education of head (10)							
8 years or less	12	5	10	11	60	2	31
9–11 years	8	4	4	19	64	1	31
12 years	5	6	3	20	65	1	34
13 years or more	2	7	2	20	68	1	47
Residence (52)							
SMSA, central city	8	7	5	19	60	1	38
SMSA, other	4	6	5	15	69	1	42
Urban, non-SMSA	7	2	3	20	67	1	32
Rural, nonfarm	4	4	3	22	66	1	31
Rural, farm	7	6	6	13	67	1	26
Total	6	6	4	18	65	1	$36

[a]Less than 0.5 percent.

[b]Includes obstetrical care including delivery. Clinics associated with a hospital which provided obstetrical care are included in Table 4–14.

[c]Not applicable.

Table 4–17. Distribution of best estimates (3) prescription drug (16) expenditures by selected characteristics and source of payment: 1970*

Characteristic	Percent Distribution by Source of Payment						Total Mean Expenditures (16) per Person
	Medicaid, welfare, free institutions	Other free care	Medicare	Voluntary insurance	Out-of-pocket	Other nonfree care	
Sex (54)							
Male	6	6	—b	6	82	a	$19
Female	9	1	—	11	79	1	26
Age (1)							
0–5	4	a	—	7	89	a	9
6–17	4	1	—	5	90	a	6
18–34	5	4	—	11	79	1	17
35–54	5	5	—	13	77	a	28
55–64	4	2	—	11	81	2	42
65 and over	17	2	—	4	78	a	56
Poverty level (26)							
Above near poverty	2	3	—	10	84	1	23
Below near poverty	25	2	—	4	69	a	23
Family income (24)							
Under $2,000	33	1	—	1	65	a	34
$ 2,000– 3,499	24	2	—	1	74	a	32
3,500– 4,999	4	2	—	8	85	a	36
5,000– 7,499	8	7	—	11	74	1	25
7,500– 9,999	2	1	—	4	93	1	16
10,000–14,999	1	4	—	11	83	1	19
15,000 and over	1	1	—	18	79	a	18

Race (49)							
White	6	3	—	9	82	1	$24
Nonwhite	28	3	—	5	63	2	16
Education of head (10)							
8 years or less	16	3	—	3	79	a	28
9–11 years	5	1	—	9	84	a	19
12 years	5	1	—	11	82	a	21
13 years or more	3	6	—	13	77	1	23
Residence (52)							
SMSA, central city	9	4	—	9	77	1	25
SMSA, other	7	3	—	9	81	a	22
Urban, non-SMSA	9	1	—	7	83	a	23
Rural, nonfarm	6	2	—	10	81	a	21
Rural, farm	8	2	—	4	86	a	21
Total	8	3	—	9	80	1	$23

*Selected observations are excluded from this table. For exclusion criteria and estimates including all observations, see Appendix Table II-13.

aLess than 0.5 percent.

bNot applicable.

Table 4-18. Distribution of best estimate (3) dental expenditures (15) by selected characteristics and source of payment: 1970*

Characteristic	Percent Distribution by Source of Payment						Total Mean Expenditures (15) per Person
	Medicaid, welfare, free institutions	Other free care	Medicare	Voluntary insurance	Out-of-pocket	Other nonfree care	
Sex (54)							
Male	4	3	—b	4	89	a	$27
Female	7	a	—	5	88	a	30
Age (1)							
0–5	6	1	—	8	85	a	3
6–17	8	1	—	2	89	a	29
18–34	5	4	—	5	86	a	33
35–54	3	a	—	7	90	a	38
55–64	3	1	—	3	93	a	27
65 and over	10	a	—	a	90	a	20
Poverty level (26)							
Above near poverty	2	1	—	5	92	a	33
Below near poverty	34	2	—	2	62	a	14
Family income (24)							
Under $2,000	29	2	—	a	69	a	14
$ 2,000– 3,499	36	1	—	3	60	a	13
3,500– 4,999	19	1	—	12	68	a	20
5,000– 7,499	6	3	—	1	90	a	23
7,500– 9,999	11	5	—	5	79	a	20
10,000–14,999	1	1	—	9	89	a	32
15,000 and over	a	a	—	1	98	1	44

Race (49)							
White	4	2	—	4	90	a	$30
Nonwhite	30	1	—	7	62	a	15
Education of head (10)							
8 years or less	13	2	—	3	82	a	20
9–11 years	10	1	—	4	85	a	24
12 years	4	1	—	8	87	a	28
13 years or more	1	2	—	3	94	1	38
Residence (52)							
SMSA, central city	10	2	—	7	81	a	26
SMSA, other	3	1	—	4	92	a	43
Urban, non-SMSA	6	1	—	3	90	a	22
Rural, nonfarm	3	1	—	5	90	1	21
Rural, farm	1	1	—	2	96	a	16
Total	5	1	—	5	88	2	$28

*Selected observations are excluded from this table. For exclusion criteria and estimates including all observations, see Appendix Table II-14.

aLess than 0.5 percent.

bNot applicable.

Table 4-19. Distribution of best estimate (3) total other (18) expenditures by selected characteristics and source of payment: 1970

Characteristic	Percent Distribution by Source of Payment						Total Mean Expenditures (18) per Person
	Medicaid, welfare, free institutions	Other free care	Medicare	Voluntary insurance	Out-of-pocket	Other nonfree care	
Sex (54)							
Male	2	5	1	17	75	a	$18
Female	6	1	2	16	74	1	24
Age (1)							
0–5	3	a	—[b]	26	71	a	5
6–17	7	2	—	14	76	1	9
18–34	5	4	—	20	70	1	21
35–54	2	4	—	17	77	a	25
55–64	9	2	—	21	68	a	38
65 and over	4	1	8	6	81	a	41
Poverty level (26)							
Above near poverty	2	3	1	18	76	a	23
Below near poverty	17	2	4	9	67	1	15
Family income (24)							
Under $2,000	22	1	5	9	63	a	19
$ 2,000– 3,499	8	3	5	6	76	2	18
3,500– 4,999	6	3	2	15	74	a	18
5,000– 7,499	11	2	3	13	70	a	21
7,500– 9,999	2	2	1	16	79	a	16
10,000–14,999	1	4	1	21	73	a	19
15,000 and more	1	2	1	19	77	a	21

Race (49)							
White	4	3	2	17	74	a	* 22
Nonwhite	12	3	1	10	73	1	11
Education of head (10)							
8 years or less	11	3	2	12	72	a	22
9–11 years	6	1	3	14	75	1	16
12 years	2	4	1	19	74	a	16
13 years or more	2	2	1	20	75	a	30
Residence (52)							
SMSA, central city	5	2	2	17	73	1	23
SMSA, other	5	4	2	17	72	a	23
Urban, non-SMSA	5	3	1	18	73	a	18
Rural, nonfarm	4	3	a	16	77	a	19
Rural, farm	1	2	3	12	82	a	16
Total	5	3	1	17	74	a	$21

*Selected observations are excluded from this table. For exclusion criteria and estimates including all observations, see Appendix Table II–15.

aLess than 0.5 percent.

bNot applicable.

Table 4-20. Best estimate (3) mean expenditures per live birth (22) by source of payment and family income level: 1970

	Source of Payment				
Family Income Level (25)	*Medicaid, welfare, free institutions*	*Voluntary insurance*[a]	*Out-of-pocket*	*Total*	
Low	$287	$124	$168	$579	(136)[b]
Middle	55	297	297	651	(112)
High	1	365	355	721	(42)
Total	$108	$264	$275	$648	(290)

[a]Includes CHAMPUS.

[b]In parentheses are the unweighted numbers of observations which can be used in combination with the procedures described in Appendix I to calculate standard errors of the 1970 estimates. Since the 1970 sample is a weighted sample, these numbers should *not* be used for weights for combining subcategories.

Table 4-21. Percent aggregate nonfree expenditures (13) for personal health services covered by aggregate health insurance benefits (29): 1953, 1958, 1963 and 1970

Expenditures Covered by Insurance Benefits

Service	All insurance 1953	All insurance 1958[b]	All insurance 1963[b]	1970 Voluntary Insurance[b]	1970 Medicare	1970 All insurance
Hospital (17)	50	58	69	66	19	84
Physician (19)	13	18	25	37	7	43
In-hospital surgery	38	48	58	66	10	76
Obstetrics	25	30	32	46	—[c]	46
Other physician	4	7	13	25	6	31
Drugs (16)	a	1	1	7	—[c]	7
Dental (15)	a	a	a	5	—	5
Other (18)	1	1	5	14	1	16
Total	15	19	27	37	9	46

[a]Less than 0.5 percent.
[b]Includes CHAMPUS.
[c]Not applicable.

Table 4-22. Mean benefits by level of nonfree expenditures for health services for insured families: 1953, 1958, 1963 and 1970

Level of Nonfree Expenditures (13) for Health Services	Mean Insurance Benefits Paid[a] (29)			
	1953	*1958*[b]	*1963*[b]	*1970*[b]
$ 1- 49	$ 2	$ 1	$ 1	$ 1	(418)[d]
50- 99	4	1	2	8	(307)
100- 199	16	10	7	14	(464)
200- 299	33	28	32	29	(318)
300- 399	67	64	49	54	(220)
400- 499	100	94	103	107	(151)
500- 749	147	156	171	199	(292)
750- 999	204	257	291	301	(180)
1,000-1,999	} 362	572	748	713 } 1396	(329)
2,000 and over				2785 }	(180)
Total[c]	$45	$ 80	$131	$ 346	(2859)

a
 These means include all insured families in the specific expenditure category whether or not they actually received any benefits.

[b]Includes CHAMPUS for 1958 and 1963. Includes CHAMPUS and Medicare for 1970.

[c]Includes a small number of families in each year with no expenditures.

[d]In parentheses are the unweighted numbers of observations which can be used in combination with the procedures described in Appendix I to calculate standard errors of the 1970 estimates. Since the 1970 sample is a weighted sample, these numbers should *not* be used as weights for combining subcategories.

Table 4-23. Aggregate benefits as a percent of aggregate nonfree expenditures for insured families by level of family expenditures: 1953, 1958, 1963 and 1970

Level of Nonfree Expenditures (13) for Health Services	Benefits as a Percent of Expenditures[a] (29)			
	1953	*1958*[b]	*1963*[b]	*1970*[b]
$ 1– 49	8	2	2	4
50– 99	6	2	3	10
100– 199	11	7	5	9
200– 299	14	11	13	12
300– 399	20	18	14	16
400– 499	23	21	23	24
500– 749	25	25	28	32
750– 999	24	30	34	-36
1,000–1,999 ⎱ 2,000 and over ⎰	23	35	45	51⎱ 71⎰ 63
Total	19	c	31	49

[a]These percentages include all insured families in the specific expenditure category whether or not they actually received any benefits.
[b]Includes CHAMPUS for 1958 and 1963. Includes CHAMPUS and Medicare for 1970.
[c]Not available.

Table 4-24. Percent insured families with specified levels of benefits (20) paid by selected magnitudes of nonfree expenditures: 1953, 1958, 1963 and 1970

| Selected Magnitude of Nonfree Expenditures (13)[c] | Percent Families with Each Level of Benefits paid as a Percent of Expenditures | | |
	20 percent or more	50 percent or more	80 percent or more
All insured families			
1953	24	9	3
1958[b]	24	10	2
1963[b]	30	14	3
1970[b]	39	24	8
Low expenditures ($100–199)			
1953	20	6	2
1958[b]	13	4	1
1963[b]	11	3	a
1970[b]	16	6	3
High expenditures ($500 or more)			
1953	49	19	2
1958[b]	56	24	4
1963[b]	64	34	12
1970[b]	69	49	17

[a]Less than 0.5 percent.
[b]Includes CHAMPUS for 1958 and 1963. Includes CHAMPUS and Medicare for 1970.
[c]Excludes families with no expenditures.

Table 4-25. Percent families receiving benefits who had 80 percent or more of charges paid for by insurance, by type of service: 1953, 1958, 1963 and 1970

| Service | Percent Families with 80 Percent or more of Charges Covered by Type of Service | | | |
	1953	1958[a]	1963[a]	1970[a]
Hospital (17)	59	61	67	70
Surgical (19)	45	53	49	54
Obstetrical-physician (19)	35	33	27	33
All services (13)	7	5	8	8

[a]Includes CHAMPUS for 1958 and 1963. Includes CHAMPUS and Medicare for 1970.

Table 4-26. Total health insurance benefits as a percent of total nonfree expenditures for all insured families by family income: 1953, 1963 and 1970

	Benefits as a Percent of Nonfree Expenditures (13)				
Family Income (24)	1953	1963[a]		1970[a]	
Under $2,000	26	30		56	
$ 2,000– 3,499	20	30		55	
3,500– 4,999	22	24		53	
5,000– 7,499	18	36		57	
7,500– 9,999		36		51	
10,000–12,499	15	26	29	42	46
12,500–14,999		23		50	
15,000 and over				45	
Total	19	31		49	

[a]Includes CHAMPUS for 1963. Includes CHAMPUS and Medicare for 1970.

Table 4-27. Percent families receiving insurance benefits which covered 80 percent or more of hospital or surgical nonfree expenditures (13) by family income: 1963 and 1970

	Percent Families Receiving Benefits[a] (29) Who Were Reimbursed for 80 Percent or more of Charges					
	For hospital charges (17)			For surgical charges (19)		
Family Income (24)	1963	1970		1963	1970	
Under $3,500	49	73		65	46	
$ 3,500– 4,999	58	72		54	56	
5,000– 7,499	71	71		52	56	
7,500– 9,999	76	73		48	48	
10,000–14,999	67	63	67	37	46	57
15,000 and over		72			72	
All families	67	70		49	54	

[a]Includes CHAMPUS for 1963. Includes Medicare and CHAMPUS for 1970.

Table 4-28. Health insurance benefits (29) as a proportion of nonfree expenditures (13) for live births (22): 1953, 1958, 1963 and 1970

	Benefits as a Percent of Expenditures			
Live Births	*1953*	*1958[a]*	*1963[a]*	*1970[a]*
Live births for which some benefits were received	53	58	63	73
All live births	30	38	43	54

[a]Includes CHAMPUS for 1958, 1963 and 1970.

Table 4-29. Distribution of families who reported that they owed money for medical care: 1963 and 1970

Characteristic	*1963*	*1970*
Percent of families reporting a debt (4)	20	17
Mean debt reported	$157	$286
Median debt reported	$ 71	$100
For those families reporting debts, percent with debt of:		
Less than $50	36	24
$ 50– 99	23	22
100–299	26	30
300 or more	15	23
All families	100	100

Table 4-30. Families with medical debt as a proportion of all families by selected family characteristics: 1963 and 1970

Characteristic	*Families with Medical Debt (4) as a Proportion of all Families*	
	1963	*1970*
Age of head (1)		
29 or less	25	24
30–44	25	25
45–64	18	13
65 and over	7	6
Major activity of main earner (37)		
Work fulltime	20	19
Other	20	13
Insurance status (34)		
Insured	19	15
Uninsured	19	24
Race (49)		
White	19	17
Nonwhite	22	19
Medical expenditures (13)		
Less than $100	8	5
$100–299	17	14
300–499	29 }	18 } 25
500 or more }		28 }
Family income (25)		
Low	17	13
Middle	22	24
High	17	15
Residence (52)		
SMSA, central city	–[a]	16
SMSA, other urban	–	15
Urban, non-SMSA	–	19
Rural, nonfarm	–	20
Rural, farm	–	15
All families	20	17

[a] Not available for 1963.

Chapter 5

Comparisons of
Social Survey Estimates
with Best Estimates

In the 1970 study an effort was made to contact all hospitals where survey respondents reported admissions, all physicians mentioned as providing medical care, and all health insurance companies and employers who provided health insurance to members of the sample. The purposes of the verification were (1) to provide additional details on diagnoses, treatments, costs and health insurance benefits which survey respondents could not be expected to report accurately; and (2) to improve the validity of respondent reported information. The information provided by the respondents in the social survey and that provided in the verification were then merged to provide what we have referred to in this volume as our "best estimates." The verification process and its results are described more fully in Appendix I. Since substantial effort went into the verification process, differences between estimates based on the social survey and the "best estimates" are of considerable methodological interest. The fundamental question addressed is: How different are the estimates that incorporate the verification information from those based only on information provided by family respondents?[1] This chapter will compare some key estimates of health services utilization, expenditures and methods of finance.

PHYSICIAN VISITS

Table 5–1 shows that the effect of the verification was to reduce the estimate of the proportion of people who saw a physician at least

[1]Additional analyses of the survey error in the 1970 study are reported in Andersen (1975), Andersen, Kasper and Frankel (1975) and Andersen, Kasper and Frankel (1976).

once during 1970 from 68 percent to 64 percent. It should be remembered that the verification was done primarily on services reported to us by respondents. Thus, while providers had an opportunity to deny services respondents had reported, there was little opportunity to discover in the verification visits to providers not reported in the social survey. While some physician contacts were discovered through physicians who were reported to have seen other members of the family and through insurance claims, the process was not ideally suited to discovering unreported contacts with physicians. Consequently, the reduction in the estimate of the proportion seeing a physician was not unexpected.

Table 5-1 also allows the examination of differential impact of the verification on various subgroups of the population. The effect of the verification was to reduce the estimates uniformly for all subgroups according to age, sex, family income, race, education and residence. If, in fact, there is differential accuracy in reporting among subgroups, we might expect the verification to have the greatest impact on the groups reporting least accurately. However, the general magnitude of change from the social survey estimates to the best estimates was fairly similar across the subgroups. The largest reductions in the best estimates appeared to be for children six to 17 and for the rural farm population while the smallest was for young adults 18 to 34.

The best estimate of mean number of visits per person per year was one-half visit less than the social survey estimate according to Table 5-2. Again, the difficulty in discovering unreported visits provides one explanation for the best estimate being lower than the social survey estimate. The magnitude of the change in the estimates for subgroups was more variable for number of visits than it was for percent seeing a physician. The groups most affected by the verification process were those 55 and over, the low income group, the least educated and urban residents who live either in central cities or outside SMSAs. One possible inference is that these are the groups reporting their visits least accurately. Another possibility is that their sources of care are less willing or able to provide accurate verification. The group estimates least influenced by the verification process were for those 18 to 34, the higher income groups and the SMSA residents who did not live in central cities.

It was suspected that respondent accuracy in reporting might differ by site of visit, and, indeed, that the accuracy and completeness of the verification information provided might vary by site. However, Table 5-3 gives no indication of such difference. The proportions of visits taking place in homes, physicians' offices, outpatient departments, emergency rooms and other sites were the same according to best estimate data as they were for social survey data.

Table 5–4 shows that the best estimate of the median number of physician visits per live birth was one-half visit less than the social survey estimate. For most social groups shown in Table 5–4 the median visits shown in the best estimate is also smaller than the corresponding social survey estimate.

HOSPITAL SERVICES

This section provides comparisons of the social survey and best estimates for hospital services. Unlike physician services, all trend tables in this volume use best estimates for 1970. This is because all previous studies also included verifications of reported hospital admissions so the most comparable data for 1970 is the best estimate data. Still, hospital utilization comparisons in this section are included to provide some indication of the effect of the verification process.

Table 5–5 suggests that the verification process had little effect on the gross hospital admission rates. While 376 admissions were rejected as a result of the verification process, 110 admissions were also discovered. While more admissions were rejected than discovered, the number of admissions per 100 person-years rounded to the nearest admission was still 14 for both the social survey and the best estimate. Table 5–5 also indicates that the verification process did not differentially affect the estimates for various subgroups. In no case did the estimate for any subgroup defined according to sex, age, family income, race or residence change by more than one admission per 100 person-years from the social survey to the best estimate.

While the verification did not influence the admission rate estimates, Tables 5–6 shows that it did affect the length of stay and total hospital day estimates. The average length of stay decreased from 8.9 days in the social survey to 7.5 days in the best estimate. Table 5–6 further indicates shorter lengths of stay for each age and sex group in the best estimate as compared to estimates from the social survey.

The number of hospital days was also smaller according to the best estimates than it was in the social survey. Hospital days per 100 persons per year is a product of the number of admissions and the length of stay. Since the number of admissions was similar in the social survey and the best estimate, the differences shown are primarily a result of the shorter lengths of stay in the best estimate. For each age and sex group the number of hospital days was less in the best estimate than in the social survey (Table 5–6).

EXPENDITURES FOR HEALTH SERVICES

This section examines the impact of the verification on hospital and physician expenditures and expenditures for all health services. Table 5–7 shows the best estimates for physician charges to be slightly less than those in the social survey. The biggest difference by type of physician service appears to be for office visits. Hospital inpatient charges appeared higher in the social survey than in the best estimate, but outpatient charges actually seemed higher in the best estimate.

Estimates of total expenditures according to income level are shown in Table 5–8. The differences are not large, but overall the estimates from the social survey appeared slightly larger. The estimates for most income groups appeared higher in the social survey for both free and nonfree expenditures.

The relationship to income appeared unclear when individual income groups were examined (Table 5–8). In general, the verification appeared to have relatively little impact on expenditure estimates of the above poverty families for either the free or nonfree component. For the below poverty groups the best estimate tended to be lower than the social survey estimate for both the free and nonfree component.

The distributions of total family expenditures according to the social survey and the best estimate are compared in Table 5–9. The distributions appear strikingly similar. This is true of free, nonfree and total distributions. Thus, it appears that the verification had little impact on the picture of family total expenditure distributions.

Table 5–10 compares family outlay for health services as a percent of family income by income level for the social survey and best estimate. Since, in general, the best estimates have been shown to be slightly lower overall than the social survey estimates, it was not surprising that aggregate outlay as a percent of income appeared slightly lower in the best estimate than in the social survey. While the best estimates were lower for most income groups, the biggest change was found for the lowest income group. This is also due to the fact that low income families were more apt to say that they had paid for care or owed money for care that was in fact provided free or paid for by Medicaid.

Tables 5–11 through 5–13 provide best estimates of expenditures by selected sociodemographic characteristics not found elsewhere in the volume. The expenditures are for all services, hospital outpatient, physician inpatient and physician outpatient. Comparable estimates from the social survey can be found in Tables 3–13 through 3–15. Comparisons of these two sets of tables suggests that the verification did not seem to have a special impact on the estimates for any of the subgroups defined according to age, sex, poverty level, education or residence. This was true for the mean estimates for the total population as well as for the mean and median estimates for those persons with expenditures.

HOW HEALTH SERVICES ARE FINANCED

The effects of the verification on estimates of individual expenditures according to source of payment are shown in Table 5–14. The best estimates appeared slightly lower than the social survey for the nonfree sources and slightly higher for the free sources. Within the nonfree component the verification reduced the out-of-pocket estimates and slightly increased estimates of payment by voluntary insurance.

SUMMARY

The effect of the best estimate was to reduce the estimates of the percent of the population seeing a doctor and the mean number of physician visits per person. The reductions were greater for some subgroups than for others. Of particular note were the reductions in estimate of mean number of visits for older people, for those with low income and for the least well educated. The verification had minimal impact on estimates of the number of hospital admissions but it did reduce the estimates of average length of stay.

The effects of the verification on expenditure estimates generally appeared to be less important than they were on utilization estimates. Best estimates of physician and hospital expenditures tended to be slightly lower than the social survey estimates. The shape of the distribution of family expenditures appeared relatively unaffected by the verification. Also, the verification seemed to have fairly similar effects on subgroups of the population defined according to age, sex, income, education and residence.

Table 5-1. Comparison of respondent reporting and best estimate of percent population seeing a physician by selected characteristics: 1970

Characteristic	Percent Population Seeing A Physician During 1970 (42)	
	As reported in social survey	*As arrived at in best estimate (3)*
Sex (54)		
Male	65	60
Female	71	68
Age (1)		
1-5	75	71
6-17	62	56
18-34	70	69
35-54	67	62
55-64	73	69
65 and over	76	72
Family income (25)		
Low	65	61
Middle	67	64
High	71	67
Race (49)		
White	70	66
Nonwhite	58	53
Education of head (10		
8 years or less	62	57
9-11 years	66	61
12 years	69	66
13 years or more	76	72
Residence (52)		
SMSA, central city	65	62
SMSA, other urban	72	69
Urban, non-SMSA	71	67
Rural, nonfarm	68	64
Rural, farm	62	55
Total	68	64

Table 5-2. Comparison of respondent reporting and best estimate of physician vistis per person-year by selected characteristics: 1970

Characteristic	*Mean Number of Physician Visits in 1970 (44)*	
	As reported in social survey	*As arrived at in best estimate (3)*
Sex (54)		
Male	3.6	3.1
Female	4.5	3.9
Age (1)		
0–5	4.2	3.8
6–17	2.2	1.7
18–34	4.2	4.1
35–54	4.0	3.3
55–64	6.3	5.1
65 and over	6.4	5.3
Family income (25)		
Low	4.9	3.9
Middle	3.9	3.6
High	3.6	3.2
Race (49)		
White	4.1	3.6
Nonwhite	3.6	2.8
Education of head (10		
8 years or less	4.2	3.4
9–11 years	3.6	3.2
12 years	3.6	3.3
13 years or more	4.5	3.9
Residence (52)		
SMSA, central city	4.2	3.4
SMSA, other urban	4.2	3.9
Urban, non-SMSA	4.4	3.4
Rural, nonfarm	3.7	3.3
Rural, farm	3.4	3.1
Total	4.0	3.5

Table 5-3. Comparison of respondent reporting and best estimate of distribution of place of physician visit: 1970

	Percent Distribution of Physician Visits	
Place of Physician Visit (45)	As reported in social survey	As arrived at in best estimate (3)
Home	2	2
Office	85	85
Outpatient department	7	7
Emergency room	2	2
Other	4	4
Total	100	100

Table 5-4. Comparison of respondent reporting and best estimate of median number of prenatal visits for live births by family characteristics of mother: 1970

	Median^a Number of 1970 Prenatal Visits (46)	
Characteristic	As reported in social survey	As arrived at in best estimate (3)
Income level (25)		
Low	9.6	9.4
Middle	12.2	11.8
High	11.0	10.5
Race (49)		
White	11.0	10.5
Nonwhite	10.5	9.9
Education (10)		
8 years or less	10.1	10.1
9–11 years	9.7	10.4
12 years	11.3	10.5
13 years or more	11.2	10.5
Residence (52)		
SMSA, central city	10.5	8.7
SMSA, other urban	11.6	10.3
Urban, non-SMSA	9.8	11.0
Rural, nonfarm	12.0	11.0
Rural, farm	b	b
Total	10.9	10.4

[a]The median is that number of visits that exceeds the number of visits made by one-half of the mothers and is less than the number made by the other half.

[b]Based on fewer than 25 unweighted cases.

Table 5-5. Comparison of respondent reporting and best estimate of hospital admissions per 100 person-years by selected characteristics: 1970

Characteristic	Hospital Admissions per 100 Person-Years (30)	
	As reported in social survey	*As arrived at best estimate (3)*
Sex (54)		
Male	11	11
Female	16	16
Age (1)		
0-5	11	11
6-17	6	6
18-34	20	19
35-54	12	12
55-64	20	19
65 and over	22	21
Family income (24)		
Under $2,000	19	19
$ 2,000- 3,499	16	15
3,500- 4,999	17	17
5,000- 7,499	16	16
7,500- 9,999	15	16
10,000-12,499	12	12
12,500-14,999	11	11
15,000 and over	9	9
Race (49)		
White	14	15
Nonwhite	11	11
Residence (52)		
Large urban	12	12
Other urban	14	14
Rural, nonfarm	15	15
Rural, farm	14	13
Total	14	14

Table 5-6. Comparison of respondent reporting and best estimate for mean length of stay and hospital days per 100 population by age and sex: 1970*

Characteristic	Mean Number of Days per Admission (32)		Hospital Days per 100 Population (31)	
	Social survey	Best estimate (3)	Social survey	Best estimate (3)
Age (1)				
0-17	5.2	4.2	38	32
18-54	8.1	6.1	127	94
55 and over	12.8	12.3	264	242
Sex (54)				
Male	10.4	8.1	113	83
Female	8.0	7.1	129	117
Total	8.9	7.5	121	100

*Selected observations are excluded from this table. For exclusion criteria and estimates including all observations, see Appendix Table II-16.

Table 5-7. Comparison of reporting and best estimate for physician and hospital inpatient and outpatient expenditures: 1970

	Mean Physician and Hospital Expenditures					
	Nonfree (13)		*Free (12)*		*Total (14)*	
Service	*Social survey*	*Best estimate (3)*	*Social survey*	*Best estimate (3)*	*Social survey*	*Best estimate (3)*
All physicians (19)						
Surgery in-hospital	$14	$13	$ 1	$ 1	$14	$14
Surgery out-of-hospital	1	1	a	a	1	1
Obstetrics	4	4	a	a	4	4
Oculist, ophthalmologist	1	1	a	a	1	1
Other physician, in hospital	7	8	1	a	8	8
Other physician, house call	1	a	a	a	1	1
Other physician, office	28	25	4	4	31	29
Hospital (17)						
Hospital inpatient	82	77	15[b]	14[b]	104	92[b]
Hospital outpatient	2	3	2	3	3	5[b]

[a] Less than 50¢.

[b] Excludes one case which accounts for more than 10 percent of the cell size. Inclusion of this case, a young man on outpatient kidney dialysis, raises the free care outpatient component to $13 and the total outpatient component to $16 in the best estimate. In the social survey, this case was included in the inpatient hospital component where it accounted for less than 10 percent of cell size in the total but was excluded from the free care component which would otherwise amount to $22.

Table 5-8. Mean expenditures for all personal health services per family by family income and poverty level from social survey and best estimate: 1970*

Income (24) and Poverty Level (26)	Mean Expenditures					
	Free (12)		Nonfree (13)		Total (14)	
	Social survey	Best estimate (3)	Social survey	Best estimate (3)	Social survey	Best estimate (3)
Under $2,000	$128	$147	$343	$313	$489	$459
$ 2,000– 3,499	180	157	403	378	583	536
3,500– 4,999	106	97	496	506	602	603
5,000– 7,499	97	97	582	623	741	721
7,500– 9,999	52	54	606	599	675	661
10,000–14,999	33	44	686	677	736	720
15,000 and over	9	13	883	859	907	894
Above near poverty	48	48	708	695	786	791
Below near poverty	194	178	432	405	626	583
Total	$ 86	$ 82	$636	$620	$744	$738

*Selected observations are excluded from this table. For exclusion criteria and estimates including all observations, see Appendix Table II-17.

Table 5-9. Percent distribution of families by source of payment and level of expenditures for all personal health services from social survey and best estimate: 1970

Level of Family Expenditures	Source of Payment of Family Expenditures					
	Free (12)		*Nonfree (13)*		*Total (14)*	
	Social survey	Best estimate (3)	Social survey	Best estimate (3)	Social survey	Best estimate (3)
None	73.8	73.4	2.8	2.6	2.0	2.0
Under $50	11.7	12.0	13.0	13.3	9.5	9.7
$ 50– 99	3.7	3.6	11.0	10.4	10.5	9.7
100– 199	3.1	3.1	14.1	15.4	13.8	15.1
200– 299	1.7	1.8	11.4	11.4	11.3	11.4
300– 399	0.9	1.2	7.6	8.2	8.0	8.4
400– 499	0.8	0.5	5.0	5.2	5.8	5.9
500– 749	1.1	1.1	10.3	9.2	10.7	10.1
750– 999	0.9	1.0	6.3	6.4	7.3	6.8
1,000–1,999	1.3	1.4	12.4	12.1	14.0	13.7
2,000–2,999	0.2	0.3	3.7	3.3	3.9	3.8
3,000–4,999	0.4	0.4	1.3	1.4	1.9	1.8
5,000 and over	0.2	0.2	1.1	1.1	1.5	1.3
Total	100.0	100.0	100.0	100.0	100.0	100.0

Table 5-10.   Aggregate family outlay for personal health services as a percent of family income from social survey and best estimate: 1970

Family Income (24) and Poverty Level (26)	Aggregate Family Outlay (39)	
	As reported in social survey	As arrived at in best estimate (3)
Under $2,000	14.5	12.5
$ 2,000- 3,499	9.3	9.3
3,500- 4,999	7.7	7.5
5,000- 7,499	6.1	5.8
7,500- 9,999	4.6	4.5
10,000-14,999	3.8	3.7
15,000 and over	3.3	3.1
Above near poverty	4.0	3.9
Below near poverty	8.9	8.3
Total	4.4	4.2

Table 5-11. Mean and median best estimate total expenditures (14) per person by selected characteristics: 1970*

Characteristic	Total Population Mean	People with Expenditures Mean	Median
Sex (54)			
Male	$210	$229	$ 61
Female	258	273	80
Age (1)			
0–5 years	105	112	42
6–17 years	96	105	39
18–34 years	246	258	80
35–54 years	236	251	87
55–64 years	376	410	134
65 years and over	428	456	142
Poverty Level (26)			
Above near poverty	256	270	74
Below near poverty	213	242	49
Education of head (10)			
8 years or less	234	262	62
9–11 years	193	209	61
12 years	208	221	66
13 years or more	295	305	85
Residence (52)			
SMSA, central city	236	255	72
SMSA, other	299	316	85
Urban, non-SMSA	190	203	65
Rural, nonfarm	199	213	57
Rural, farm	181	201	56
Total	$246	$264	$ 69

*Selected observations are excluded from this table. For exclusion criteria and estimates including all observations, see Appendix Table II-18.

NOTE: Data for the social survey equivalent of this table are found in Table 3–13.

Table 5-12. Mean and median best estimate total (14) hospital outpatient (17) expenditures per person by selected characteristics: 1970*

Characteristic	Total Population	People with Expenditures	
	Mean	Mean	Median
Sex (54)			
Male	$ 5	$48	$25
Female	4	55	24
Age (1)			
0–5 years	4	44	31
6–17 years	3	38	20
18–34 years	5	53	23
35–54 years	3	48	28
55–64 years	4	41	21
65 years and over	3	71	37
Poverty level (26)			
Above near poverty	4	43	23
Below near poverty	6	65	40
Education of head (10)			
8 years or less	5	55	25
9–11 years	4	50	23
12 years	3	38	25
13 years or more	4	45	23
Residence (52)			
SMSA, central city	8	68	30
SMSA, other	4	38	23
Urban, non-SMSA	1	26	21
Rural, nonfarm	3	36	16
Rural, farm	1	24	13
Total	$ 4	$51	$25

*Selected observations are excluded from this table. For exclusion criteria and estimates including all observations, see Appendix Table II-19.

NOTE: Data for the social survey equivalent of this table are found in Table 3–14.

Table 3-13. Mean and median best estimate (3) total (14) physician expenditures per person by selected characteristics: 1970*

Characteristic	Physician Inpatient, Including Surgery (20)			Physician Outpatient (21)		
	Total Population	People with Expenditures		Total Population	People with Expenditures	
	Mean	Mean	Median	Mean	Mean	Median
Sex (54)						
Male	$ 22	$305	$142	$ 29	$ 53	$ 26
Female	22	267	182	42	67	31
Age (1)						
0–5 years	11	143	89	32	47	30
6–17 years	7	180	135	15	31	16
18–34 years	17	229	139	46	75	30
35–54 years	22	272	197	35	61	30
55–64 years	38	338	287	53	82	42
65 years and over	42	298	168	54	79	48
Poverty level (26)						
Above near poverty	24	290	174	38	60	30
Below near poverty	17	259	130	29	60	30
Education of head (10)						
8 years or less	23	264	175	31	60	31
9–11 years	15	215	159	31	55	28
12 years	20	263	133	34	54	24
13 years or more	22	302	187	46	70	34
Residence (52)						
SMSA, central city	19	301	201	38	69	35
SMSA, other	25	332	209	42	66	30
Urban, non-SMSA	20	208	108	32	50	24
Rural, nonfarm	18	206	122	31	52	25
Rural, farm	18	220	147	26	48	23
Total	$ 22	$284	$161	$ 36	$ 60	$ 30

*Selected observations are excluded from this table. For exclusion criteria and estimates including all observations, see Appendix Table II-20.

NOTE: Data for the social survey equivalent of this table are found in Table 3-15.

Table 5-14. Mean expenditures per person for all personal health services by source of payment from social survey and best estimate: 1970

Source of Payment	Mean Expenditures	
	As reported in social survey	As arrived at in best estimate (3)
Nonfree (13)	$213	$208
Voluntary insurance	73	76
Out-of-pocket	116	109
Medicare	21	21
Other nonfree	3	3
Free (12)	36	39
Medicaid, Welfare, free institutions	27	31
Other free	9	8
Total	$248	$246

Chapter 6

The Utilization and Expenditure Experience of People with Varying Kinds of Health Insurance Coverage

This chapter provides a picture of the utilization and expenditure experience of people with no health insurance or with varying types of health insurance. The data used are best estimates for hospital and physician services. The tables in this chapter provide some control for age and income level. Individuals 65 and over are separated from the rest of the population because of the virtual universal coverage this group has under Medicare and because of their special health needs. The rest of the population is divided into those in families above and below the near poverty level. People below the near poverty level receive most of the current Medicaid benefits and have the greatest difficulty meeting the rest of their medical care costs. Differences in people's medical care experience are examined according to the presence of insurance and whether this insurance is supplementary to Medicare for the aged; or basic, major medical or prepaid group practice for the younger population.

Many of the optional coverages examined in this chapter are proposed in one or another of the national health insurance bills. Documentation of the experiences of people who already have such coverage and comparison of these experiences with those of people who do not might prove of assistance in attempting to assess the impacts of the various proposals. While the differences between the insured and the uninsured shown in this chapter can be suggestive of changes in behavior that might be anticipated by new insurance legislation, we are not assuming that those without coverage would act exactly like those with coverage if insurance were extended. The people with and without coverage differ in other ways, such as in desire for and access to services, which also influence their utilization. Further, if everyone had coverage, prevailing conditions under which people seek and obtain services would change (i.e., appointment queues, and office waiting time). Some of these additional problems in estimating change in demand for health services with new health insurance legislation are considered in analyses by Phelps (1975) using data from the 1970 study.

UTILIZATION DIFFERENCES

Table 6-1 provides an overall view of the utilization experience of subgroups in the U.S. defined according to age, income and type of health insurance coverage. First, for people 65 and over it seems that those with insurance supplementary to Medicare generally use more services than those without additional voluntary insurance coverage. Those with supplementary coverage appeared more likely to see the physician, enter the hospital, have surgical procedures performed in the hospital and use prescribed drugs. An exception is that the "Medicare only" elderly do *not* have fewer visits to the doctor than those with supplementary coverage. It should also be noted that those with supplementary coverage are more likely to see a dentist than those without, even though supplementary coverage seldom includes dental coverage. This suggests that the elderly with supplementary coverage are different from those without in ways other than insurance coverage which also may influence their utilization of health services. For example, they may be better educated or have a prior history of higher use which makes them more apt to purchase the supplementary coverage.

Turning to those under 65, we find that people below the near poverty level without voluntary insurance are the least likely of any group to see a physician (Table 6-1). However, those who do see a physician have as many visits on average as any other group under 65. They are also relatively heavy users of hospitals, but the surgical use rate and use of drugs and dentists is below average. The poor with voluntary insurance appear more likely than the poor without insurance to see a physician but have fewer visits per person and may use the hospital less frequently.

The nonpoverty group without insurance appear more likely to see a physician than the poor but seem less likely to do so than other nonpoor with insurance (Table 6-1). Like the poor without insurance, however, those who do see the physician have a relatively high mean number of visits. They differ from the poor in that they have a very low hospital admission rate.

Among the nonpoor groups with insurance, those with only major medical coverage appear to be among the lowest utilizers—particularly with respect to mean number of physician visits and use of prescribed drugs (Table 6-1). The exception is seeing the dentist, for which the "major medical only" group has the greatest proportion of any group seeing the physician. Since it is unlikely that many of these people have dental insurance, this finding suggests that this group differs from the others by characteristics other than insurance which also influence their utilization pattern. Individuals with major medical coverage are of higher income than other insured groups and so may not see the necessity for first dollar coverage. High income is, of course, highly correlated with high use of dental services.

Those persons with basic insurance only have the highest rates (except for the elderly) of hospital admissions and inpatient surgical procedures (Table 6-1). These are, of course, the services which are insured by basic insurance.

People with both basic and major medical coverage are high in percent seeing a physician and percent using prescribed drugs (Table 6-1). However, they hold an intermediate position for mean number of visits and hospital admissions.

The use of physicians by persons in prepaid group practices does not appear to be particularly distinct from other nonpoverty groups with insurance (Table 6-1). As might be expected from the literature on prepaid groups, their hospital admission rate is low. Their rate of prescribed drug use is relatively high but similar to that for persons with basic and major medical coverage.

EXPENDITURE DIFFERENCES

Table 6-2 shows the total health care expenditures for each of the groups discussed in the previous section. This total includes the free as well as the nonfree component. It thus includes payments by Medicaid and welfare as well as those by Medicare, voluntary insurance, payment made out-of-pocket and estimates of the value of services provided under prepaid group practice when exact amounts could not be provided by families or the plans.

As expected, the expenditures were considerably higher for the elderly than for the rest of the population (Table 6-2). The expenditures for the elderly with supplementary insurance seem higher than expenditures for those with Medicare only but sampling error could account for the difference.

The poor under 65 had relatively low total expenditures (Table 6–2). The poor with insurance had higher total expenditures than those without.

Among the nonpoverty groups under 65 the prepaid group practice people and the uninsured appeared to have the lowest total expenditures (Table 6–2). The expenditures for the group with major medical only also appeared to be relatively low. The group with the highest expenditures were those covered with basic insurance only.

To provide some idea of the direct financial impact of medical care costs, Table 6–3 shows the out-of-pocket costs according to age, income and insurance status. Even though the elderly have a relatively high percentage of their expenses paid for by a third party, their total expenditures are of such a magnitude that they still have above average out-of-pocket expenses. Further, the elderly with supplementary insurance spend slightly more on their own than those without additional insurance.

The out-of-pocket expenses for those below the near poverty level are low (Table 6–3). Those poor persons with insurance have higher expenses than those without. As was the case with the aged, the people who buy insurance have total expenses that are still higher than those who do not purchase insurance, so that even with insurance benefits their out-of-pocket expenses are higher than the expenses of those without insurance. One possible interpretation is that those poor people with insurance are employed and are not eligible for Medicaid or charity care to cover costs not covered by insurance.

Among the nonpoor below 65, the uninsured and those with basic insurance appear to have relatively high out-of-pocket expenses (Table 6–3). Persons with prepaid group practice and those with major medical plus basic insurance have relatively low out-of-pocket expenses.

UTILIZATION AND EXPENDITURE DIFFERENCES FOR PEOPLE WITH SPECIAL TYPES OF INSURANCE COVERAGE

In this section we will examine the utilization and expenditure experiences of persons who have types of coverage that are currently uncommon but that are considered for possible inclusion under some proposals for national health insurance. These forms include coverage for physician visits, for prescribed drugs and for dental services.

Physician Visit Coverage

Doctor visit coverage includes, in addition to first dollar coverage for physician visits, certain other kinds of coverage which cover doctor visits after a deductible has been met. These include Medicare, Part B, and major medical coverage. Table 6-4 shows that persons with doctor visit coverage are more likely to see the doctor than those without among the elderly, the poor under 65 and the nonpoor under 65. While physician visit coverage is associated with an increased tendency to see the physician within a certain time period, the *mean number* of visits for those who do see the doctor is consistently as high or higher for the people *without* doctor visit coverage.

Hospital admissions are also examined, since there is some conjecture that coverage of outpatient services might reduce the emphasis on in-hospital care. However, only among the poor under 65 years of age does the admission rate for persons with doctor visit coverage appear lower than for the people without doctor visit coverage. The expenditure data in Table 6-4 show that physician outpatient expenditures are generally higher for people with doctor visit coverage than without it. While it is difficult to make comparisons for physician inpatient charges and hospital expenses due to the instability of some of the estimates, the available results do not suggest lower inpatient hospital expenditures for those with doctor visit coverage.

Drug Coverage

Prescribed drug coverage includes coverage which pays something for prescribed drugs after an initial deductible has been paid by the family. Table 6-5 shows those with drug coverage were slightly more likely than those without to purchase prescribed drugs during the survey year. The difference was greatest for those under 65 and above the near poverty level. The mean total drug expenditure did not appear closely related to whether or not people had drug coverage.

Dental Coverage

Table 6-6 suggests that people with dental insurance are more likely to see the dentist within a year's time period than those with no dental coverage. The data suggest that the difference may be greater for those below the near poverty level than it is for those above that level. For those seeing the dentist, the mean number of visits seems to be higher for those with dental coverage among people below the near poverty level but not for those above the near poverty level. The only available comparison of mean dental expenditures suggests that for people above the near poverty level, expenditures are higher for those with insurance than for those without coverage.

SUMMARY

The elderly with supplementary coverage are more likely to use health services but the coverage does not result in decreased out-of-pocket expenditure.

Poor people under 65 with voluntary coverage are more likely to see the physician and have surgery performed than the poor without voluntary insurance coverage. However, the insured poor average more visits once an initial contact has been made. The poor with insurance spend much more out-of-pocket than the poor without voluntary insurance.

Among the nonelderly nonpoor, those without voluntary insurance are low on most all utilization measures, but they report a high number of physician visits once a physician is seen. Among the insured nonpoor those with major medical only generally appear to be low utilizers. Persons in prepaid group practices have low hospital admission rates but higher relative rates for the use of physicians and drugs. Generally, the highest utilization rates, particularly for hospital services, are found for people with basic insurance only and for those with major medical plus basic.

People with doctor visit insurance appear more likely to see a doctor than those without but they do not appear to average more visits after the initial contact is made. Those with prescribed drug insurance appear slightly more likely to use drugs than those without such coverage but their overall expenditures for drugs do not appear appreciably higher, except possibly for the elderly. People with dental insurance are more likely to see the dentist than those without and appear to have somewhat higher dental expenditures.

In summary, the relationship of type of health insurance coverage to utilization of health care is extremely complex and not always in the direction that might be expected. Even when the relationship is in the expected direction, the reason may not be entirely the insurance benefit per se but rather characteristics associated both with having the insurance benefit and with higher use—better than average income or education, for example, or a prior history of heavy use. Nevertheless, it is probably safe to say that covering a benefit under national health insurance will increase its use and providing first dollar coverage will probably increase it even more. The case of prepaid group practice indicates, however, that even with first dollar coverage, certain utilization—i.e., inpatient hospital—can be kept low if the structure of the system under which care is delivered is altered. This may be one possible way to increase coverage without increasing actual use but it would, of course, involve some major changes in the American system.

Table 6-1. Health care utilization by age, family income and type of financing: 1970

Age (1), Family Income (25) and Type of Financing (2) (36)	Best Estimate (3) Utilization Measure						
	Percent seeing MD (42)	Mean MD visits for those with visits (44)	Hospital admissions per 100 population (30)	In-hospital surgical procedures per 100 population (56)	Percent using prescribed drugs (16)	Percent seeing a dentist (6)	Estimated number of persons in group (in millions)
Age 65 and over							
Medicare only	71 ± 2[a]	7.7 ± 0.4[a]	20 ± 2[a]	6.7 ± 1.1[a]	61 ± 2[a]	22 ± 2[a]	11.8
Medicare plus supplemental insurance	76 ± 2	7.3 ± 0.5	24 ± 2	8.5 ± 1.3	64 ± 2	33 ± 3	7.8
Age less than 65, below near poverty							
Without voluntary insurance	49 ± 2	5.6 ± 0.2	14 ± 1	4.7 ± 0.9	30 ± 2	27 ± 2	23.8
With voluntary insurance	53 ± 2	4.7 ± 0.4	13 ± 1	5.6 ± 0.7	33 ± 3	38 ± 2	12.6
Age less than 65, above near poverty							
Without voluntary insurance	57 ± 2	5.6 ± 0.8	9 ± 1	4.4 ± 0.7	37 ± 2	39 ± 3	21.9
Major medical insurance only	66 ± 5	4.4 ± 0.7	*	*	37 ± 6	64 ± 5	6.0
Basic insurance only	67 ± 2	5.0 ± 0.3	15 ± 2	7.5 ± 0.9	40 ± 1	50 ± 2	40.6
Major medical plus basic insurance	70 ± 2	4.8 ± 0.2	12 ± 1	6.0 ± 0.7	47 ± 2	56 ± 2	64.2
Prepaid group practice	65 ± 4	5.1 ± 0.5	9 ± 2	*	45 ± 4	47 ± 4	12.1
Total	64 ± 1	5.3 ± 0.2	13 ± 1	6.0 ± 0.4	43 ± 1	46 ± 1	200.8

[a]The numbers following the estimates in Tables 6-1 through 6-6 are estimates of the associated standard errors.
*Coefficient of variation ≥.25. This coefficient used in Tables 6-1 through 6-6 is defined as the standard error of the estimate divided by the estimate.

Table 6–2. Total health care expenditures by age, family income and type of financing: 1970

Age (1), Family Income (25) and Type of Financing (2) (36)	Best Estimate Mean Expenditures Per Person (3) (14)					
	Hospital (17)	Physician (19)	Drugs (16)	Dental (15)	Other (18)	Total
Age 65 and over						
Medicare only	$200 ± 31[a]	$ 90 ± 8[a]	$71 ± 5[a]	$16 ± 3[a]	$43 ± 10[a]	$420 ± 42[a]
Medicare plus supplemental insurance	217 ± 30	112 ± 10	66 ± 5	24 ± 4	39 ± 8	458 ± 39
Age less than 65, below near poverty						
Without voluntary insurance	81 ± 11	30 ± 3	20 ± 1	12 ± 1	12 ± 3	155 ± 15
With voluntary insurance	*	45 ± 5	22 ± 3	17 ± 2	13 ± 2	193 ± 30
Age less than 65, above near poverty						
Without voluntary insurance	*	40 ± 4	30 ± 4	28 ± 5	17 ± 3	*
Major medical insurance only	44 ± 10	54 ± 12	*	51 ± 12	*	209 ± 37
Basic insurance only	115 ± 25	71 ± 7	30 ± 4	32 ± 4	20 ± 2	267 ± 32
Major medical plus basic insurance	83 ± 15	57 ± 5	27 ± 2	34 ± 3	22 ± 2	224 ± 20
Prepaid group practice	*	58 ± 10	27 ± 5	37 ± 8	17 ± 3	184 ± 26
Total	$107 ± 14	$ 58 ± 2	$31 ± 1	$28 ± 2	$21 ± 1	$246 ± 16

[a]Estimates are followed by the associated standard error estimates.
*Coefficient of variation ≥ .25.

Table 6-3.   Out-of-pocket (13) health care expenditures by age, family income and type of financing: 1970

Age (1), Family Income (25) and Type of Financing (2) (36)	Best Estimate Mean Expenditures Per Person (3) (13)					
	Hospital (17)	Physician (19)	Drugs (16)	Dental (15)	Other (18)	Total
Age 65 and over						
Medicare only	*	$38 ± 3[a]	$55 ± 4[a]	$13 ± 2[a]	*	$148 ± 14[a]
Medicare plus supplemental insurance	*	42 ± 3	58 ± 5	23 ± 4	32 ± 8	166 ± 10
Age less than 65, below near poverty						
Without voluntary insurance	7 ± 1	12 ± 1	14 ± 1	5 ± 1	*	45 ± 4
With voluntary insurance	*	23 ± 3	20 ± 2	13 ± 1	10 ± 2	83 ± 10
Age less than 65, above near poverty						
Without voluntary insurance	24 ± 4	30 ± 3	28 ± 4	24 ± 5	12 ± 2	118 ± 12
Major medical insurance only	*	25 ± 3	21 ± 5	*	17 ± 3	115 ± 17
Basic insurance only	*	39 ± 5	29 ± 4	31 ± 4	15 ± 1	131 ± 15
Major medical plus basic insurance	*	27 ± 2	25 ± 2	32 ± 3	16 ± 1	109 ± 7
Prepaid group practice	*	31 ± 5	21 ± 3	*	10 ± 2	97 ± 12
Total	$12 ± 3	$29 ± 1	$27 ± 1	$25 ± 2	$16 ± 1	$109 ± 5

[a]Estimates are followed by the associated standard error estimates.
*Coefficient of variation ≥ .25.

Table 6–4. Physician and hospital utilization and expenditures by age, family income and presence of doctor visit insurance: 1970

Age (1) and Family Income (25)	Physician visit insurance (43)	Best Estimate Utilization (3)			Best Estimate Mean Expenditures Per Person (3) (14)		
		Percent seeing MD (42)	Mean MD visits for those with visits (44)	Hospital admissions per 100 population (30)	Physician outpatient (21)	Physician inpatient (20)	Hospital (17)
65 and over	NO	65 ± 4[a]	7.5 ± 1.0[a]	22 ± 6[a]	$40 ± 6[a]	*	$166 ± 32[a]
	YES	73 ± 1	7.4 ± 0.3	24 ± 2	57 ± 3	44 ± 6	212 ± 29
Under 65, below near poverty	NO	49 ± 2	5.5 ± 0.2	15 ± 1	23 ± 2	10 ± 2	84 ± 10
	YES	55 ± 3	4.4 ± 0.4	12 ± 2	28 ± 6	*	*
Under 65, above near poverty	NO	63 ± 2	5.2 ± 0.4	13 ± 2	34 ± 3	22 ± 5	*
	YES	69 ± 2	4.9 ± 0.2	14 ± 1	38 ± 2	22 ± 3	81 ± 11
TOTAL		64 ± 1	5.3 ± 0.2	15 ± 1	$36 ± 2	$22 ± 2	$108 ± 14

[a]Estimates are followed by the associated standard error estimates.
*Coefficient of variation ≥ .25.

Table 6-5. Prescribed drug utilization and expenditures by age, family income and presence of prepaid drug insurance: 1970

Age (1) and Family Income (25)	Prescribed Drug Insurance (9)	Percent Using Prescribed Drugs (16)	Mean Prescribed Drug Expenditures Per Person (16) (14)
65 and over	NO	59 ± 5[a]	$52 ± 6[a]
	YES	62 ± 2	57 ± 4
Under 65, below near poverty	NO	31 ± 2	15 ± 1
	YES	32 ± 4	14 ± 3
Under 65, above near poverty	NO	40 ± 2	22 ± 3
	YES	46 ± 2	19 ± 1
Total		43 ± 1	$23 ± 1

[a]Estimates are followed by the associated standard error estimates.

Table 6-6. Dental care utilization and expenditures by age, family income and presence of dental insurance: 1970

Age (1) and Family Income (25)	Dental Care Insurance (5)	Utilization		Mean Dental Expenditures Per Person (16) (14)
		Percent seeing dentist (6)	Mean dentist visits for those with visits (7)	
65 and over	NO	26 ± 1[a]	3.3 ± 0.2[a]	$20 ± 2[a]
	YES	*	*	*
Under 65 below near poverty	NO	30 ± 2	2.8 ± 0.1	13 ± 1
	YES	41 ± 8	3.2 ± 0.7	*
Under 65, above near poverty	NO	50 ± 1	3.3 ± 0.1	32 ± 2
	YES	57 ± 3	3.1 ± 0.2	37 ± 6
Total		45 ± 1	3.2 ± 0.1	$28 ± 2

[a]Estimates are followed by the associated standard error estimates.
*Coefficient of variation ≥ .25.

Chapter 7

Observations and Conclusions

The foregoing chapters have presented in detail the patterns and trends in health care use of four household surveys conducted by the Center for Health Administration Studies and the National Opinion Research Center for 1953, 1958, 1963 and 1970. In this concluding chapter we will attempt to select the highlights of the findings.

Solutions to problems of public policy in health care delivery, particularly the currently debated problem of national health insurance, are dependent upon knowledge of currently existing patterns of care and reimbursement. This should be the case for public policy decisions in all areas. In many instances, however, adequate and valid information simply does not exist. In this instance, the United States has had more information available than any other country on the expenditure and use patterns of personal health services of families and third party source of funding. Trend data are also in good supply. This country, thus, has the opportunity to tailor-make a national health insurance program in relation to the documented problems of families rather than some a priori assumption of such problems.

The first nationwide household survey was conducted during the period 1928 to 1931. It was part of the study by the Committee for the Costs of Medical Care and was funded by six philanthropic foundations (Falk, 1933). The four major surveys described in this book are direct descendants of this first study. All these surveys have been referred to frequently in public policy discussions and debates on the problems of organizing and financing personal health services.[1]

The overwhelming impression one gets from reviewing the trends in personal health services use is that for the most part they have been in the desired direction. More people are using more services as measured by visits to physicians and dentists and admissions to hospitals and use of preventive services. Indeed, there is now concern with "overuse." More people are being covered by some kind of health insurance, either private or governmental. In addition, health insurance is gradually paying for increasingly larger portions of total health service expenditures, particularly hospital care expenses. The trend is toward extensive coverage of physician services and a start is being made in covering other health goods and services. Further, and an extremely important consideration given the now official policy of considering health services a right, the use of services by lower income groups is increasing in relation to those of higher incomes.

From the standpoint of equitable public policy, there have also been undesirable trends. A serious one is the decrease in physicians in inner city low income areas and rural areas. This particular trend is not documented in our surveys but has an important effect on the use of services reported in them. Another is the great increases in expenditures for services, particularly hospital care, which have made it difficult for health insurance benefits to keep up with the costs of services. This, of course, results in the consumer having to pay the balance out-of-pocket, usually at a time when he is ill-prepared to do so.

Despite the undesirable trends, the forces operating in the health field have still been ones pervasively directed toward expansion of use, health insurance coverage and health insurance benefits. This expansion has occurred with only limited governmental intervention thus far: Medicare for the elderly and Medicaid for the poor. Inevitably, gaps have appeared: some people are not covered by any third party payer; many people are inadequately covered and experience high out-of-pocket costs for expensive medical episodes; Medicaid coverage smacks of charity because of its means test and leads in many cases to a dual standard of care because of inadequate government reimbursement. Gaps between need and use of services remain, particularly for the poor, although these are narrowing.

Inevitably, it is suggested that government must close these gaps by some form of universal and comprehensive health insurance and by some method of control over prices and use. The primary ques-

---

[1]See Appendix V for a listing of the uses of the current survey.

tion continues in this country to be one of the appropriate mix of the private and public sectors in the financing and organization of health services. In order to close these gaps, does the government need to fund and control the entire health services enterprise, or can there be a judicious mix of private and public efforts, a mix which has been evolving for many years? We are approaching the time when the nature of this mix needs serious thought. The range of health insurance bills now being considered in Congress reflects the concern with the nature of the financial mix. Professional Standards Review Organization (PSRO) legislation, which would monitor federally funded patients, reflects the concern with use.

We now wish to point out what we regard as more specific highlights from the details of the previous chapters and to provide interpretations and implications for public policy.

WHERE AND WHY PEOPLE RECEIVE HEALTH SERVICES

The proportion of the population that named a place such as a hospital outpatient department or a health center rather than a particular doctor as a regular source of care in 1963 and in 1970 increased considerably for so short a period, from 11 percent to 18 percent. By 1970, about one-half of all low income, central city children had a clinic as their regular source of care. The trend is apparently toward some organizational type of health services delivery that will blur the traditional concept of a regular and known physician for each individual. It is likely that higher income groups will demand a regular physician. As long as the health services delivery system remains relatively open, there will be a variety of arrangements possible according to demands and opportunities of different segments of the population. Legislation for national health insurance will likely respect the general openness of the American health services mix. It must do this in order to be politically feasible.

There was a general increase in the tendency of people to see a doctor for most symptoms between 1963 and 1970. When reasons for seeing a doctor were classified by seriousness—i.e., (1) mandatory, (2) mixture of mandatory and elective, and (3) elective only—it was found that patients fell into approximately equal thirds for each grouping. Those who were most likely to delay in seeing a doctor tended to be treated for more severe conditions when they did see a doctor. As expected, the poor were more likely to be classified as mandatory than those with higher incomes, but the differences, although persistent, were not large. As measured by disability days, however, high income individuals had considerably more physician contact per 100 disability days than did the poor.

The fitting of need to use is a very difficult public policy problem given the current crudeness of the methodology for measuring this fit. In the 1963 and 1970 surveys we are, however, trying to formulate methodology for this purpose. If the concept of equal access to health services could be applied to its optimum, it should be concerned with matching need and use. The crude and largely implicit current standard is that low income use should approximate high income use. It is reasonable to assume, however, that a portion of high income use can be classified as "luxury" or "unnecessary" use. It would be a major accomplishment in itself for national health insurance to first eliminate the gap in use between the poor and the better off and in due course work toward increasingly sophisticated methods of relating actual need to use, as measured both by number of visits and by type of practitioner providing the care.

Between 1963 and 1970 there was an appreciable increase in the proportion of the population receiving preventive examinations for any reason. This occurred for most major population segments and is a very interesting and significant trend because of the increased use of resources implied. There is by no means unanimity among experts as to the value of preventive examinations. In all likelihood, if the trend continues, it will stimulate critical analysis of the effectiveness of preventive examinations in relation to proper allocation of resources.

TYPE AND VOLUME OF SERVICE

The long term trend has been for an increasing proportion of the population to see a physician during a year. From 1958 through 1963 there was little change in the proportion of the population who saw a physician, but between 1963 and 1970 there was a small increase. The increase was not spread evenly over all age groups; much of it was accounted for by older people.

A substantially greater proportion of the low income population was seeing a physician in 1970 compared with 1963, 65 percent and 56 percent, respectively. The higher income groups remained constant, although, as expected, at a higher proportion, 71 percent. As to residence, between 1963 and 1970, the percent of the population seeing a doctor increased for each group including the rural farm population that traditionally has had and continues to have least access to physicians.

Among children from one to five years of age the proportion

seeing a doctor in the low income groups is considerably lower than for children in the middle and high income categories. However, this difference by income level appeared to decrease between 1963 and 1970.

Access to dental care continues to reveal the greatest differential between income groups, although the gap is narrowing over time. Considering an accepted standard of at least one visit to a dentist during a year, for prophylaxis if for no other reason, the population is seeking dental services far below the recommended optimum. Only 45 percent of the population saw a dentist in 1970. Still, this is appreciably higher than the 38 percent figure in 1963.

The percentage of physicians visits classified as home visits continued to decrease. It is now down to only 2 percent of all visits. Obviously, given the current interest in encouraging care in the home, such a movement will have a difficult time appreciably reversing a long term trend even if paramedical personnel are used rather than physicians.

In view of the great absolute increase in the use of emergency medical services during recent years, it is of interest that they account for only 2 percent of all visits to physicians. It is a very visible 2 percent, however, since the hospitals bear the entire brunt of this pressure and a large proportion of patients in emergency departments are not there for true emergency reasons.

It is of great interest, given the concern with quality in surgery and medical care generally, that the proportion of surgery performed by physicians who were board-certified for surgery increased from 37 percent in 1953 to 60 percent in 1970. These figures exclude those who are regarded as board-eligible. It may be remarked that this shift in the proportion of surgery performed by board-certified surgeons took place before there were any direct attempts by government funding agencies to influence quality through certain criteria. The entire health services delivery system itself was improving its quality base by raising professional standards. It would seem, therefore, that the most official agencies can do regarding the improvement in standards is to stimulate the trends already in motion. If the general level of quality is not good, external standards imposed on a profession not in tune with these standards will be difficult to implement.

A generally accepted professional standard for prenatal care is that the pregnant woman see a physician within the first trimester. From 1953 to 1970 the percent of low income women having live births who saw a physician within the first trimester increased from 42 percent to 66 percent. Those in the middle income third increased from 66 percent in 1953 to 86 percent in 1963 and increased further to 92 percent in 1970. The high income third remained at about 90 percent during that 17 year period. Undoubtedly, if these contacts with physicians during the first trimester were standardized for quality, there would be a clear differentiation between low and high income—i.e., the high income mothers would be more likely to have board-certified obstetricians.

What is again of interest from a public policy standpoint is that these improvements in access would appear to be greater over a relatively short period than is warranted by environing changes in health service delivery systems or public health programs for mothers and infants during the same period. General maternal and infant mortality rates have fallen to respectably low points, although they are still higher than those in countries with more homogeneous populations.

The foregoing observations are, of course, based on gross averages by broad income and residential categories. There are large pockets of underserviced rural and urban areas where maternal and child health programs for targeted problems could reduce certain types of maternal and infant mortality related to environmental conditions, particularly communicable and infectious diseases. Improvements in these areas would not be significantly reflected in the national rates, but significantly lowered rates would be visible in the target areas.

EXPENDITURES FOR PERSONAL HEALTH SERVICES

Currently, public policy is concerned more with the rising expenditures for personal health services and the extent to which families have to pay out-of-pocket for high cost medical episodes than with problems of access as such. The two prominent methods to measure financial impact on families are percent of family income paid out-of-pocket for health care services in a year and the proportion of families who experience costs above certain magnitudes regardless of how these costs are financed.

On average between 1958 and 1970 the percent of aggregate income spent out-of-pocket for personal health services dropped from 5.5 percent in 1958 to 4.2 percent in 1970. This means that, despite increased use and rising prices, voluntary health insurance and government programs did reduce the out-of-pocket expenses of families measured as a proportion of family income. The irony, however, is that although the overall average dropped between 1958 and 1970, the proportion of expenditures for low income groups as a percent of family income did not show such a reduction. The differential between low and high income families continues to be very wide, from 12.6 percent of family income for those under $2,000 a year to 3.5 percent for those with incomes of $10,000 and over in 1970. Clearly, the burden of the cost continues to be shared very unequally, although, of course, higher income families spend more out-of-pocket in total dollars.

A more precise measure of impact on family financial burden is the concept of economic "catastrophe." It was found that 8.5 percent of the families or 5.5 million families had outlays of $1,000 or more in 1970. Ten percent (about seven million families) had outlays which equaled at least 15 percent of their incomes. The trend has been that families with catastrophic illnesses are taking a larger share of the medical care dollar. In 1963 the top 1 percent of the families in terms of expenditure magnitudes accounted for 17 percent of the total and the top 5 percent accounted for 43 percent of the expenditures. In 1970, the top 1 percent accounted for 23 percent of the total and the top 5 percent of the families accounted for 48 percent of the expenditures.

The foregoing data are exceedingly pertinent to public policy directed toward the concept of national health insurance for catastrophes. A national health insurance plan designed to reduce high family outlays for personal health services, without taking into account family income level, would benefit a very different group of families than would a plan which seeks primarily to reduce outlay as a proportion of family income. In the interest of equity, a national health insurance plan directed to catastrophic expenditures should relate them to proportion of family income. Otherwise, the differential between low and high income families will actually be made worse than it is now. An explicit public policy could equalize the burden of high cost illness episodes among family income levels in a way not feasible in voluntary health insurance. A philosophical difficulty with this proposal, of course, is that it involves a means test unless first dollar coverage is provided for all groups.

It is assumed that a governmentally funded and operated health service system is better able to allocate resources toward certain objectives than can the private sector. There is justification for this assumption, of course, if a government program is given the effective power and the resources to do so. It would seem that an implicit if not explicit public policy would support increased allocations to both the young and the old in the event of a national health insurance program. Both are relatively high users of services, although of a different mix of services. The average annual percent use increase for all services for 1963–1970 as compared with 1953–1963 was highest for the age groups five and under and 55 and over. It seems reasonable to assume that part of this increase can be attributed to Medicare and Medicaid. Even before 1963, however, there is evidence that resources were beginning to be differentially allocated to the young and the old for physician services, the primary entry point to the health care system. We make this observation to indicate that even prior to explicit government programs, the trends these programs were to influence were already underway. It seems reasonable to assume that they were accelerated by these programs. Whether or not a national health insurance plan will be designed so as to allocate resources toward target problems cannot be automatically assumed. There will be pressure group politics within a national health insurance plan just as there are without one.

Methods to control use and the price of services continue to be exceedingly crude; even methods to measure the degree to which use and price contribute to overall cost increases are crude. This series of surveys has contributed some perspective to the relative importance of use and price in the increases in expenditures over 17 years. Even allowing for possible errors in measurement, it is clear that increased use has contributed much less to rising expenditures than has price.

A public policy implication, of course, is that in order to contain rising cost it is logical to concentrate on price rather than use. It seems, however, that current methodology is directed more to containing use (e.g., PSRO review and certificate-of-need) than to price. Politically, methods of reimbursement are a much more sensitive area than methods of controlling use. Eventually, there will undoubtedly be more attention paid to price as well, a concern already evident in rate regulations for hospitals. Thus far, this has been limited to federally funded programs such as Medicaid and Medicare, but the trend is toward rate setting for private reimbursement as well. Control of physician services will be in the form of negotiated or arbitrarily set fee schedules, capitation methods of payment, straight salaries and combinations of these.

INSURANCE COVERAGE

It is a reasonable observation that voluntary health insurance has reached the saturation level for hospital care. Ten years ago it was relieved of the problem of covering hospitalization for the aged segment of the population with the advent of Medicare. Remaining deficiencies in coverage are to be expected, since most of the population lacking coverage are not in employee groups yet have incomes too high to be eligible for Medicaid. This population poses a small but persistent problem for hospitals, and the economic effect on a family whose insurance runs out or who has too high an income for charity is frequently little short of devastating.

It is also a reasonable observation that voluntary health insurance has not yet reached a saturation point for other than hospital services. Because of this, the proportion of family expenditures paid by insurance, particularly for high cost illness episodes, is not as high as in other countries. In 1970 the public payed out directly 44 percent of all costs of services. The rest was covered by governmental programs and voluntary health insurance. Even with Medicare, people 65 and over payed directly for 36 percent of all expenditures. Still, given the rapidly rising expenditures for health services, it is significant that voluntary health insurance largely supported by combined employee and employer funding expanded its coverage from 15 percent of all private expenditures in 1953 to 37 percent in 1970. When Medicare is added, mediated through the private insurance payment mechanism, the overall percentage was 46 percent in 1970.

Throughout the period, the hospital component was most likely to be financed by insurance of various kinds. The proportion of hospital expenses increased from 50 percent in 1953 to 84 percent in 1970. In-hospital surgery follows, with an increase from 38 percent to 76 percent for the same period. Among physician components, home and office calls are last, with an increase from 4 percent to 31 percent. In 1970, drugs and dental care were still not covered to any significant extent.

The trends, thus, have been clearly in the direction of insurance paying for an increasing proportion of high magnitude expenditures. This implies that voluntary health insurance (and Medicare) have reflected an American propensity toward health insurance as a risk concept rather than as a provision of service concept. This is not to say that the United States will settle for a risk or catastrophic concept in the long run; but high cost episodes are very visible, though relatively few, and the mitigation, if not the elimination, of high cost out-of-pocket episodes appears to have a high priority in public policy formulation.

There is abundant evidence for the logic of the catastrophe approach as documented earlier. In general, since 1953, it appears that the proportion of expenditures covered by insurance has increased for relatively high cost episodes (the rough breakoff point appears to be $500 or more a year for a family) and decreased for lower magnitudes. In 1953, disregarding inflation, families with expenditures in excess of $1,000 had 24 percent of such expenditures paid by voluntary insurance. In 1970 the proportion paid by voluntary insurance and Medicare had increased to 63 percent. Indeed, in 1970 (no comparable previous data), families with expenditures of over $2,000 had 71 percent of such expenditures paid by voluntary insurance and Medicare. It thus appears that the most dynamic aspect of health insurance in this country is that of catastrophic coverage. It seems reasonable to infer that the growth of major medical coverage has accounted for the foregoing trends. Currently, 41 percent of the population is covered by some form of high cost illness episode insurance. Clearly, though, the health insurance industry has far from achieved the saturation point for this type of insurance.

A final observation on health insurance benefit levels is that, as expected, the lower the income (and the more likely a family resides in a rural farm area), the lower the proportion of their health care expenditures paid for by health insurance. Again, the private sector finds it inherently difficult to cover those segments of the population. The government does not find it easy either, but, given a policy with mechanisms for implementation, the government can more easily fill these deficiency gaps.

As an indication of the strong reliance on employee fringe benefits as the means of financing voluntary health insurance, there has been a steady increase in cost sharing on the part of the employers. In fact, for over 90 percent of employees having group coverage the employer pays at least part of the premiums and for 39 percent the employer pays all. Given the strong tradition for this type of financing and the reluctance to shift the burden to general taxation, it is likely that payroll deduction will continue to be the major source of funding for national health insurance. Medicare is a precedent. Employer contributions under such a scheme would then continue to be a bargaining point between labor and management.

As for the relative strength of insurers as measured by enrollment of various types of insurance agencies, it appears the Blue Cross hospital plans and Blue Shield medical plans are more or less even with the private insurance carriers. The Blue Cross and Blue Shield plans, however, particularly Blue Cross, are better able to operate as a national federation relative to the great number of private insurance companies selling health insurance. If permitted, the Blue Cross and Blue Shield plans may well function as bargaining giants for the providers, with that even bigger giant, the federal government, logically representing the public.

Another health service delivery type, prepaid group practice plans, continues to be a very small segment of the health insurance field given its seeming general support as a means of containing costs.

Such plans still cover only 5 percent or so of the population. If this country is to have a diversity of health service delivery options, similar to the diversity in other sections of the economy, clearly the group practice plans need to increase in number and geographical distribution so that these options are real.

IMPLICATIONS FOR STRUCTURING THE HEALTH SERVICES SYSTEM

These surveys were not directed to health services delivery systems but to the trends in use, expenditures patterns and sources of payment for the general population. Obviously, however, the data have implications for the structuring of health services delivery systems.

An attempt was made to make these implications more explicit by surveying the attitudes of the population toward aspects of medical care that do have implications for changes in the delivery system (Andersen, Kravits and Anderson, 1971). Three-quarters of the heads of families in 1970 agreed with the statement: "There is a crisis in health care in the United States." Rarely is there as large a majority in the general population in agreement on any political issue. Clearly, there was a felt crisis in the body politic. Something was wrong. On further querying into the dimensions of this crisis, an appreciable minority of the population, approximately 40 percent, were dissatisfied with access to physicians. Thirty-seven percent were dissatisfied with the length of waiting time in offices or clinics, and 43 percent were dissatisfied with the availability of medical care at night and on weekends.

Only 13 percent of the population, however, expressed dissatisfaction with the ease and convenience of getting to a doctor from their homes. Geographic availability of doctors was apparently less of a problem than was access to doctors. This average of 13 percent, however, obscures the relatively high proportion (as high as 38 percent) of low income segments of the population who were dissatisfied.

About two-fifths of the population expressed dissatisfaction with out-of-pocket costs. It will be recalled that, on average, the population pays out 44 percent of total costs of all health services directly. It will also be recalled that visible percentages of the households have relatively high expenditures as well, a great deal of which are not covered by insurance.

Clearly, the issues as seen by the public are to improve access to physicians and to reduce out-of-pocket expenditures, rather logical perceptions given the data. Interestingly, however, and contrary to much popular opinion, only 10 percent of the population expressed dissatisfaction with the overall quality of care and only 8 percent were dissatisfied with the courtesy of physicians and nurses.

The range of health insurance proposals now in Congress deal with these issues as seen by the public in various ways. Increasing the supply of physicians would, of course, not automatically improve access unless physicians would also operate their practices so as to minimize waiting time and inaccessability at night and on weekends. There is no inherent reason why physicians cannot improve the ease with which patients can see them within a private practice, fee for service system. More highly structured practice systems are not inherently more accessible unless they are organized to be so.

Unpopular areas for physicians to go to, such as inner city ghettos and remote rural counties, are a somewhat separate problem requiring a different outreach policy of some kind. Various methods are contemplated and in operation, such as a national service corps. Other countries also have these problems, and no country has as yet completely solved them.

The method of insuring against high cost illness episodes is in essence an actuarial problem given a deliberate public policy. It appears that a catastrophic type of insurance would be popular. One basic issue involves whether the same dollar amount expended would be considered a catastrophe for everyone. Whether solved with a means test or by arbitrarily using the same expenditure for all, this might well be the opening wedge in national health insurance.

Although not documented in this study, it seems that high deductibles and co-insurance methods of controlling use are unpopular with the public. These are not always popular with the providers either, as they are sometimes difficult to collect. Precedents in other countries point to such controls being a constant issue politically. Out-of-pocket expenditures of any magnitude seem simply to be disliked by the public.

In sum, the main issues concerning national health insurance are comprehensiveness of benefits and controls on patients and/or providers. The organization of services is an issue which will become more apparent as previous issues are settled. Universality has an egalitarian ring to it, and universality is now politically acceptable because the broad middle income groups seem to favor national health insurance as a means of correcting the deficiencies in the current system that have been documented in this book. Universality in itself may not, however, be the most equitable manner for deploying services to low income groups, inner city ghettos and remote rural areas unless the legislation is so formulated as to work in that direction.

Even under the best type of legislation, it is reasonable to predict that universality will obscure the deficient care given the low income groups in ghetto areas. The broad middle class will likely get and take more of the resources within the national system under the illusion that universality in itself leads to equal access. In order to be equitable, a national health insurance system must be deliberately and heavily weighted toward those with low incomes. Universality does not guarantee this and may, in fact, obscure pockets of deprivation under the assumption that universality is by itself automatically equitable.

Appendix I

Methodology

Martha J. Banks and Ronald Andersen

SAMPLE DESIGN

The data presented in this book are based on results of area probability samples conducted by the Center for Health Administration Studies and the National Opinion Research Center of the University of Chicago for the calendar years 1953, 1958, 1963 and 1970.

The universe sampled in these studies was the total noninstitutionalized population of the United States. This universe excludes the following individuals:

1. residents in medical, mental, penal, religious or other institutions who were not residents of a private dwelling at any time during the calendar year;
2. residents on military reservations (the latter three studies included, however, personnel in the armed forces living off base with their families or in other civilian households); and
3. transient individuals having no usual or permanent residence.

The 1953 and 1963 studies were self-weighting samples using data for 8,874 and 7,803 persons respectively. The 1958 and 1970 studies were not self-weighting samples. Rather, they stressed persons and families of special concern in health policy formulation. Families with high medical care expenditures were oversampled in 1958. In 1970 those families with low incomes living in central cities, the rural population, and persons 66 and over were emphasized. The 1958 sample size was 9,546; in 1970 it was 11,619.

In order to obtain a sample with the special characteristics of interest in the 1970 study, four separate subsamples were drawn:

1. a sample (U) selected from 73 special urban segments in the NORC master sample. These segments were so designated because of the presence of a high proportion of low income urban families according to 1960 Census data;
2. a sample (A) selected from the remaining segments in the NORC national probability sample;
3. a sample (S) consisting of families either classified as low income[1] or containing a person 66 years or older obtained by screening households in all NORC segments; and
4. a sample (R) obtained from 30 additional rural primary sampling units drawn especially for this study. Only families thought to be living in rural areas of these PSUs were interviewed. No screening procedure was involved for this sample.

Given the complex sampling design of this study, a weighting scheme must be applied before estimates and tabulations can be produced. Weighting is necessary to correct the different probabilities of selection among sample observations. Adjustment is also made for the varying completion rates among the various subsamples. A final poststratification adjustment in the weights was employed to make the sample more closely representative of the actual U.S. population and, thus, to reduce sampling variance. The control factor is the ratio of estimates from the Current Population Survey (U.S. Bureau of the Census, 1971a: 30–32) to estimates based on the NORC sample for some 16 population classes defined by family size, family income, race and whether or not the family dwelling unit is in a Standard Metropolitan Statistical Area.

1. A family was included as a "low income" family if they reported their gross income to be less than the following amounts for a given family size:

Family Size	Yearly	Monthly	Weekly
1	$2,600	$220	$ 50
2	3,700	310	70
3	4,500	370	85
4	5,700	470	110
5	6,600	550	130
6	7,500	620	145
7	9,100	760	175

VERIFICATION

In all four studies, an attempt was made to verify all hospital admissions reported by families in the social survey. In the last two studies, health insurance coverage through Blue Cross–Blue Shield, private insurance companies and independent plans was checked through insurers and, in the case of group coverage, employers. In the most recent study, verification was expanded to cover physicians or clinics where visits reportedly occurred and to cover payments made for health services by health insurers.

The dual purpose of these procedures was to determine if the family reports were accurate and to get more precise information than the families were likely to give on diagnosis, cost, kinds of treatment and sources of payment for services. Verifying information was not obtained on some hospital and physician services and insurance coverage reported in the social survey. Approximately 10 percent of the families in the social survey refused to sign the permission forms that were needed to obtain information from doctors, hospitals and insurers. For some families that did sign the permission form, not enough information was available on certain names and addresses to contact the sources.

The verification studies picked up some unreported utilization and expenditures, particularly for people who reported contact with a physician or hospital but underreported the number of visits or admissions. However, the verifications were not optimally designed to identify respondents who incorrectly reported no visits to physicians, hospital admissions or insurance coverage, since verification was not attempted on these "false negatives." Medical services or insurance coverage not mentioned by the respondent were discovered only if a source that was mentioned reported it. For example, an insurance company identified by the respondent might report a claim for a hospitalization not reported by the respondent, or a hospital confirming a reported hospitalization might indicate that surgery was performed by a physician not reported as having provided care by the respondent.

Table I–1 shows the effects of the verifications on number of hospital admissions, physicians seeing members of the sample and health insurance policies. Column 1 shows the total number of each as reported by families. Column 2 indicates those reported admissions, physicians seen and policies for which verification was not attempted because permission was refused, identifying information was inadequate, etc. The number of cases for which verification was attempted but no conclusive judgment was made due to nonresponse or refusal of the verification source is given in Column 3. Observations initially reported by the family for which verifying information was obtained are shown in Columns 4 and 5. If this verifying information denied that the service had been provided or indicated that it occurred outside of calendar year 1970 and was judged reliable by the coding staff, the observation was rejected and is found in Column 4. If, however, the verifying source confirmed the family report or was not judged by the coding staff to conclusively refute the family claim, it was accepted (Column 5). An example of the latter case would be one in which the respondent reports services for which he has documented records while the provider appears to have inadequate records or have made an incomplete records check. Column 6 shows new admissions, physician contacts and policies that were discovered as a result of the verification process. The final column (7) is a sum of all observations that were accepted in the best estimate analysis, including those for which no verification was attempted or completed, those that were positively verified, and those that were newly discovered in the verification process.

ESTIMATING PROCEDURES

The same general methods of processing the data and deriving estimates for the population as had been employed in the earlier studies were used in 1970. For cases in which necessary quantitative information was not obtained at all in the interview, or in which it was not obtained in sufficiently precise terms, estimates were made by the study staff during the processing stage. In the 1953 study, some cases were assigned ultimately to an "indeterminant" category. In the 1958 and 1963 studies, however, all cases were made "determinant" with respect to charges for major categories of goods and services, utilization in these major categories, and family money income. The 1970 procedure was similar to that followed in 1958 and 1963, but, in addition, the monetary value of care that had been defined as 'free care" in the earlier studies was also estimated. Sources used for estimating included tabulations from the American Hospital Association's annual survey of hospitals, the American Medical Association's periodic survey of physicians and the California Medical Association's relative value studies (1969).

Table I-2 provides information on specific utilization and independent variables that were estimated in part and also indicates how often these estimating procedures were used.

FACTORS INFLUENCING
SAMPLE ESTIMATES

There are two types of errors possible in an estimate based on a sample survey—sampling and nonsampling. Sampling errors occur because observations are made only on a sample, not on the entire population. Nonsampling errors can be attributed to many sources: inability to obtain information about all cases in the sample; definitional difficulties; differences in the interpretation of questions; inability or unwillingness to provide correct information on the part of respondents; mistakes in recording or coding the data obtained; and other errors of collection, response, processing, coverage and estimation for missing data. Nonsampling errors also occur in complete censuses. The "accuracy" of a survey result is determined by the joint effects of sampling and nonsampling errors.

Nonsampling Errors

Noninterview Error. Table I–3 shows the completion rates for each of the subsamples in the 1970 study. The estimates in the report are based only on those families interviewed. The amount of discrepancy between these estimates and the figures that would have been obtained with full response depends, for any characteristic being estimated, on how different the families not interviewed were from those who were interviewed with respect to this characteristic. While we are unable to make any direct comparisons regarding health behavior, Table I-4 shows some basic locational characteristics of interviewed and noninterviewed families in 1970. Persons living in large cities and apartment dwellers were less likely to be interviewed than were persons living elsewhere.

Table I–5 provides the overall results of each assigned case in 1970. The reasons given by nonrespondents for not participating in the study are shown in Table I–6. In many instances the interviewer did not agree that the reason given by the respondent was the true reason for the refusal. Therefore, interviewer explanations for the refusals are also included if given. The reason most often given by both nonrespondents and interviewers is a lack of interest on the part of the family. The second most frequent reason given by the nonrespondents was that they were too busy and did not have time. However, interviewers generally did not agree with this interpretation. The second most frequent reason recorded by interviewers was that the respondent was suspicious of the study or its motives or just didn't like strangers. These results are consistent with results in previous studies (Andersen and Anderson, 1967).

In order to derive estimates pertaining to a period as long as a year from a single wave survey, it is necessary to compensate for the absence on the interview date of individuals who had been members of the population at some time during the year but had left it before the interview date. This is of special importance for a study of this type because of the generally high utilization and expenditures of individuals who died or were institutionalized during the survey year.

An attempt was made to include in the survey at least those decedents and other former members of the population who had, at some time during the survey year, lived with a relative who was still a population member at the end of the survey year. Precautions were taken, however, to make sure that each person who had left the population could be counted as a former member of only one family, thus giving him exactly the same probability of falling in the sample as an individual who was still a member of the population.

Using this method of asking proxies about the medical care of decedents, it appears that slightly over half of the people in the U.S. population who died during the year were represented in the sample data. The actual coverage was somewhat higher, however, because many people who died in the United States during 1970 were residents of institutions and thus not part of the survey universe. All individuals dying during 1970 who had been living alone or only with individuals who were also to leave the population were automatically excluded, since there was no one who could be interviewed on their behalf.

Errors in the Interviewing Process. Estimates may differ from the population characteristics because there are discrepancies between the collected data on utilization and expenditure and the actual experience of the sample. The data are valid to the extent that they accurately reflect the sample's behavior. However, distortions can occur between the time of the behavior itself and the description of that behavior in the final report. Distortions can be due either to respondent error or to interviewer error.

It was anticipated that many families would have little detailed information on their health service use and health insurance readily available. Consequently, letters explaining the study and the information sought were sent to all sample families in advance of the interviewer's visit. These letters, as well as the interviewers themselves, urged respondents to consult any documents such as insurance policies, membership cards, medical bills or tax records that could provide reliable information. Interviewers reported that over 40 percent of the families consulted at least one document in the 1970 study.

The interviewer was instructed on first contact to make an appointment for a time when the family members who knew most about family use of health services and health insurance would be available. During the interview, the main respondents were urged to consult other family members who might be better informed than they about some questions asked. If important information could not be obtained during the interview, interviewers were instructed to phone later or make additional calls in person to obtain the missing information. It was recognized that in instances of change in family composition (other than by birth) during the year, or in families consisting of several related but unmarried adults, it was unlikely that a single member respondent could give accurage information for the entire year about all family members. In these cases, as many family members as necessary were interviewed separately.

Considerable effort was devoted to quality control of the field work in the 1970 study. Each interviewer was instructed to edit the questionnaire as soon as possible after the interview was done. If important information had not been obtained, she was instructed to phone the family or make a return visit if necessary. If addresses or names of doctors and hospitals were not clear, she was instructed to look these up in local telephone directories. Other checks on the validity of the interviews were done by the field supervisors in the primary sampling unit. In the NORC central office, a list of critical items was used to determine when a call-back was necessary.

Processing Errors. Distortions can also result from inaccurate coding, keypunching, data processing, analyzing and writing of the report.

Coding was divided into specialized coding sections. A general coding section handled the basic questionnaire material. Special coding sections were established to deal with the coding of insurance information, all hospitalizations, all diagnostic coding and all estimating. The study staff itself was intimately involved in all special coding procedures. In addition, the diagnostic coding drew heavily upon advice from two medical consultants, both in setting up the original codes and in coding difficult or unusual cases.

Merging of data from the verifications with data from the social survey results in a "best estimate" for many of the variables used in the social survey. For years prior to 1970, best estimates are available only for hospitalization data. Thus, in tables in the text giving trend data, best estimates are given only for hospitalization data; social survey estimates are given for the rest. In tables in which only 1970 data are presented, best estimate data are provided.

Differences Between the 1970 and Earlier Studies. While the emphasis was on comparability between the 1970 survey and the earlier surveys, certain questions were altered and other questions were added in the current study to meet the changing situation with respect to the delivery of medical care in this country and to facilitate some specially planned analyses. Changes in the 1970 questionnaire included a new emphasis on defining regular source of care, questions concerning waiting time and travel time with respect to regular source of care, questions on Medicare coverage, more specification regarding site of physician visits, more detailed questions on third party payment sources (particularly for those categories of third party payment that in previous studies has been classified as "free care"), and more detailed treatment of "unearned income" in order to locate those individuals in the sample who were eligible for Medicaid or welfare payments for the medical care that they received. A special section was also added to the attitude section of the questionnaire dealing with people's perceptions of the health care system. While the length of the interview varied a great deal according to family size and amount of services used, the average length was about one and one-half hours.

Sampling Errors

For each year, the particular sample used was one of a large number of all possible samples of the same size that could have been selected using the sample design. Estimates derived from the different samples would differ from each other. The deviation of a sample estimate from the average of all possible samples is called the sampling error. The standard error of a survey estimate is a measure of the variation among the estimates from the possible samples and thus is a measure of the precision with which an estimate from a particular sample approximates the average result of all possible samples.

As calculated for this report, the standard error also partially measures the effect of nonsampling errors but does not measure any systematic biases in the data. Bias is the difference, averaged over all possible samples, between the estimate and the desired value. Obviously, the accuracy of a survey result depends upon both the sampling and nonsampling error measured by the standard error, and the bias and other types of nonsampling error, not measured by the standard error.

The generalized standard error tables given in this appendix provide approximations to the standard errors of various estimates shown in Chapters One through Five. The tables in Chapter Six contain the actual standard errors computed for estimates in those tables. In order to derive standard errors that would be applicable to a wide variety of items and could be prepared at a moderate cost, a number of approximations were required. As a result, the tables of standard errors provide an indication of the order of magnitude of the standard errors rather than the precise standard error for any specific item.

The computation of standard errors for estimates based on these samples is complex because the families were geographically clustered and because stratification was used in the selection of the units. The computation was complicated further in 1958 and 1970 by differential weighting schemes. The method used to compute standard errors, the collapsed strata method, tends to provide slightly conservative results, i.e., overestimates of the magnitudes of standard errors (Kish, 1965: 283–86).

The sample estimate and an estimate of its standard error permit us to construct interval estimates with prescribed levels of confidence that the interval includes the average result of all possible samples. To illustrate, if all possible samples were selected, each of these were surveyed under essentially the same conditions, and an estimate and its estimated standard error were calculated from each sample, then:

1. approximately two-thirds of the intervals from one standard error below the estimate to one standard error above the estimate would include the average value of all possible samples. We call an interval from one standard error below the estimate to one standard error above the estimate a 68 percent confidence interval.
2. approximately nine-tenths of the intervals from 1.6 standard errors below the estimate to 1.6 standard errors above the estimate would include the average value of all possible samples. We call an interval from 1.6 standard errors below the estimate to 1.6 standard errors above the estimate a 90 percent confidence interval.
3. approximately nineteen-twentieths of the intervals from two standard errors below the estimate to two standard errors above the estimate would include the average value of all possible samples. We call an interval from two standard errors below the estimate to two standard errors above the estimate a 95 percent confidence interval.
4. almost all intervals from three standard errors below the sample

estimate to three standard errors above the sample estimate would include the average value of all possible samples.

Thus, for a *particular* sample, one can say with specified confidence that the average of all possible samples is included in the constructed interval.[2]

For simplicity's sake, we will use only the 68 percent and the 95 percent confidence intervals in further discussion.

Cautionary Remark: The 68 percent confidence interval will exclude the expected value (the average value of all possible samples) 32 percent of the time, on the average. Similarly, the 95 percent confidence interval will exclude the expected value 5 percent of the time. Thus, when examining a number of estimates, one out of 20 can be expected to appear at the 95 percent confidence level to be different from a hypothesized value, even though none of them actually are different. Consequently, in order to avoid any inference that sample results are significant when they are not, traditional statistical theory demands that hypotheses be made before examining the data. Not doing so increases the likelihood of accepting false hypotheses. Goodman (1969) discusses a method which avoids this problem by applying factors to individual estimates of standard errors.

Standard Errors for 1970 Data. *Standard errors of percents for certain basic demographic groups.* In about half the tables in this report that present estimated percents, certain standard demographic groups are used as the base for these percents. Table I–7 contains a list of these basic demographic groups followed by a letter code. Table I–8 contains a list of these codes followed by a set of standard errors.

Illustration: Table 1–1 estimates show that about 6 percent of all persons aged one to five had no source of regular care in 1970. Table I–7 gives the code for persons aged one to five as "I." Table I–8 estimates the standard error for 5 percent as 1.2 percentage points and for 10 percent as 1.6 percentage points. Linear interpolation results in a standard error for 6 percent as

$$1.2 \; + \; \left[\left(\frac{6-5}{10-5}\right) \; (1.6-1.2)\right]$$

2. The above general discussion of standard errors draws heavily upon U.S. Bureau of the Census (1974) information.

or about 1.3. Two standard errors is 2.6, which rounds to 3, so we can conclude with 95 percent confidence that the average estimate of the percentage of children aged one to five with no regular source of care derived from all possible samples would be between 3 percent and 9 percent (6±3). We can conclude with 68 percent confidence that the average estimate would be between 5 percent and 7 percent.

Standard errors of percents for most other groups. For most other groups, we can estimate the standard error using Table I–11 if we know the number of sample cases the estimated percent is based upon. Tables I–9 and I–10 provide the number of sample cases for many groups. Other numbers of sample cases are to be found as part of the text tables. The standard errors shown in Table I–8 also can be calculated using Tables I–9, I–10 and I–11. However, Tables I–7 and I–8 provide a simpler means of calculating these errors for some of the most commonly used estimates in the study.

Illustration: Table 1–2 estimates that about 14 percent of all rural low income persons have no source of regular care. Table I–9 shows that 1,417 rural low income persons were in the sample. Two way linear interpolation in Table I–11 gives an estimated standard error of 2.4 percentage points on a 14 percent estimate with a 1,417 base. Two standard errors is about 5 percentage points. The 68 percent confidence interval is 14±2. The 95 percent confidence interval is 14±5, i.e., from 9 percent to 19 percent.

Standard errors of means. The sampling variability of an estimated mean depends on the form of the distribution as well as on the number of sample cases. An approximate method for measuring the reliability of a mean is to divide the estimated mean by the number of sample cases and multiply the square root of the result by the appropriate factor in Table I–12 or Table I–13.

This method applies because the variance of a mean tends to be approximately proportional to the mean in this study and always is inversely proportional to the sample size. The factors were obtained by grouping the data by distribution shape and computing the standard errors of a number of means in each group.

Illustration: Table 3–13 shows that the mean medical expenditure for persons 65 and over with expenses is $456, while Table I–10 show that 1,401 such persons were in the sample:

$$\frac{\$\ 456}{1,401} = \$0.571$$

Table I-12 shows the correct factor to be 33:

$$\$0.571 \times 33 = \$18.8$$

Thus, the 68 percent confidence interval extends from $437 to $475 ($456 ± $19); while the 95 percent confidence interval extends from $419 to $494 ($456 ± 38).

Standard errors of medians. The sampling variability of a median, like that of a mean, depends heavily upon the form of the distribution of the characteristic, as well as upon the number of sample cases upon which the median is based. Since the median value is the value that divides all the cases in half, bounds of the confidence interval around a median are related to the standard error of 50 percent of the given number of cases.

If x represents the standard error of 50 percent of k where k is the number of cases a median is based upon, the 68 percent confidence interval around the median can be obtained by finding the $(50+x)$ percent value and the $(50-x)$ percent value (Kish, 1965: 495-96 and Hansen, Hurwitz and Madow, 1953:448-49). It can be seen that the median will not be in the center of the confidence interval if the distribution is not symmetrical, and that the width of each two standard error confidence interval need not be equal to that of twice its corresponding one standard error interval.

Tables I-14 and I-15 provide factors that approximate the ratios of the confidence intervals to the median values. To obtain an estimated confidence interval, multiply the appropriate factor by the median value.

Illustration: Table 3-2 shows the estimated median family expenditure as $326. This estimate was based upon all 3,880 sample families. Linear interpolation in Table I-14 gives the factor for the lower bound of the 68 percent confidence interval as 0.940; while Table I-15 gives the corresponding factor for the upper bound as 1.065.

$$\$326 \times 0.940 = \$306 \text{ and } \$326 \times 1.065 = \$347.$$

Thus, the 68 percent confidence interval ranges from $306 to $347; that is, from $326 - $20 to $326 + $21. Similarly, the 95 percent confidence interval ranges from $286 to $372, or from $326 - $40 to $326 + $46.

Standard errors of rates or ratios. The manner in which standard errors of rates or ratios are estimated depends both on whether or not the numerator is a subclass of the denominator and on whether or not the denominator is a number of persons or families. If both are the case, the ratio is a percent whose standard error can be estimated using the method described on pages 212-13. For example, the ratio of 4.223 sample persons below poverty with medical expenses to 4,973 total sample persons below poverty converts to 85 percent.

A ratio where the numerator is not a subclass of the denominator but the denominator is a number of persons or families can be converted to a mean whose standard error can be estimated using the method described on pages 213-13. For example, 83 hospital days per 100 males is converted to a mean of 0.83 hospital days per man.

The standard error (σ) of a ratio (A/B) where the denominator is not a number of persons or families can be obtained from the formula:

$$\sigma \frac{A}{B} = \frac{A}{B} \sqrt{\left(\frac{\sigma_A}{A}\right)^2 + \left(\frac{\sigma_B}{B}\right)^2 - \frac{2\rho\sigma_A\sigma_B}{AB}}$$

where ρ is the correlation between A and B. When the numerator is a subclass of the denominator, $\rho = A\sigma_B/B\sigma_A$. Therefore, the standard error formula becomes

$$\frac{A}{B} \sqrt{\left(\frac{\sigma_A}{A}\right)^2 - \left(\frac{\sigma_B}{B}\right)^2}$$

The ratio of the mean medical expenditure for persons below near poverty to mean medical expenditure for all persons is an example of a ratio of this kind.

When the numerator is not a subclass of the denominator, using a value of zero for ρ usually will result in only a slight overestimate for the standard error of a ratio of this kind. The ratio of the mean medical expenditure for persons below near poverty to the mean medical expenditure for persons above near poverty is such a ratio.

Illustration: We have previously calculated the standard error of the mean medical expenditure of all persons 65 and over with expenditures. The mean and standard error are $456 and $18.8. For persons under six years old, the corresponding figures are $114 and $10.5. The mean for persons 65 and over is 4.00 times as large as the mean for persons under six years old.

We can estimate the standard error of the 4.00 ratio of means to be about

$$\frac{456}{114} \sqrt{\left(\frac{18.8}{456}\right)^2 + \left(\frac{10.5}{114}\right)^2} = 0.4036$$

This rounds to 0.40, and two standard errors rounds to 0.8l. The 68 percent confidence interval ranges from 3.60 to 4.40; while the 95 percent confidence interval is 3.19 to 4.81.

Standard errors of differences. For a difference between two sample estimates (A and B), the standard error is obtained from the formula:

$$\sigma_{A-B} = \sqrt{\sigma_A^2 + \sigma_B^2 - 2\rho\sigma_A\sigma_B}$$

As with the formula above for ratios, assuming a value of zero for ρ (the correlation between A and B) usually will result in only a slight overestimate of ρ_{A-B}, except for differences between two estimates based on the same observations. For example, the difference between mean family expenditures for hospital services and mean family expenditures for physician services involves estimates based on the same observations.

Illustration: We have previously calculated that the estimated $456 mean medical expenses for persons 65 and older with expenses (Table 3-13) has a standard error of about $18.8. For persons 55 to 64 the mean and standard error are $415 and $21.9, respectively. Thus, the standard error of the apparent $41 difference is

$$\sqrt{(\$21.9)^2 + (\$18.8)^2} = \$28.9$$

or about $29.

The 68 percent confidence interval ranges from a $12 to a $70 difference between the mean expenses for these age groups. The 95 percent confidence interval ranges from −$17 to +$99. Therefore, it cannot be said with 95 percent confidence that the mean medical expenses for persons 55 to 64 with expenses differs from the mean for persons 65 and older.

Standard Errors for Years Prior to 1970.

General Discussion.   A major purpose of this report has been to examine changes taking place over time. Each estimated change should be studied in light of both the substantive significance of the change and its statistical significance.

Standard errors of selected 1963 data appear in Andersen and Anderson (1967:168-70) and in Tables 14 to 43 of Andersen, Smedby and Anderson (1970). For standard errors of 1953 data, see Anderson and Feldman (1956:218-22). Standard errors for 1953, 1958 and 1963 may also be estimated by following the procedures discussed above for 1970 data and applying a factor of 1.2 for persons having moderate to high medical use or expenses; a factor of 0.5 for persons with low medical use or expenses; a factor of 1.1 for nonwhites, persons 65 and older, and persons with low incomes; and a factor of 0.7 for everything else. These conversion factors are based on comparison of available calculated errors for the various studies and must be considered broad approximations.

Standard errors of annual percent changes. Annual percent changes are presented in a number of tables, since they make it easier to compare time periods which differ in length. If a figure is B at the beginning of a k year period and A afterward, with an i percent average annual increase, then

$$B\left(1.00 + \frac{i}{100}\right)^k = A \quad \text{and} \quad 100\left(\sqrt[k]{\frac{A}{B}} - 1.00\right) = i$$

Therefore, the process of calculating the standard error of i begins by finding the standard error of the ratio A/B and then determining the desired confidence interval around this ratio. Then find the kth roots of the upper and lower values of the confidence interval, subtract 1.00 from each, and convert the answers to percents. The results will give the confidence interval around the average annual percent increase.

Illustration: Table 3–9 indicates that the mean nonfree medical expenditure per person was $112 in 1963 and $209 in 1970. This represents an 8.9 average annual percent increase during this seven year period, since

$$100\left(\sqrt[7]{\frac{209}{112}} - 1.00\right) = 8.9 \ .$$

The 68 percent confidence interval of the ratio 209/112 = 1.866 ranges from 1.692 to 2.040. Since the seventh root of 1.692 is 1.078, 7.8 percent is the lower limit of the 68 percent confidence interval. Since the seventh root of 2.040 is 1.107, the upper limit is 10.7 percent. The 95 percent confidence interval ranges from 6.1 percent to 12.0 percent.

COMPARABILITY OF SAMPLE ESTIMATES WITH INDEPENDENT ESTIMATES

This section provides some ideas of how sample estimates compare to estimates from other sources for the year 1970. CHAS social survey and best estimates are compared with independent national estimates of health service use, expenditures and insurance coverage. These independent estimates are provided by the National Center for Health Statistics (NCHS), the American Hospital Association (AHA), the Social Security Administration (SSA) and the Health Insurance Association of America (HIAA). NCHS estimates are based on nationwide household interview surveys, while estimates from the other sources come from data collected from providers of care and insuring agencies.

Table I-16 compares estimates of use from CHAS with those from NCHS and AHA. Admission rates to short term hospitals are similar for each source. CHAS social survey estimates of length of stay and total hospital days appear slightly higher than those from NCHS and AHA. The CHAS "best estimates" of length of stay and total days are somewhat lower than the other sources.

There are a number of differences between the CHAS and NCHS studies that might affect the estimates. (1) The NCHS estimate is based on hospital discharges reported to have occurred within six months of the week of the interview, while CHAS social survey estimates are based on reports for the full 12 months of 1970. The AHA estimate is based on mail questionnaire data from hospitals generally covering a period from October 1, 1969 to September 30, 1970. Since there is some evidence that underreporting of hospitalization increases with an increasing time interval between discharge and the interval, this difference might tend to make the CHAS estimates relatively lower than they might have been with a shorter recall (NCHS, 1965a). (2) The CHAS interviewing technique picked up the hospital experiences of those people who died during the survey year but were living prior to their death with someone in our sample who reported their hospital experiences. The AHA estimates include the experience of *all* decedents who have been in short term hospitals. The NCHS estimates include only the experience of persons living at the time of the interview. Since decedents tend to be heavy utilizers of hospitals, this difference would tend to make NCHS estimates lower than that of CHAS or AHA. (3) The verification process for the CHAS study eliminated much of the "overreporting" of hospitalization but was probably less successful in discovering "underreporting." The verification, in addition, provided independent information on length of stay. People have a tendency to overreport length of stay (NCHS, 1965a). Consequently, the verification would tend to make the CHAS best estimates lower than the NCHS estimates, which were not verified through an independent source, and the AHA estimates, which are based on provider records and are, thus, not subject to the problems of patient "underreporting."

The estimates of percent seeing a physician produced by CHAS appear lower than those provided by NCHS. Again, the difficulty in discovering unreported care in the verification while eliminating incorrect reports of service may account for the lower CHAS best estimate. The NCHS survey included no physician verification.

The CHAS social survey estimate and that of NCHS are the same for mean number of physician visits. The NCHS estimate for number of visits is based on a two week recall period, while the CHAS estimate is based on a year recall period. Given the shorter recall period of NCHS, it might be expected that the NCHS estimate would exceed the CHAS estimate. However, the CHAS interview includes separate questions about physician visits for each illness experienced, while NCHS asks about number of visits only once. The multiple question approach of CHAS might increase the number of visits reported. The CHAS best estimate of mean number of visits is one-half visit less than the NCHS and CHAS social survey estimates.

The estimates of percent seeing a dentist and mean number of dental visits are similar for NCHS and CHAS despite the fact that mean number of visits is calculated on the basis of a two week recall period for NCHS and a one year recall period for CHAS.

Table I–17 provides some comparisons of individual expenditures provided by NCHS and the Social Security Administration (SSA) with those from the CHAS sample. The comparisons with NCHS are limited to out-of-pocket expenditures, while the comparisons with SSA are for total expenditures for personal health services including all sources of payment.

The NCHS estimates are based on the responses to a self-enumerated questionnaire mailed in April 1971 to some 11,970 households comprising a representative sample of the nation's households. Information was requested on out-of-pocket expenditures for hospital, doctor, dental or optical services; prescribed medicines; and other medical expenses for each family member. Differences in the definitions of various expenditure categories between NCHS and NORC are noted in Table I–17.

The NCHS estimate (Table I–17) is considerably higher than that produced by CHAS. The physician component shows the largest discrepancy. The reason for this discrepancy is not clear. One possibility is that expenses that are reported as out-of-pocket in the NCHS study are attributed to some third party payer in the CHAS study. In addition, the self-enumeration method used by NCHS produces estimates of expenditures somewhat higher than the interview technique used by CHAS (NCHS, 1963). This expected difference has been reported to be greatest for physician expenditures.

The SSA procedures for producing estimates of total personal expenditures (Table I-17) differ from the CHAS approach in important respects. The SSA estimates are for the institutionalized as well as the noninstitutionalized population. Further, the SSA estimates are not based on consumer reports but rather on total producer income data including an aggregate of all hospitals' operating budgets and all physicians' practice-related incomes.

Table I-17 shows that per capita expenses for health care as estimated by SSA were $49 higher than that produced by CHAS data. This difference is accounted for almost entirely by the hospital and nursing home category. An analysis of the discrepancy done in an earlier report showed that the difference was largely explained by hospital and nursing home expenditures for the institutionalized population 65 and over which are included in the SSA estimates but excluded in the CHAS estimates (Andersen et al., 1973: 63-68).

Table I-18 provides comparative estimates of voluntary health insurance coverage as provided by CHAS, NCHS and the Health Insurance Association of America. The CHAS and NCHS estimates are both based on consumer reports. NCHS estimates of percent of the population covered appear higher. One reason for this is that insurance coverage reported in the CHAS survey was verified through insurer and employer. As a result of this process, 5 percent of the policies reported by respondents were rejected because they were found not to be health insurance or not to be in effect during the survey year, while considerably fewer unreported policies were discovered (see Table I-1). Consequently, the verification reduced the estimates of percent covered in the CHAS data. The HIAA estimates are based on surveys of insuring agencies and show a higher proportion of the population with insurance than either the CHAS or NCHS estimates.

Table I-1. Verification of hospital admissions, physicians seen and health insurance policies: 1970[a]

Unit of Observation	Total [1]	Reported in Social Survey				Discovered during Verification [6]	Accepted in Best Estimate[b] [7]
		Verification attempted?					
		No [2]	*Yes*				
			Verification completed?				
			No [3]	*Yes*			
				Observation accepted?			
				No [4]	Yes [5]		
Hospital admissions	1,771	143	70	163	1,395	110	1,718
Physicians seen	10,981	1,678	1,567	1,639	6,097	168	9,510
Health insurance policies in effect	3,635	356	298	181	2,800	65	3,519

[a]All data are unweighted.
[b]The "Accepted in the Best Estimate" column [7] is the sum of columns [2] + [3] + [5] + [6].

Table I-2. Extent to which selected utilization and independent variables used in this report were estimated in social survey data: 1970

Variable	Type of Estimating Done	Percent of Unweighted Observations for Which an Estimate was Made
Dentist visits, mean number	If the dentist was seen in 1970 but number of visits was not stated, visits were estimated.	1.1 percent
Family income	All families who did not answer this question had income estimated for them. Earned family income for at least one family member was estimated for 402 families. Other family income was estimated for 268 families.	3.4 percent earned income; 2.3 percent other income. Since some families had both earned and other income estimated, the percentage of families with any portion of their income estimated lies between 3.4 and 5.7 percent.
Physician visits, some estimated in following types of episode		
Hospitalized illness	These are physician visits outside of the hospital in conjunction with an illness for which the patient was hospitalized.	8.6 percent of episodes have visits estimated
Major illnesses	These are physician visits outside of the hospital for a chronic or expensive illness.	1.3 percent of episodes have visits estimated
Pregnancies terminating in 1970	These are prenatal care visits and include the delivery and inhospital visits. They include, in addition to live births, still births, miscarriages and abortions, both legal and illegal.	2.9 percent of episodes have visits estimated
Minor illnesses, routine checkups, shots, tests, and routine visits to an opthalmologist for eye refraction	In order to be counted as a doctor visit, the test must have been administered in a doctor's office.	2.2 percent of episodes have visits estimated
Hospital days per admission	If number of days was unknown but expenditure was given, the per diem for that hospital was divided into expenditure to obtain total days. If neither days nor expenditure was known, number of days was based on diagnosis combined with age. If diagnosis was not known, number of days was based on age, sex and race.	0.9 percent of stays have days estimated

Table I-3. Final interviewing results: 1970

Category	A	U	R	$S_1{}^a$	$S_2{}^a$	$Total^b$
(1) Number of dwelling units listed in the original sampling frame.	1,515	2,068	810	2,887	2,451	7,280
(2) Dwelling units which were vacant during the interviewing period or had been torn down between the time of listing and the time of interviewing.	176	415	126	407	—	1,124
(3) Dwelling units where respondents' and interviewers' race did not match. Applicable only in some urban segments.	5	43	—	9	—	57
(4) Indicates not qualified. Applicable only in the S sample, where families were screened out if they were nonpoor or had no member 66 or over.	—	—	—	—	1,539	1,594^c
(5) Indicates extra family units. These units were added when multiple family dwelling units were discovered at the time of interview or multiple dwelling units within the same structure had originally been listed as single units.	42	72	15	68	—	197
(6) Net assignment; categories (1)-(2)-(3)-(4)+(5).	1,376	1,682	699	2,539	912	4,702^c
(7) Number of completed interviews.	1,119	1,376	601	2,451	784	3,880
(8) Noninterview reports. They include "refusals," "breakoffs," "no one home after repeated calls," "language problems," "respondent too ill to be interviewed," etc.	257	306	98	88	128	822^c
(9) Completion rate; categories (7) ÷ (6).	0.813	0.818	0.860	0.965	0.860	0.825^c

[a]The report on the S sample is divided into two parts. S_1 refers to the screening operation. S_2 refers to the regular interviewing.

[b]Includes S_1 figures for categories (1) through (3) and S_2 figures elsewhere.

[c]Figure based on the assumption that a portion of the S samples noninterview reports are not qualified.

Table I-4. Comparisons of interviewed and noninterviewed families: 1970[a]

Characteristic of Population	Families	
	Percent of the interviewed	Percent of those not interviewed
Location[b]		
Northeast	27	31
North Central	27	22
South	30	25
West	16	22
Sample		
A	62	70
U	8	7
R	12	8
S	18	16
Type of dwelling[c]		
Located on farm	7	3
Nonfarm: single family house	65	60
Nonfarm: duplex or two family structure	10	11
Nonfarm: multiunit structure (e.g., apartment)	18	26
Community[d]		
Inside largest city in the primary unit	45	57
In a suburb of the largest city in a primary sampling unit	24	21
In the outskirts (including in all other towns in the primary sampling unit)	22	18
In open country	9	4
Residence		
Urban	71	75
Rural	29	25
Total	100	100
N	(3,880)	(876)

[a]Computed using weighted data.
[b]Same divisions used by the United States Bureau of the Census.
[c]Excludes 186 interviewed and 153 noninterviewed families with "no answer."
[d]Excludes 160 interviewed and 71 noninterviewed families with "no answer."

Table I-5.   Results of interviewing attempts for all sample families: 1970

Result	*Percent of Families*	
Interviewed	82	
Not interviewed	18	
Refused		13
Broke off		1
Not at home after repeated calls		2
Other (language problem, respondent too ill to be interviewed, etc.)		1
Temporarily unavailable for entire field period		1
All sample families	100	
N	(4,756)	

Table I-6. Reasons given by nonrespondents and interviewers for refusals, break-offs and other losses:[a] 1970

Reason for Respondent Loss	Percent of All Reasons Given by	
	Nonrespondents	Interviewers
Reasons coded for both nonrespondents and interviewers		
Not interested enough to be interviewed	47	32
Too busy—doesn't have time	23	10
Information is too personal	20	15
Illness or death in family	13	7
Someone else persuaded main respondent to say "no"	9	5
Language barrier	1	2
Antigovernment, felt survey only done in low income areas	3	5
Against surveys, doesn't like this particular survey	11	3
Reasons coded for nonrespondents only		
They aren't "appropriate" for study (e.g., no medical costs)	7	–
No reason given (e.g., slammed door)	4	–
Afraid to let people into house	*	–
Reasons coded for interviewers only		
Respondent is suspicious of study (e.g., thinks we are selling something)	–	15
Respondent doesn't feel he will know how to answer the questions	–	1
Respondent never really refused—continually broke or postponed appointments	–	2
Respondent drunk, high, incompetent, unbalanced, couldn't participate, noncommunicative	–	5
Total percent	138[b]	102[b]
Total cases	(647)[c]	(470)[d]

*Indicates less than 0.5 percent.
[a]Excludes families not at home after repeated calls.
[b]Total exceeds 100 because more than one reason given for some cases.
[c]Excludes 20 cases with "no answer."
[d]Excludes 179 cases where interviewer gave no additional reason for respondent refusal.

Table I-7. Basic demographic groups and their standard error codes: 1970

Characteristic	Code	Characteristic	Code	Characteristic	Code
Families—total	D	Education of head		Income of head	
Persons—total	A	0–6	K	Low	E
White	B	0–8	F	Middle	F
Nonwhite	K	7–8	J	High	H
Male	B	9–11	I	Less than $2,000	M
Female	B	9–12	D	$2,000–3,499	K
		12	H	$3,500–4,999	L
		13 or more	J	$5,000–7,499	I
Age 0–5	G			$7,500–9,999	J
0–17	C	Residence—Urban	C	$10,000–12,499	L
1–5	I	SMSA, central city	D	$12,500–14,999	N
1–17	C	SMSA, other	K	$15,000–17,499	P
6–17	D	Urban, non-SMSA	M	$15,000+	L
18–34	E	Rural, nonfarm	G	$17,500+	O
18–64	C	Rural, farm	L	Below near poverty	E
35–54	F			Above near poverty	D
55–64	I				
65 and over	G				

Table I-8. Standard errors of estimated percents: 1970

	Estimated Percent									
Code	*2 or 98*	*5 or 95*	*10 or 90*	*15 or 85*	*20 or 80*	*25 or 75*	*30 or 70*	*35 or 65*	*40 or 60*	*50*
A	0.3	0.5	0.7	0.8	1.0	1.0	1.1	1.1	1.2	1.2
B	0.4	0.6	0.8	1.0	1.1	1.2	1.2	1.3	1.3	1.3
C	0.4	0.6	0.9	1.1	1.2	1.3	1.4	1.4	1.5	1.5
D	0.5	0.8	1.1	1.3	1.4	1.5	1.6	1.7	1.7	1.8
E	0.6	0.9	1.2	1.4	1.6	1.7	1.8	1.9	1.9	2.0
F	0.6	1.0	1.3	1.6	1.8	1.9	2.0	2.1	2.2	2.2
G	0.7	1.0	1.4	1.7	1.9	2.1	2.2	2.3	2.3	2.4
H	0.7	1.1	1.5	1.8	2.0	2.2	2.3	2.4	2.5	2.6
I	0.8	1.2	1.6	1.9	2.2	2.3	2.5	2.6	2.6	2.7
J	0.9	1.3	1.8	2.2	2.4	2.6	2.8	2.9	3.0	3.1
K	0.9	1.5	2.0	2.4	2.7	2.9	3.1	3.2	3.3	3.4
L	1.1	1.7	2.3	2.7	3.0	3.3	3.5	3.6	3.7	3.8
M	1.2	1.9	2.6	3.1	3.5	3.8	4.0	4.2	4.3	4.4
N	1.3	2.0	2.8	3.3	3.7	4.1	4.3	4.5	4.6	4.7
O	1.4	2.2	3.0	3.6	4.1	4.4	4.6	4.8	5.0	5.1
P	1.7	2.6	3.6	4.2	4.8	5.1	5.4	5.7	5.8	5.9

Table I-9. Number of interviewed persons; age by family income, race and residence: 1970

			Race		*Residence*		
Age and Income		*Total*	*White*	*Non-white*	*SMSA, central city*	*Other urban*	*Rural*
	Under $2,000	28 ⎫					
	$ 2,000–4,999	69 ⎬	56	64	73	25	22
	5,000–5,999	23 ⎭					
0	6,000–9,999	91 ⎫	62	36	49	23	26
	10,000–10,999	7 ⎭					
	11,000–14,999	21 ⎫	27	5	10	10	12
	15,000 and over	11 ⎭					
	Under $2,000	56 ⎫					
	$ 2,000–4,999	266 ⎬	156	256	270	63	79
1	5,000–5,999	90 ⎭					
to	6,000–9,999	331 ⎫	271	126	168	76	153
5	10,000–10,999	66 ⎭					
	11,000–14,999	145 ⎫	178	46	80	58	86
	15,000 and over	79 ⎭					

Age and Income	Total	Race		Residence		
		White	Non-white	SMSA, central city	Other urban	Rural
6 to 17						
Under $2,000	189 }					
$ 2,000–4,999	807 }	493	773	761	177	328
5,000–5,999	270 }					
6,000–9,999	956 }	762	363	475	194	456
10,000–10,999	169 }					
11,000–14,999	447 }	624	151	311	185	279
15,000 and over	328 }					
18 to 34						
Under $2,000	141 }					
$ 2,000–4,999	479 }	432	387	485	150	184
5,000–5,999	199 }					
6,000–9,999	772 }	642	269	386	183	342
10,000–10,999	139 }					
11,000–14,999	413 }	563	126	276	186	227
15,000 and over	276 }					
35 to 54						
Under $2,000	121 }					
$ 2,000–4,999	364 }	381	288	336	108	225
5,000–5,999	184 }					
6,000–9,999	624 }	520	233	329	138	286
10,000–10,999	129 }					
11,000–14,999	413 }	674	130	323	222	259
15,000 and over	391 }					
55 to 64						
Under $2,000	122 }					
$ 2,000–4,999	270 }	335	151	199	94	193
5,000–5,999	94 }					
6,000–9,999	243 }	227	68	114	52	129
10,000–10,999	52 }					
11,000–14,999	134 }	209	29	102	58	78
15,000 and over	104 }					
65 and over						
Under $2,000	364 }					
$ 2,000–4,999	616 }	888	222	443	281	386
5,000–5,999	130 }					
6,000–9,999	221 }	225	31	108	69	79
10,000–10,999	35 }					
11,000–14,999	60 }	130	10	52	49	39
15,000 and over	80 }					
All Ages						
Under $2,000	1,021 }					
$ 2,000–4,999	2,871 }	2,741	2,141	2,567	898	1,417
5,000–5,999	990 }					
6,000–9,999	3,238 }	2,709	1,126	1,629	735	1,471
10,000–10,999	597 }					
11,000–14,999	1,633 }	2,405	497	1,154	768	980
15,000 and over	1,269 }					

Table I-10. Number of interviewed persons: sex, age, education, residence and poverty level by type of medical expense: 1970

Characteristics	All persons	All Persons with Medical Expenditures									
		Total	In-patient hospital	Out-patient hospital	In-patient physician	Out-patient physician	Pre-scribed drugs	Nonpre-scribed drugs	Dental	Non-MD practitioner	Tests, glasses etc.
Sex											
Male	5,515	4,830	509	559	388	2,600	1,900	3,588	1,730	644	828
Female	6,104	5,549	811	641	452	3,292	2,624	4,186	2,090	800	1,110
Age											
0-5	1,283	1,126	101	173	65	725	714	829	130	22	12
6-17	3,166	2,642	163	292	115	1,127	502	1,958	1,252	283	401
18-34	2,419	2,214	399	309	152	1,286	941	1,713	974	293	404
35-54	2,226	2,056	240	217	162	1,177	947	1,614	836	368	483
55-64	1,019	940	145	97	119	603	509	692	289	199	275
65 and over	1,506	1,401	272	112	227	974	911	968	339	279	363
Education of head											
8 years or less	3,898	3,364	440	384	303	1,773	1,453	2,496	901	486	665
9-11 years	2,718	2,349	301	329	163	1,224	940	1,711	767	298	399
12 years	2,931	2,694	341	291	215	1,590	1,155	2,092	1,101	370	450
13 years or more	2,072	1,972	238	196	159	1,305	976	1,475	1,051	290	424
Residence											
SMSA, central city	5,350	4,589	564	793	273	2,278	1,919	3,445	1,492	607	838
SMSA, other	1,560	1,426	179	162	111	903	685	1,031	648	193	286
Urban, non-SMSA	841	789	121	41	93	530	378	575	309	125	153
Rural, nonfarm	2,799	2,603	335	171	265	1,602	1,113	2,014	988	355	463
Rural, farm	1,069	972	121	33	98	579	429	709	383	164	198
Poverty level											
Above near poverty	6,646	6,156	749	573	546	3,840	2,828	4,660	2,655	982	1,281
Below near poverty	4,973	4,223	571	627	294	2,052	1,696	3,114	1,165	462	657
Total	11,619	10,379	1,320	1,200	840	5,892	4,524	7,774	3,820	1,444	1,938

Table I–II. Standard errors[a] of estimated percentages: 1970

	Estimated Percent									
Number of Sample Cases	2 or 98	5 or 95	10 or 90	15 or 85	20 or 80	25 or 75	30 or 70	35 or 65	40 or 60	50
25	7.2	11.2	15.4	18.3	20.5	22.2	23.5	24.5	25.1	25.7
40	5.7	8.8	12.2	14.5	16.2	17.6	18.6	19.3	19.9	20.3
70	4.3	6.7	9.2	10.9	12.3	13.3	14.1	14.6	15.0	15.3
100	3.6	5.6	7.7	9.2	10.3	11.1	11.8	12.2	12.6	12.8
150	2.9	4.6	6.3	7.5	8.4	9.1	9.6	10.0	10.3	10.5
250	2.3	3.5	4.9	5.8	6.5	7.0	7.4	7.7	7.9	8.1
400	1.8	2.8	3.8	4.6	5.1	5.6	5.9	6.1	6.3	6.4
700	1.4	2.1	2.9	3.5	3.9	4.2	4.4	4.6	4.8	4.8
1,000	1.1	1.8	2.4	2.9	3.2	3.5	3.7	3.9	4.0	4.1
1,500	0.9	1.4	2.0	2.4	2.6	2.9	3.0	3.2	3.2	3.3
2,500	0.7	1.1	1.5	1.8	2.1	2.2	2.4	2.4	2.5	2.6
4,000	0.6	0.9	1.2	1.4	1.6	1.8	1.9	1.9	2.0	2.0
7,000	0.4	0.7	0.9	1.1	1.2	1.3	1.4	1.5	1.5	1.5
10,000	0.4	0.6	0.8	0.9	1.0	1.2	1.2	1.2	1.3	1.3

[a]For nonwhite persons, multiply by 1.6.
For family data, multiply by 0.85.

Table 1-12.   Factors used in obtaining standard errors for mean expenditures: 1970

| | Health Expenditures Category | | | |
| | Total Physician; Physician Outpatient; Drugs, Dental and Other Expenditures and Their Subcategories | | All Other | |
Demographic Category	Free care and its subcategories	Total and nonfree care and subcategories	Free care and its subcategories	Total and nonfree care and subcategories
Nonwhite persons	90	25	180	80
Persons by educational or income category	60	17	150	55
Persons by narrow (5–10 year) age category	36	10	90	33
Families, general	48	13	120	44
Persons, general	55	16	140	50
Live births	90	35	90	35

Table I-13. Factors used in obtaining standard errors for all other mean values: 1970

Table	Characteristic	Factor	Table	Characteristic	Factor
1-9, 1-10	All	2.5	2-7, 2-8	Visit per person seeing MD, middle income nonwhites	3.1
2-6	Low income, nonwhites, education less than nine years, SMSA central city	10.4	2-7, 2-8	Visit per person seeing MD, all other nonwhite categories	5.8
2-6	All other	6.0	2-7, 2-8	Visit per person seeing MD, middle income total and white	4.1
2-7, 2-8	Visits per person-year, middle income nonwhites	3.6	2-7, 2-8	Visit per person seeing MD, all other	5.3
2-7, 2-8	Visits per person-year, all other nonwhite categories	7.0	2-9, 2-10, 2-12	All	1.6
2-7, 2-8	Visits per person-year, middle income total and white	4.7	2-11	All	7.7
2-7, 2-8	Visits per person-year, all other	6.0	2-21	Visits per person-year	6.0
			2-21	Visits per person seeing dentist	5.3

Table I-14.   Factors to apply to medians to obtain lower confidence bounds: 1970

| | Factors for Lower Confidence Bounds | | | | | | | |
| | Tables 2-17, 2-18, 3-21 | | Table 3-2 | | Table 3-13 | | Tables 3-14 through 3-18 | |
Number of Interviewed Persons or Families	68 percent factor	95 percent factor	68 percent factor	95 percent factor	68 percent factor	95 percent factor	68 percent factor	95 percent factor
25	0.80	0.42	0.42	0.03	0.33	0.01	0.59	0.01
40	0.84	0.69	0.53	0.13	0.43	0.12	0.67	0.34
70	0.87	0.77	0.62	0.34	0.55	0.25	0.77	0.52
100	0.89	0.80	0.67	0.42	0.61	0.33	0.82	0.59
150	0.901	0.84	0.72	0.51	0.67	0.42	0.86	0.66
250	0.926	0.87	0.78	0.60	0.74	0.52	0.89	0.75
400	0.939	0.89	0.82	0.67	0.79	0.61	0.913	0.82
700			0.87	0.75	0.83	0.70	0.936	0.87
1,000			0.88	0.78	0.85	0.74	0.945	0.89
1,500			0.905	0.82	0.88	0.78	0.961	0.907
2,500			0.925	0.86	0.904	0.82	0.966	0.928
4,000			0.941	0.88	0.931	0.85	0.977	0.945
7,000					0.946	0.89	0.983	0.960
10,000					0.955	0.906	0.984	0.966
11,619					0.958	0.913	0.987	0.968

Table I-15. Factors to apply to medians to obtain upper confidence bounds: 1970

	Factors for Upper Confidence Bounds							
Number of Interviewed Persons or Families	Tables 2-17, 2-18 and 3-21		Table 3-2		Tables 3-13 and 3-16		Tables 3-14, 3-15, 3-17 and 3-18	
	68 percent factor	95 percent factor	68 percent factor	95 percent factor	68 percent factor	95 percent factor	68 percent factor	95 percent factor
25	1.27	1.91	2.48	a	2.92	a	1.84	a
40	1.21	1.47	1.99	a	2.20	a	1.59	3.50
70	1.16	1.34	1.66	2.91	1.84	3.84	1.42	2.20
100	1.13	1.27	1.52	2.48	1.68	2.92	1.33	1.84
150	1.11	1.21	1.40	2.02	1.57	2.30	1.27	1.61
250	1.082	1.16	1.29	1.71	1.42	1.90	1.18	1.44
400	1.067	1.13	1.22	1.52	1.33	1.68	1.15	1.33
700			1.16	1.37	1.25	1.53	1.11	1.24
1,000			1.14	1.29	1.20	1.42	1.083	1.18
1,500			1.11	1.23	1.16	1.34	1.066	1.15
2,500			1.079	1.17	1.11	1.27	1.034	1.11
4,000			1.064	1.14	1.088	1.20	1.028	1.083
7,000					1.058	1.14	1.014	1.041
10,000					1.046	1.11	1.012	1.034
11,619					1.041	1.10	1.011	1.034

a5.00 or larger.

Table I-16. Health services utilization, 1970[a]: comparison of estimates from the CHAS sample with independent estimates

Health Services Utilization	CHAS		NCHS[b]	AHA[c]
	Social survey	Best estimate		
Short term hospital				
Admissions per 100 persons per year	14	14	13[e]	14[g]
Mean length of stay	8.9	7.5	8.6	8.3
Total hospital days per 100 persons per year	121	100	114	120
Physician				
Percent seeing a physician within the year	68	64	72	—
Number of visits per person per year	4.0	3.5	4.0[f]	—
Dentist				
Percent seeing a dentist within the year	45	d	47	—
Number of visits per person per year	1.4	d	1.5	—

[a]CHAS data is for calendar year 1970; AHA estimates represent year ending September 30, 1970, or individual hospital fiscal year; portions of NCHS data range from calendar 1969 to 1970.
[b]NCHS (1972a:19, 24-26).
[c]AHA (1971:447).
[d]There was no verification of dental services in CHAS study.
[e]Hospital discharges.
[f]This estimate excludes telephone calls to maximize comparability with CHAS estimates. With telephone calls included the NCHS estimate is 4.6.
[g]AHA hospital data excludes stays in VA and other federal short term hospitals which are included in CHAS and NCHS estimates.

Table I-17. Expenditures for personal health services, 1970: comparison of estimates from CHAS sample with independent estimates

Mean Expenditure per Person	*Out-of-Pocket*			*Total*		
	CHAS		*NCHS[a]*	*CHAS*		*SSA[b]*
	Social survey	*Best estimate*		*Social survey*	*Best estimate*	
Total	$116[e]	$109	$135	$248[e]	$248[e,h]	$297
Hospital[c]	17[e]	12[e]	21	107[e]	108[e,h]	149[e]
Physician	31	29	47	60	58	65
Drugs	27	f	27[g]	32	f	35
Dental	25	f	29	28	f	21
Other[d]	16	f	15[e]	21	f	27

[a]NCHS (1974:2). Component expenditures do not sum to "total" because "total" category excludes cases with incomplete data.
[b]Cooper and Worthington (1972:5). Data shown are the averages of estimates for fiscal years 1970 and 1971.
[c]Includes outpatient care.
[d]Includes "other professional services," eyeglasses and appliances, and "other health services."
[e]Includes nursing home care.
[f]There was no verification of drugs, dental and "other" expenditures in the CHAS study.
[g]Excludes nonprescribed drugs.
[h]Includes one case whose weighted expenditures account for more than 10 percent of the size of this cell. Exclusion of this case reduces the mean total hospital expenditures to $96.

Table I-18. Voluntary health insurance coverage, 1970: Comparison of estimates from the CHAS sample with independent estimates[a]

Voluntary Insurance Coverage	CHAS	NCHS[b]	HIAA[c]
Percent of total population with:			
Hospital insurance	71	75	79
Surgical insurance	68	72	75

[a]All data excludes Medicare and CHAMPUS.
[b]NCHS (1972b:3, 7).
[c]Health Insurance Institute (1976:22–23). Health Insurance Association of America data revised from earlier estimates.

Appendix II

Estimates Including Extreme Values

Given the sampling design and weighting system used in this study, certain observations account for extremely high weighted units of use or expenditures and substantially influence the estimates in the table cells where they are found. Consequently, in the text tables where this occurs the estimates exclude the highly weighted case or cases. The general exclusion criterion is that an observation accounts for 10 percent or more of the total weighted utilization units or expenditures in a given cell. These appendix tables show the estimates including all observations. Estimates in parentheses have one or more observations omitted from the corresponding text table.

Table II-1. (Corresponds to Table 2-11) Mean length of stay and hospital days per 100 population by age and sex: 1953, 1963 and 1970[a]

Age and Sex	Mean Number of Days per Admission			Hospital Days per 100 Population		
	1953	1963	1970	1953	1963	1970
Age						
0–17	5.3	4.9	4.2	41	30	32
18–54	6.8	6.6	6.1	96	108	94
55 and over	11.9	11.9	(13.8)	148	208	(277)
Sex						
Male	8.3	8.0	(9.3)	71	83	(98)
Female	7.0	7.1	7.1	101	108	117
Total	7.4	7.4	(8.0)	87	96	(107)

[a]Table 2–11 excludes one case: A 62 year old man with a brain tumor who had four continuous hospital stays in different hospitals accounting for 221 unweighted days. While this observation does not account for 10 percent of the total observations or days in the "total" row, the observation is excluded from all cells in Table 2–11 because of its unique characteristics.

NOTE: Figures in parentheses include all cases but have had one or more cases excluded in Table 2–11.

Table II-2. (Corresponds to Table 3-9) Mean nonfree expenditures per person by age, sex and income: 1953, 1963 and 1970

Characteristic	Mean Nonfree Expenditures		
	1953	1963	1970
Sex			
Male	$ 51	$ 92	$187
Female	80	131	231
Age			
0–5	28	47	(129)
6–17	38	56	(96)
18–34	70	124	212
35–54	80	151	209
55–64	96	165	(412)
65 and over	102	184	387
Income			
Low	a	95	205
Middle	a	105	191
High	a	128	228
Total	$ 65	$112	$209

[a]Not available for 1953.

NOTE: Figures in parentheses include all cases but have had one or more cases excluded in Table 3–9.

Table II-3. (Corresponds to Table 3–13) Mean and median total expenditures per person by selected characteristics: 1970

Characteristic	Total Population Mean	For People with Expenditures	
		Mean	Median
Sex			
Male	$213	$232	$ 62
Female	260	275	79
Age			
0–5	(140)	(150)	47
6–17	(111)	(121)	41
18–34	246	260	80
35–54	244	259	89
55–64	(445)	(485)	135
65 and over	429	456	135
Poverty level			
Above near poverty	243	256	75
Below near poverty	217	246	50
Education of head			
8 years or less	238	265	63
9–11 years	197	213	64
12 years	209	223	67
13 years or more	298	307	86
Residence			
SMSA, central city	236	256	71
SMSA, other	301	318	88
Urban, non-SMSA	195	207	69
Rural, nonfarm	202	216	60
Rural, farm	184	203	55
Total	$238	$254	$ 70

NOTE: Figures in parentheses include all cases but have had one or more cases excluded in Table 3–13.

Table II-4. (Corresponds to Table 3–14) Mean and median total hospital expenditures per person by selected characteristics: 1970

Characteristic	Inpatient Hospital			Outpatient Hospital		
	Total population	People with expenditures		Total Population	People with expenditures	
	Mean	Mean	Median	Mean	Mean	Median
Sex						
Male	$ (82)	$ (951)	$461	$ 4	$(55)	$26
Female	101	764	451	3	60	28
Age						
0–5	(54)	(611)	279	(4)	(46)	30
6–17	(33)	(642)	308	(3)	(41)	24
18–34	94	602	396	(5)	(59)	23
35–54	75	741	507	4	(76)	34
55–64	(211)	(1527)	(839)	3	(50)	25
65 and over	199	1209	796	(4)	(83)	32
Poverty level						
Above near poverty	89	816	451	3	44	25
Below near poverty	101	906	478	(7)	(88)	35
Education of head						
8 years or less	98	904	58	5	(73)	30
9–11 years	74	701	482	5	(67)	27
12 years	78	722	397	2	38	27
13 years or more	(115)	(1008)	442	4	53	25
Residence						
SMSA, central city	86	874	537	(7)	(74)	32
SMSA, other	(128)	(1132)	526	3	(47)	24
Urban, non-SMSA	65	503	320	1	a	a
Rural, nonfarm	(76)	(686)	397	2	39	21
Rural, farm	75	736	385	(1)	(34)	15
Total	$ 92	$ 837	$455	$ 4	$ 57	$27

[a]Fewer than 25 unweighted cases in cell.

NOTE: Figures in parentheses include all cases but have had one or more cases excluded in Table 3–14.

Table II-5. (Corresponds to Table 3-15) Mean and median total physician expenditures per person by selected characteristics: 1970

Characteristic	Inpatient, Including Surgery			Outpatient[a]		
	Total population	People with expenditures		Total population	People with expenditures	
	Mean	Mean	Median	Mean	Mean	Median
Sex						
Male	$22	$294	$140	$33	$55	$26
Female	21	261	178	46	70	30
Age						
0–5	(21)	(294)	85	36	50	32
6–17	(8)	(192)	125	18	33	16
18–34	19	246	123	48	76	31
35–54	22	277	253	43	70	31
55–64	(46)	(369)	287	58	87	41
65 and over	41	291	162	55	79	45
Poverty level						
Above near poverty	23	284	167	42	63	30
Below near poverty	17	248	112	33	64	28
Education of head						
8 years or less	23	253	161	34	61	29
9–11 years	16	228	157	35	59	29
12 years	20	259	140	36	56	25
13 years or more	(27)	(362)	190	53	75	33
Residence						
SMSA, central city	17	269	189	43	75	33
SMSA, other	28	359	240	46	69	30
Urban, non-SMSA	20	201	99	36	55	28
Rural, nonfarm	(22)	(255)	135	32	52	25
Rural, farm	(19)	(236)	129	28	48	23
Total	$21	$277	$156	$40	$63	$30

[a]Includes all obstetrical care including delivery.

NOTE: Figures in parentheses include all cases but have had one or more cases excluded in Table 3-15.

Table II-6. (Corresponds to Table 3-16) Mean and median total drug expenditures per person by selected characteristics: 1970

Characteristic	Prescribed Drugs			Nonprescribed Drugs		
	Total population	People with expenditures		Total population	People with expenditures	
	Mean	Mean	Median	Mean	Mean	Median
Sex						
Male	$19	$49	$17	$ 9	$12	$ 5
Female	26	56	24	9	13	6
Age						
0-5	9	19	10	6	9	5
6-17	6	20	10	6	8	5
18-34	17	40	16	9	12	5
35-54	28	62	27	10	14	7
55-64	(49)	(98)	50	14	21	10
65 and over	56	92	52	12	18	10
Poverty level						
Above near poverty	23	51	20	9	13	6
Below near poverty	23	60	22	7	12	5
Education of head						
8 years or less	28	69	29	8	13	5
9-11 years	19	47	19	8	11	5
12 years	21	47	20	9	13	6
13 years or more	23	50	17	9	13	6
Residence						
SMSA, central city	25	60	20	9	13	5
SMSA, other	22	47	20	8	12	7
Urban, non-SMSA	23	51	20	9	13	5
Rural, nonfarm	21	51	20	9	12	5
Rural, farm	21	54	29	8	12	5
Total	$23	$53	$20	$ 9	$13	$ 5

NOTE: Figures in parentheses include all cases but have had one or more cases excluded in Table 3-16.

Table II-7. (Corresponds to Table 3-17) Mean and median total dental expenditures per person by selected characteristics: 1970

| | Dental | | |
| | Total population | People with expenditures | |
Characteristic	Mean	Mean	Median
Sex			
Male	$27	$65	$25
Female	30	70	26
Age			
0-5	(5)	(33)	17
6-17	29	54	22
18-34	33	66	27
35-54	38	83	29
55-64	27	84	31
65 and over	20	80	28
Poverty level			
Above near poverty	33	70	25
Below near poverty	14	54	20
Education of head			
8 years or less	20	74	25
9-11 years	24	66	25
12 years	28	61	24
13 years or more	38	69	26
Residence			
SMSA, central city	26	68	25
SMSA, other	43	86	30
Urban, non-SMSA	22	53	20
Rural, nonfarm	21	54	22
Rural, farm	16	43	18
Total	$28	$67	$25

NOTE: Figures in parentheses include all cases but have had one or more cases excluded in Table 3-17.

Table II-8. (Corresponds to Table 3-18) Mean and median total other expenditures per person by selected characteristics: 1970

	Non-MD Practitioners			Tests, Glasses, Other Goods and Services		
	Total population	People with expenditures		Total population	People with expenditures	
Characteristic	*Mean*	*Mean*	*Median*	*Mean*	*Mean*	*Median*
Sex						
Male	$ 5	$33	$14	$13	$47	$33
Female	(7)	(45)	14	17	51	32
Age						
0-5	(1)	a	a	(6)	(47)	20
6-17	2	(19)	12	7	35	28
18-34	(5)	(34)	13	16	44	30
35-54	5	30	14	20	55	36
55-64	(11)	(42)	16	27	62	40
65 and over	(19)	(92)	14	22	57	35
Poverty level						
Above near poverty	6	40	14	16	50	33
Below near poverty	(4)	(34)	14	11	48	32

Education of head					
8 years or less	(7)	(41)	14	16	55	34
9–11 years	3	(24)	13	13	46	32
12 years	4	28	14	12	41	30
13 years or more	(9)	(60)	14	20	55	35
Residence					
SMSA, central city	6	37	14	17	52	33
SMSA, other	(7)	(52)	15	16	51	31
Urban, non-SMSA	(5)	(34)	15	13	46	33
Rural, nonfarm	(5)	(37)	12	14	48	32
Rural, farm	4	24	13	12	41	32
Total	$ 6	$39	$14	$15	$50	$32

aFewer than 25 unweighted cases in cell.

NOTE: Figures in parentheses include all cases but have had one or more cases excluded in Table 3–18.

Table II-9. (Corresponds to Table 4-12) Best estimate expenditures for all personal health services by selected characteristics and source of payment: 1970

	Source of Payment						Total Mean Expenditures per Person
Characteristic	Medicaid, welfare, free institution	Other free care	Medicare	Voluntary insurance	Out-of-pocket	Other nonfree care	
Sex							
Male	$(36)	$14	$ 19	$ 66	$ 98	$1	$(234)
Female	26	2	22	85	119	4	258
Age							
0–5	12	a	—	(69)	(54)	a	(135)
6–17	(14)	(2)	—	(31)	(63)	a	(110)
18–34	(74)	10	—	88	117	8	(296)
35–54	20	13	—	82	121	a	236
55–64	23	(10)	a	(211)	(197)	4	(445)
65 and over	26	13	204	32	153	a	428
Poverty level							
Above near poverty	23	8	14	88	120	3	256
Below near poverty	57	8	42	34	70	2	213
Family income							
Under $2,000	88	9	83	23	98	1	302
$ 2,000– 3,499	63	13	63	28	90	2	259
3,500– 4,999	32	9	29	73	111	1	256
5,000– 7,499	23	12	30	83	105	2	255
7,500– 9,999	10	8	5	74	89	2	186
10,000–14,999	(50)	7	11	75	104	5	(252)
15,000 and over	5	4	6	(103)	(140)	2	(260)

Race							
White	29	8	21	81	116	3	258
Nonwhite	45	8	15	40	53	2	162
Education of Head							
8 years or less	32	11	42	52	96	1	234
9–11 years	22	4	20	55	89	2	193
12 years	(56)	5	14	75	98	2	(249)
13 years or more	9	11	9	116	146	5	295
Residence							
SMSA, central city	30	11	21	73	99	1	235
SMSA, other	(61)	8	22	101	145	5	(342)
Urban, non-SMSA	16	5	17	57	94	2	190
Rural, nonfarm	12	5	18	70	93	2	199
Rural, farm	11	9	29	44	86	2	181
Total	$ 31	$ 8	$ 21	$ 76	$109	$3	$ 248

[a]Less than 50¢.

NOTE: Figures in parentheses include all cases but have had one or more cases excluded in Table 4–12.

Table II-10. (Corresponds to Table 4–13) Best estimate of hospital inpatient expenditures by selected characteristics and source of payment: 1970

Characteristic	Source of Payment						Total Mean Expenditures per Person
	Medicaid, welfare, free institutions	Other free care	Medicare	Voluntary insurance	Out-of-pocket	Other nonfree care	
Sex							
Male	$ 6	$ 7	$ 15	$(42)	$(11)	$1	$(82)
Female	15	1	17	55	11	2	101
Age							
0-5	6	a	—	(45)	3	a	(54)
6-17	(8)	a	—	(19)	(5)	1	(33)
18-34	14	3	—	58	15	5	94
35-54	13	7	—	47	8	a	75
55-64	12	(5)	—	(153)	(40)	1	(211)
65 and over	7	11	160	14	7	—	199
Poverty level							
Above near poverty	5	3	11	56	12	2	89
Below near poverty	30	6	34	24	8	1	101
Family income							
Under $2,000	49	6	66	14	13	a	148
$ 2,000- 3,499	31	10	50	19	9	a	119
3,500- 4,999	(16)	5	19	(52)	13	1	(106)
5,000- 7,499	13	4	24	(54)	11	a	(106)
7,500- 9,999	4	5	4	51	9	1	73
10,000-14,999	4	3	10	42	7	3	68
15,000 and over	(5)	1	4	(68)	(18)	1	(97)

Race							
White	9	4	17	51	12	1	94
Nonwhite	(24)	5	12	(28)	2	a	(72)
Education of head							
8 years or less	15	7	33	35	7	a	98
9-11 years	12	2	16	34	9	2	75
12 years	10	2	11	47	7	1	78
13 years or more	(6)	5	6	(75)	(20)	3	(115)
Residence							
SMSA, central city	16	5	16	43	5	a	86
SMSA, other	(11)	3	17	(70)	(24)	3	(128)
Urban, non-SMSA	7		13	33	7	1	65
Rural, non-farm	7	2	14	(44)	8	1	(76)
Rural, farm	6	6	24	29	9	1	75
Total	$11	$ 4	$ 17	$48	$11	$1	$92

aLess than 50¢.
NOTE: Figures in parentheses include all cases but have had one or more cases excluded in Table 4-13.

Table II-11. (Corresponds to Table 4–14) Best estimate of hospital outpatient expenditures for all personal health services by selected characteristics and source of payment: 1970

Characteristic	Source of Payment						Total Mean Expenditures per Person
	Medicaid, welfare, free institutions	Other free care	Medicare	Voluntary insurance	Out-of-pocket	Other nonfree care	
Sex							
Male	$(25)	a	a	$1	$1	a	$(27)
Female	1	a	a	1	1	a	4
Age							
0–5	2	a	—	1	1	a	4
6–17	1	a	—	(2)	1	a	(4)
18–34	(53)	a	—	1	1	a	(55)
35–54	1	a	—	(2)	1	a	(4)
55–64	1	a	—	1	1	a	4
65 and over	(2)	a	(2)	a	1	a	(5)
Poverty level							
Above near poverty	(16)	a	a	2	1	a	(19)
Below near poverty	(5)	a	a	a	1	a	(6)
Family income							
Under $2,000	(9)	a	a	a	1	a	(10)
$ 2,000– 3,499	(3)	a	a	a	2	a	(7)
3,500– 4,999	3	a	a	1	1	a	(7)
5,000– 7,499	1	a	a	1	1	a	(3)
7,500– 9,999	(1)	a	a	1	1	a	3
10,000–14,999	(45)	a	a	2	1	a	(48)
15,000 and over	___	a	a	2	(2)	a	4

Race						
White	(14)	a	a	1	1	a	(16)
Nonwhite	4	a	a	1	2	a	7
Education of head						
8 years or less	2	a	a	1	1	a	5
9–11 years	(3)	a	a	1	1	a	(5)
12 years	(41)	a	a	1	1	a	(43)
13 years or more	(a)	a	a	2	2	a	4
Residence						
SMSA, central city	3	a	a	2	2	a	8
SMSA, other	(44)	a	a	2	1	a	(47)
Urban, non-SMSA	a	a	a	a	a	(a)	1
Rural, nonfarm	a	a	a	1	1	a	(4)
Rural, farm	a	a	a	a	a	a	a
Total	$(13)	a	a.	$1	$1	a	$(16)

[a]Less than 50¢.

NOTE: Figures in parentheses include all cases but have had one or more cases excluded in Table 4–14.

Table II-12. (Corresponds to Table 4-15) Best estimate of physician inpatient expenditures for all personal health services by selected characteristics and source of payment: 1970

Characteristic	Source of Payment						Total Mean Expenditures per Person
	Medicaid, welfare, free institutions	Other free care	Medicare	Voluntary insurance	Out-of-pocket	Other nonfree care	
Sex							
Male	a	a	$2	$13	$6	a	$22
Female	1	a	2	12	5	1	22
Age							
0-5	a	a	–	(15)	3	a	(19)
6-17	1	a	–	(5)	2	a	(8)
18-34	1	a	–	(12)	(6)	2	(20)
35-54	1	a	–	15	5	a	22
55-64	1	a	–	(31)	(17)	1	(49)
65 and over	1	a	24	8	9	a	42
Poverty level							
Above near poverty	a	a	2	15	6	1	24
Below near poverty	3	a	5	5	4	a	17
Family income							
Under $2,000	3	a	(10)	5	(7)	a	(24)
$ 2,000– 3,499	4	a	7	4	6	a	22
3,500– 4,999	1	a	3	(9)	5	a	(19)
5,000– 7,499	1	a	4	(15)	(9)	a	(29)
7,500– 9,999	1	a	1	(11)	5	a	(18)
10,000–14,999	a	a	1	13	5	1	21
15,000 and over	a	a	1	(17)	(5)	a	(23)

Race							
White	1	a	3	14	6	1	24
Nonwhite	1	a	(1)	(5)	(2)	a	(9)
Education of head							
8 years or less	2	a	5	8	7	a	23
9–11 years	1	a	2	9	3	a	15
12 years	1	a	1	13	5	1	(20)
13 years or more	a	a	1	(19)	(7)	1	(29)
Residence							
SMSA, central city	1	a	2	13	3	a	19
SMSA, other	a	a	3	(15)	(9)	1	(29)
Urban, non-SMSA	2	a	3	11	4	a	20
Rural, nonfarm	1	a	2	(12)	6	a	(21)
Rural, farm	(1)	a	3	8	5	a	18
Total	$1	a	$2	$13	$6	a	$22

aLess than 50¢

NOTE: Figures in parentheses include all cases but have had one or more cases excluded in Table 4–15.

Table II-13. (Corresponds to Table 4-17) Best estimate of prescription drug expenditures for all personal health services by selected characteristics and source of payment: 1970

Characteristic	Source of Payment						Total Mean Expenditures per Person
	Medicaid, welfare, free institutions	Other free care	Medicare	Voluntary insurance	Out-of-pocket	Other nonfree care	
Sex							
Male	$ 1	$1	–	$1	$16	a	$19
Female	2	a	–	3	21	a	26
Age							
0–5	a	a	–	1	8	a	9
6–17	a	a	–	a	6	a	6
18–34	1	1	–	2	14	a	17
35–54	1	1	–	4	21	a	28
55–64	2	1	–	5	(41)	1	(49)
65 and over	9	1	–	2	44	–	56
Poverty level							
Above near poverty	1	1	–	2	19	a	23
Below near poverty	6	1	–	1	15	a	23
Family income							
Under $2,000	11	a	–	a	22	a	34
$ 2,000– 3,499	8	1	–	a	24	a	32
3,500– 4,999	1	1	–	3	31	a	36
5,000– 7,499	2	2	–	3	18	a	25
7,500– 9,999	a	a	–	1	15	a	16
10,000–14,999	a	1	–	2	16	a	19
15,000 and over	a	a	–	3	(17)	a	(21)

Race							
White	1	1	–	2	19	a	24
Nonwhite	4	a	–	1	10	a	16
Education of head							
8 years or less	4	1	–	1	22	a	28
9–11 years	1	a	–	2	16	a	19
12 years	1	a	–	3	17	a	21
13 years or more	1	1	–	3	18	a	23
Residence							
SMSA, central city	2	1	–	2	20	a	25
SMSA, other	2	1	–	2	18	a	22
Urban, non-SMSA	2	a	–	2	19	a	23
Rural, nonfarm	1	a	–	2	17	a	21
Rural, farm	2	a	–	1	18	a	21
Total	$ 2	$1	–	$2	$18	a	$23

a Less than 50¢.

NOTE: Figures in parentheses include all cases but have had one or more cases excluded in Table 4–17.

Table II-14. (Corresponds to Table 4-18) Best estimate of dental expenditures for all personal health services by selected characteristics and source of payment: 1970

Characteristic	Source of Payment						Total Mean Expenditures per Person
	Medicaid, welfare, free institutions	Other free care	Medicare	Voluntary insurance	Out-of-pocket	Other nonfree care	
Sex							
Male	$1	$1	–	$1	$24	a	$27
Female	2	a	–	1	26	a	30
Age							
0–5	a	a	–	a	(4)	a	(5)
6–17	2	a	–	1	26	a	29
18–34	2	1	–	2	28	a	33
35–54	1	a	–	3	34	a	38
55–64	1	a	–	1	25	a	27
65 and over	2	a	–	a	18	–	20
Poverty level							
Above near poverty	1	a	–	2	30	a	33
Below near poverty	5	a	–	a	8	–	14
Family income							
Under $2,000	4	a	–	–	(11)	–	(15)
$ 2,000– 3,499	5	a	–	a	8	–	13
3,500– 4,999	4	a	–	2	(16)	a	(22)
5,000– 7,499	1	1	–	a	20	a	23
7,500– 9,999	2	1	–	1	16	a	20
10,000–14,999	a	a	–	3	28	a	32
15,000 and over	a	a	–	1	44	a	44
Race							
White	1	a	–	1	27	a	30

	4	a	–	1	9	a	15
Nonwhite	4	a	–	1	9	a	15
Education of head							
8 years or less	3	a	–	1	16	–	20
9–11 years	2	a	–	1	21	–	24
12 years	1	a	–	2	24	a	28
13 years or more	a	1	–	1	36	a	(38)
Residence							
SMSA, central city	3	1	–	2	21	a	26
SMSA, other	1	1	–	2	40	a	43
Urban, non-SMSA	1	1	–	1	20	–	22
Rural, nonfarm	1	a	–	1	19	a	21
Rural, farm	a	a	–	a	15	–	16
Total	$1	a	–	$1	$25	a	$28

[a]Less than 50¢.

NOTE: Figures in parentheses include all cases but have had one or more cases excluded in Table 4–18.

Table II-15. (Corresponds to Table 4-19) Best estimate of total other expenditures for all personal health services by selected characteristics and source of payment: 1970

Characteristic	Source of Payment						Total Mean Expenditures per Person
	Medicaid, welfare, free institutions	Other free care	Medicare	Voluntary insurance	Out-of-pocket	Other nonfree care	
Sex							
Male	a	$1	a	$3	$13	a	$18
Female	2	a	a	4	18	a	24
Age							
0-5	a	a	–	(2)	(4)	–	(7)
6-17	1	a	–	1	7	a	9
18-34	1	1	–	4	15	a	21
35-54	1	1	–	4	19	a	25
55-64	3	1	–	8	26	a	38
65 and over	2	a	3	2	33	a	41
Poverty level							
Above near poverty	1	1	a	4	17	a	23
Below near poverty	3	a	1	1	10	a	15
Family income							
Under $2,000	4	a	1	2	12	–	19
$ 2,000- 3,499	(3)	1	1	1	(16)	a	(22)
3,500- 4,999	1	1	a	3	14	a	18
5,000- 7,499	2	a	1	3	15	a	21
7,500- 9,999	a	a	a	3	13	a	16
10,000-14,999	a	1	a	4	14	a	19
15,000 and over	a	1	a	5	21	a	27
Race							
White	1	1	a	4	17	a	22

	1	a	a	1	8	a	11
Nonwhite	1	a	a	1	8	a	11
Education of head							
8 years or less	2	1	a	3	16	a	22
9–11 years	1	a	1	2	12	a	16
12 years	a	1	a	3	12	a	16
13 years or more	1	1	a	6	22	a	30
Residence							
SMSA, central city	1	1	a	4	17	a	23
SMSA, other	1	1	a	4	17	a	23
Urban, non-SMSA	1	a	a	3	13	a	18
Rural, nonfarm	1	a	a	3	14	a	19
Rural, farm	a	a	a	2	13	a	16
Total	$1	$1	a	$3	$16	a	$21

aLess than 50¢.

NOTE: Figures in parentheses include all cases but have had one or more cases excluded in Table 4–19.

Table II-16. (Corresponds to Table 5-6) Comparison of respondent reporting and best estimate for mean length of stay and hospital days per 100 population by age and sex: 1970

Characteristic	Mean Number of Days per Admission		Hospital Days per 100 Population	
	Social survey	Best estimate	Social survey	Best estimate
Age				
0–17	5.2	4.2	38	32
18–54	8.1	6.1	127	94
55 and over	(14.5)	(13.8)	(300)	(277)
Sex				
Male	(11.7)	(9.3)	(128)	(98)
Female	8.0	7.1	129	117
Total	(9.4)	(8.0)	(128)	(107)

NOTE: Figures in parentheses include all cases but have had one or more cases excluded in Table 5-6.

Table II-17. (Corresponds to Table 5-8) Mean expenditures for all personal health services per family by family income and poverty level, from social survey and best estimate: 1970

| | Mean Expenditures | | | | | |
| | Free | | Nonfree | | Total | |
Income and Poverty Level	Social survey	Best estimate	Social survey	Best estimate	Social survey	Best estimate
Under $2,000	($146)	$147	$343	$313	$489	$459
$ 2,000– 3,499	180	157	403	378	583	536
3,500– 4,999	106	97	496	506	602	603
5,000– 7,499	97	97	(644)	623	741	721
7,500– 9,999	(69)	(62)	606	599	675	661
10,000–14,999	(153)	(205)	686	677	(839)	(882)
15,000 and over	(24)	(36)	(999)	(971)	(1,024)	(1,006)
Above near poverty	(78)	(96)	708	695	786	791
Below near poverty	194	178	432	405	626	583
Total	($108)	($117)	$636	$620	$744	$738

NOTE: Figures in parentheses include all cases but have had one or more cases excluded in Table 5-8.

Table II-18. (Corresponds to Table 5-11) Mean total expenditures per person by selected characteristics: 1970

Characteristic	Total Population Mean	People with Expenditures Mean
Sex		
Male	$(234)	$(254)
Female	258	273
Age		
0-5 years	(136)	(145)
6-17 years	(110)	(121)
18-34 years	(296)	(312)
35-54 years	236	251
55-64 years	(445)	(485)
65 years and over	428	456
Poverty level		
Above near poverty	256	270
Below near poverty	213	242
Education of head		
8 years or less	234	262
9-11 years	193	209
12 years	(249)	(264)
13 years or more	295	305
Residence		
SMSA, central city	235	255
SMSA, other	(342)	(361)
Urban, non-SMSA	190	203
Rural, nonfarm	199	213
Rural, farm	181	201
Total	$246	$264

NOTE: Figures in parentheses include all cases but have had one or more cases excluded in Table 5-11.

Table II-19. (Corresponds to Table 5-12) Mean total hospital outpatient expenditures per person by selected characteristics: 1970

Characteristic	Total Population Mean	People with Expenditures Mean
Sex		
Male	$(28)	$(297)
Female	4	55
Age		
0–5 years	(5)	(48)
6–17 years	(4)	(45)
18–34 years	(56)	(545)
35–54 years	(4)	(53)
55–64 years	4	41
65 years and over	(4)	(90)
Poverty level		
Above near poverty	(19)	(220)
Below near poverty	(7)	(77)
Education of head		
8 years or less	5	55
9–11 years	(6)	(64)
12 years	(43)	(553)
13 years or more	(5)	(52)
Residence		
SMSA, central city	8	(75)
SMSA, other	(47)	(476)
Urban, non-SMSA	(2)	(28)
Rural, nonfarm	3	36
Rural, farm	1	(32)
Total	$(16)	$(186)

NOTE: Figures in parentheses include all cases but have had one or more cases excluded in Table 5-12.

Table II-20. (Corresponds to Table 5-13) Mean total physician expenditures per person by selected characteristics: 1970

Characteristic	Inpatient, Including Surgery		Outpatient	
	Population Mean	People with Expenditures Mean	Population Mean	People with Expenditures Mean
Sex				
Male	$22	$305	$29	$53
Female	22	267	42	67
Age				
0–5 years	(19)	(229)	32	47
6–17 years	(8)	(206)	15	31
18–34 years	(20)	(269)	46	75
35–54 years	22	272	35	61
55–64 years	(49)	(424)	53	82
65 years and over	42	298	54	79
Poverty level				
Above near poverty	24	290	38	60
Below near poverty	17	259	29	60
Education of head				
8 years or less	23	264	31	60
9–11 years	15	215	31	55
12 years	20	263	34	54
13 years or more	(29)	(383)	46	70
Residence				
SMSA, central city	19	301	38	69
SMSA, other	(29)	(378)	42	66
Urban, non-SMSA	20	208	32	50
Rural, nonfarm	(21)	(239)	31	52
Rural, farm	18	220	26	48
Total	$22	$284	$36	$60

NOTE: Figures in parentheses include all cases but have had one or more cases excluded in Table 5-13.

Definitions of Variables

This appendix provides definitions for the variables used in the text and appendix tables.

1. **Age**
   For the first three studies, this is age as of the actual date of the interview. For the 1970 study, it is age as of the last day of the study year, that is, December 31, 1970.

2. **Basic Health Insurance**
   Hospital and/or surgical medical insurance that is not major medical insurance. Generally, it provides first dollar coverage for hospital and inpatient surgical procedures but has lower maximum benefits than major medical insurance. As used in this report, basic insurance also excludes prepaid group practice plans.

3. **Best Estimate**
   This is a final figure arrived at for hospital and physician utilization and expenditures and health insurance coverage by merging verifying data from hospitals, physicians, insurance companies and employers with the social survey data supplied by the respondent. The best estimate is usually but not always the verifying data when this is available.

4. **Debt for Medical Care**
   This is money still owed by the family for medical bills incurred in the survey year or before, whether the money is owed to a

tion is based upon responses at the time of the social survey interview, so that money that was later written off in the 1970 verifications as a bad debt or as charity care is included as owed here. Conversely, money discovered as owed in the verification that had not been acknowledged by the respondent is not included here. This was done in order to make a comparison possible between 1963 and 1970.

5. **Dental Insurance**
    This is insurance which pays for all or part of the cost of out-patient dentistry. It can be either a separate plan limited to dentistry or part of a larger plan, such as a prepaid group practice. Plans that pay only for the accidental injury of teeth or for dentistry only when it is performed in a hospital are *not* considered dental insurance. Individuals covered by CHAMPUS are considered to have dental insurance.

6. **Dentist, Percent Seeing**
    Proportion of the sample seeing the dentist at least once during the survey year. This variable excludes all persons who were not in the universe for all 12 months of the survey year.

7. **Dentist Visits, Mean Number**
    Based on response to question: "Did (PERSON) have any dental care such as teeth cleaned, x-rayed, filled or pulled, or any bridge work done last year?" and the followup question: "How many times did (PERSON) visit a dentist's office during the past year?"

    The mean number of dentist visits for those with visits is the mean for sample members who had at least one visit. Person-year is defined in 40.

8. **Disability Days—1971**
    The sum of days reported in response to the questions: "Within the last two weeks, how many days did (PERSON) stay in bed all or part of the day because (he/she) was not feeling well?" and "(Apart from the days (PERSON) stayed in bed) how many days within the last two weeks was (PERSON) not able to do the things (he/she) usually does because (he/she) was not feeling well?"

9. **Drug Insurance**
    This is insurance that pays for all or part of the cost of prescribed drugs. Major medical insurance that pays for prescribed drugs only for a specified illness and/or only when a deductible

has been met is considered to be drug insurance in this definition. Individuals covered by CHAMPUS are considered to have drug insurance.

10. **Education**

a. *of Head*—This variable is attributed to all family members. It is based on the response to the question: "What is the highest grade or year (PERSON) has completed in school?" Interviewers were instructed not to include trade schools, business colleges, correspondence courses and the like in the calculation of years of formal education. Family head is defined in 27.

b. *of Mother*—Defined as in 10a.

11. **Enrollment for Health Insurance**

This is the method through which individuals and families purchase health insurance. The two categories used in this study are:

a. *Group*—Enrollment through an organization, usually an employer group, covered by one general health insurance policy. This includes Medicare and CHAMPUS.

b. *Nongroup*—Enrollment by direct purchase of a single policy covering individual or family from an insurer or insurance agent. This includes conversions from a group.

12. **Expenditures, Free**

Expenditures for medical goods and services provided to the family at no direct cost or at substantially reduced rates and without benefits being provided by any type of health insurance plan. These expenditures have been estimated in 1970 for all free care as described in Appendix I. This variable consists of care that had no monetary value attached to it in the previous studies. Its two subdivisions are:

a. *Medicaid, Welfare, Free Institutions*—This includes expenditures for medical care made by public aid departments on behalf of their recipients and includes as well expenditures for those people not on welfare but with incomes sufficiently low to qualify them for payment of some or all of their medical bills (Medicaid). Eligibility requirements vary widely from state to state for both of these programs. The main distinction between them is that welfare recipients receive a monthly check while Medicaid recipients do not. Also included here is the estimated monetary value of care provided by locally tax-supported hospitals and institutions, including city and county hospitals, state mental and tuberculosis hospitals, and board of health clinics.

All of the care contained in this variable can be considered free care because of inability to pay.

b. *Other Free Expenditures*—This variable includes all expenditures that had no monetary value attached to them in the previous studies but that are not included in Medicaid, welfare and free institutions above. This care, while free, generally does not have stringent income requirements for eligibility and thus is treated separately. Included here is care provided by Veteran's Administration hospitals, care provided to armed forces members, workmen's compensation, care provided by certain governmental agencies such as federally funded crippled children's programs, and care paid for by liability insurance carried by a non-family member.

13. **Expenditures, Nonfree**
    These are generally considered to be expenditures for care that the consumer pays for himself, either directly or through some third party to which he pays premiums or has premiums paid on his behalf. This variable consists of care that had a monetary value attached to it in the previous studies. Its four subdivisions are:

    a. *Voluntary Insurance*—This is health insurance carried either directly by the patient or by his employer on his behalf. Insurance that pays for accidental injuries only is excluded.

    b. *Medicare*—This insurance is funded through Social Security payments for people 65 and over. Part A, which covers inpatient hospital care, requires no additional payment. Part B, which covers physician care, requires a monthly premium paid by those who carry it. Medicare is considered as nonfree care in this report because there are no income restrictions on eligibility for its use and because in large part it replaces voluntary health insurance carried by people 65 and over in 1963.

    c. *Out-of-Pocket Expenditures*—These are expenditures made directly either at time of service or to pay off medical bills incurred previously during the year. Out-of-pocket expenditures also include money owed but not yet paid for care received in 1970.

    d. *Other Nonfree Expenditures*—This variable consists of two items that are not voluntary health insurance but that had expenditures associated with them in the 1963 study. One is CHAMPUS, insurance provided by the armed forces for dependents of members. The other is payments made by accident and liability insurance carried by some member of the patient's family.

14. **Expenditures, Total**
Sum of free (12) and nonfree (13) expenditures.

15. **Expenditures for Dental Care**
Charges by the dentist for his services and those of his auxiliary personnel such as a dental hygienist and for dental appliances. Includes also expenditures to cover charges made to him by dental laboratories and dental manufacturers for work done at his request. Excludes in-hospital extractions and other surgery (included under physician surgery [19a]).

16. **Expenditures for Drugs**
This is the sum of the following two components of drug expenditures:

a. *Prescribed Drugs*—Charges for drugs and medicines prescribed at some time by the physician, other medical practitioner or dentist and purchased by the consumer directly from a pharmacy or elsewhere. It excludes drugs administered by the physician or dentist and charged for on his bill as well as drugs received from a hospital and included in the hospital bill. Any person with free or nonfree expenditures for prescribed drugs is considered to be "using" prescribed drugs.

b. *Nonprescribed Medicines and Drugs*—Charges for all medicines, tonics, vitamins, aspirin, lotions, etc. that are "over the counter" purchases rather than being prescribed.

17. **Expenditures for Hospital Care**
This is the sum of the following two components of hospital care expenditures:

a. *Hospital Inpatient*—Charges incurred in connection with an inpatient admission. They include room and board charges, laboratory fees, drugs, x-rays, operating and delivery room fees, and the usual "extras." They include charges for pathologist, radiologist and anesthesiologist if these are included in the hospital bill rather than being billed privately. Charges for special duty nursing are always excluded (included under nonmedical practitioners [18a]).

b. *Hospital Outpatient*—These are charges for services given in a hospital outpatient clinic or emergency room by a salaried physician or technician in the employ of a hospital. Excluded are charges made by a private physician who attends a patient in the outpatient department or emergency room (included in other physician care [19d] or surgery [19a] depending upon the nature of the service).

18. **Expenditures for Other Medical Care**
This is the sum of the following two components:

a. *Nonmedical Practitioners*—Charges for private duty nursing in the hospital, services of an optometrist or optician excluding glasses (included in other medical care [18b]), and charges by physical therapists, practical and registered nurses in the home, midwives, psychologists, podiatrists, Christian Science practitioners and chiropractors.

b. *Other Medical Care*—Charges for appliances (except for dental appliances, which are included under dental care [15]) and for prostheses such as eye glasses, hearing aids, crutches, wheelchairs, braces, artificial limbs, orthopedic shoes and vaporizers. Also includes ambulance fees, charges for oxygen if not billed by a hospital or doctor directly, and charges for diagnostic tests and x-rays given by a nonhospital laboratory for which the patient was billed directly.

19. **Expenditures for Physician Care**
This is the sum of the following four subcomponents of physician care expenditures:

a. *Surgery*—Physicians' charges for all cutting procedures except caesarian sections (included in obstetrics [19b]) and circumcision of the newborn and suturing (not considered surgery). All setting of dislocations and fractures is included. Both inpatient and outpatient physician charges are included. In general, the expenditures consist of the charge for the operation only, but in a few instances they include charges for preoperative and postoperative care when these could not be distinguished from the charge for the operation itself. All charges by assistant surgeons and anesthesiologists are included here as well as charges by dentists operating in the hospital.

b. *Obstetrics*—Physicians' charges in connection with prenatal care and delivery or termination of the pregnancy regardless of when in the survey year this occurred. Included are charges for a caesarean section, for circumcision when performed right after birth, for a D and C in connection with a miscarriage or abortion and for anesthesiologist charges for an obstetrical procedure.

c. *Ophthalmologist*—Physicians' charges for routine eye refractions. Excluded are charges for eye surgery (included under surgery [19a]), treatment for eye conditions other than those requiring refractions (included under other physician [19d]), refractions done by an optometrist (included under nonmedical practitioners [18a]) and glasses (included under other medical care [18b]).

d. *Other Physician*—Includes physician charges in the hospital that are not included in surgery and all physician care rendered on an outpatient basis except for obstetrics and routine eye refractions. Includes charges for care by the practitioner himself and for special tests and x-rays, treatments, drugs and medications when the physician himself bills the patient for such services without necessarily performing them himself.

20. **Expenditures for Physician Care—Inpatient**
This is the sum of expenditures for inpatient surgery plus all other physician care delivered to an inpatient in the hospital. It excludes *all* charges for obstetrical care, including the delivery charge and the anesthesiologist. Because of the large prenatal care component of these charges, they are included in Expenditures for Physician Care—Outpatient (21).

21. **Expenditures for Physician Care—Outpatient**
This is expenditures for all physician care delivered outside of the hospital except for salaried physicians in a hospital outpatient department or emergency room. It also includes the entire charge of obstetrical care, including the delivery and the anesthesiologist connected with the delivery.

22. **Expenditures Per Live Birth**
These are all expenditures in connection with a live birth occurring during the survey year even if the expenditures themselves were incurred or paid during a previous year. To compensate for using expenditures from a previous year, all expenditures for survey year pregnancies that did not terminate until the following year have been excluded.

Included are the hospital charge for both mother and infant, all physician charges including circumcision of the newborn and any charge for checking the baby out of the hospital, and all drugs and tests connected with pregnancy and delivery. If the baby stayed in the hospital after the mother went home, its further charges are excluded from this category.

23. **Family**
One person or a group of persons living together and related to each other by blood, marriage or adoption. More informal arrangements are also recognized as long as the respondents con-

sider themselves a family (i.e., common law marriages, foster children). When there were two related married couples living in a single dwelling unit, each married couple and its unmarried children were considered a separate family. Any person unrelated to anyone else in the dwelling unit, such as a roommate, boarder or live in housekeeper, was considered a separate family.

A "small" family is defined as one to three members. A "medium-sized" family has four to five members. A "large" family includes six or more members.

24. **Family Income**
    Total family money income before taxes for the survey year. Income from wages, salaries, own business or farm, professional work or trade, pensions, rents, welfare agencies, unemployment compensation, alimony, regular contributions from friends or relatives, dividends, interest, and similar sources are included. Income in kind—the value of free rent or noncash benefits—is excluded. In the 1958 and 1963 studies, data on income were obtained through a series of questions covering the earned income of each worker in the family and unearned and other income for the family as a whole. In the 1970 study, the questions covered the earned and unearned income of each individual 14 or older in the family. Total family income is the sum of these components.

25. **Family Income Level**
    These designations of income were altered in each study to allow for inflation. For each study, approximately one-third of the families surveyed fell into the following low, middle and high categories.

	Incomes Represented by Each Family Income Level		
Year	Low	Middle	High
1953	$0–2,999	$3,000– 4,999	$ 5,000 and over
1958	0–3,499	3,500– 5,999	6,000 and over
1963	0–3,999	4,000– 6,999	7,000 and over
1970	0–5,999	6,000–10,999	11,000 and over

26. **Family Income, Near Poverty**
    A family was considered to be at the near poverty level or below if they reported their income to be less than the following amounts for a given family size for 1970:

Family Size	Monthly	Yearly	Weekly
1	$220	$2,600	$ 50
2	310	3,700	70
3	370	4,500	85
4	470	5,700	110
5	550	6,600	130
6	620	7,500	145
7 or more	760	9,100	175

Near poverty income adjusted for family size was determined using Bureau of Labor Statistics figures for 1969 updated for 1970.

27. **Head of Family**
Self-defined by family respondents, with one exception—the male member of a married couple was always coded head. If respondent was unable to decide who was family head, the person owning the dwelling unit, the one who signed the mortgage or lease, or the one mainly responsible for rent was coded head.

28. **Health Insurance**
Any plan specifically designed to pay all or part of the health expenses of an insured individual or family. Includes rare disease policies for all four survey years; CHAMPUS for 1958, 1963 and 1970; and Medicare for 1970. Accident insurance, workmen's compensation, Medicaid, and disability or loss of income insurance are excluded from the definition of health insurance.

29. **Health Insurance Benefits**
Benefits paid by a plan defined as health insurance for care rendered within the survey year. Excludes payments made within the survey year for care rendered prior to that year. Includes payments made after the survey year for care rendered prior to the end of the year. For pregnancies terminating during the survey year, includes all benefits connected with the pregnancy, regardless of when the care occurred.

30. **Hospital Admissions**
Overnight stay in or surgery performed in hospitals classified as short term by the American Hospital Association and in hospitals not listed by the AHA but not clearly long term. Excluded are admissions to hospitals classified as long term, mental and

tuberculosis hospitals. Only admissions beginning during the survey year are included. The delivery admission for an obstetrical case is counted as one admission for the mother and none for the infant. If the infant stays in the hospital after the mother goes home or if the infant is readmitted after being discharged, a separate admission is counted for the infant. Person-year is defined in 40.

31. **Hospital Days**
Total number of days spent in short term hospitals during the survey year. For stays beginning before the survey year or ending after the survey year, only those days actually occurring during the survey year are included. Person-year is defined in 40.

32. **Hospital Days Per Admission**
Total number of days spent in short term hospitals during the survey year for all stays regardless of when they began or ended divided by number of admissions occurring during the year. This denominator excludes admissions prior to the survey year but extending into the year. It includes admissions that extended into the year following the survey year. For terminated pregnancies, it includes all admissions and days regardless of when they occurred.

33. **Hospital Insurance**
This is health insurance designed to pay all or part of the inpatient hospital bill for the insured person. The hospital bill includes only the bill submitted by the hospital itself, not that submitted by the doctor who treated the patient in the hospital nor those submitted by any private duty nurses. Flat rate insurance that pays a given amount for every day the person is hospitalized is considered hospitalization insurance. Major medical insurance is considered hospital insurance. Medicare, Part A, and CHAMPUS are considered hospital insurance.

34. **Insured Family**
Family in which one or more members were covered by some type of health insurance (unless a particular type is indicated in the text) on the last day of the survey year.

35. **Insured Person**
Individual covered by any type of health insurance (unless a particular type is indicated in the text) on the last day of the survey year, or on the last day individual was in the population for sample individuals leaving population during the survey year (e.g., those dying or becoming institutionalized). In calculating percentages of persons insured for various types of services,

people for whom information on coverage was not provided in the interview and could not be determined by our verification procedures were included in the base (treated as not insured). This practice differed from the usual procedure of excluding no answers from the base. This was done because of the thorough verification procedure used to obtain coverage information. Using this alternate method of calculating insurance coverage resulted in at most a 1 percent difference in the 1963 survey.

36. **Insurer**
These are organizations providing reimbursement for the cost of health care in return for premiums. Five types of insurers are distinguished in this study:

a. *Blue Cross–Blue Shield*—This is a federation of not for profit plans that write policies on both a group and nongroup basis and that usually reimburse the hospital or physician directly.

b. *Private Insurance*—This category consists of all for profit insurance companies that write health insurance policies on both a group and nongroup basis, either exclusively or in connection with other types of insurance. They may reimburse the hospital or physician directly or may pay the policyholder directly.

c. *Independent Plans*—These consist mainly of prepaid group practices but also include union-administered plans and self-insured employers. They are almost always not for profit and tend to provide a wider range of benefits than either Blue Cross–Blue Shield or private insurance companies. Enrollment is almost always on a group basis.

d. *CHAMPUS*—This is the coverage provided for dependents of armed forces members. It provides a wide range of benefits and is by definition available only on a group basis.

e. *Medicare*—This is coverage provided by the federal government for virtually all U.S. citizens 65 or over. Medicare, Part A, covers hospitalization; Part B covers physician care both in and out of the hospital. It should be noted that Blue Cross–Blue Shield and private insurance companies are the fiscal intermediaries for this program so that percent of population covered by type of insurer tends to understate the number of people covered by these two groups when Medicare is used as a category. Supplementary to Medicare plans are those that pay for the Medicare deductible and co-insurance as well as filling other gaps. They may be written by Blue Cross–Blue Shield, private insurers or independents.

"Voluntary insurance" as used in this report includes insurance provided by a, b and c above.

37. **Main Earner in Family**

Every family was defined as having a main earner who must have been a family member on the last day of the survey year. The main earner was determined as follows:

a. *One Person Family*—Individual automatically coded main earner.

b. *Family Includes Two Adults (14 or over) Who Are a Married Couple*—(1) Male coded main earner unless not in labor force (retired, disabled, unable to work). Even if male head was currently unemployed, or only part time worker, he was coded main earner. (2) If male head not in labor force but wife was in labor force, wife was coded main earner. (3) If neither male nor female was in labor force, male was coded main earner.

c. *Family Includes Three or More Adults Including a Married Couple*—(1) With adult children, none of whom was in the labor force, coded as in b above. (2) With adult children or other adult relatives in labor force, husband, if working full time, coded main earner. (3) In all other (c) situations, the family member earning the most money coded as main earner.

d. *Family Includes Two or More Adults None of Whom Is Married*—(1) If only one adult in labor force, he was coded main earner. (2) If two or more adults in labor force, the one earning the most money was coded main earner. (3) If no adults in labor force, that person judged to have the greatest potential earning power, or having largest past earnings, was coded main earner.

38. **Major Medical Insurance**

This is health insurance that is designed to cover the heavy medical expenses resulting from a particular catastrophic or prolonged illness. It typically includes a deductible (e.g., $100), co-insurance (e.g., 20 percent) and a maximum payment (e.g., $25,000 to $100,000). Within these limits, it covers most out of hospital as well as in-hospital expenses associated with the particular illness.

Major medical insurance can be carried either alone or in combination with a basic hospital-surgical plan which it supplements.

39. **Outlay for Personal Health Services**

Computed as follows: total charges for health services received during the survey year; plus prepayment and insurance premiums for insurance designed specifically to cover charges for personal health services (including family but excluding employer contributions); plus payments by the family for personal health services received by persons not family members; minus health insurance benefits covering personal health services received during the survey year; minus amounts still owed for personal health services; minus accident or liability insurance benefits covering personal health services received during the survey year; minus payments from friends and relatives outside the family toward charges for personal health services incurred by family members during the survey year.

40. **Person-Years**
Person-years were computed by summing the total months by sample members in the population universe during the survey year and dividing this sum by 12. The purpose of this base is to adjust for sample members who were not in the population the entire survey year, such as those who died, were institutionalized or were born during the year.

41. **Physician Contact—1971**
Based on response to question: "Within the last two weeks did (PERSON) visit or talk on the phone to a doctor about (his/her) health?" and the followup question: "How many times?"

42. **Physician, Percent Seeing**
Proportion of the sample who reported at least one physician visit during the survey year. Excluded are all persons not in the universe for all 12 months of the survey year.

43. **Physician Visit Insurance**
This is insurance that pays for all or part of the cost of seeing the physician in his office for nonsurgical procedures. Major medical insurance that pays for physician office visits for a specified illness and when a deductible has been met is considered to be physician visit insurance in this definition. Individuals covered by CHAMPUS are considered to have physician visit insurance.

44. **Physician Visits, Mean Number**
Sum of all visits related to hospitalized illness, other major nonhospitalized illness, pregnancy, other minor illness and routine checkups, shots, tests, and ophthalmologist visits for the survey year. Includes seeing either a doctor or osteopath or his nurse or technician at the following sites: patient's home, doctor's office or private clinic, hospital outpatient department or emergency

room; industrial, school, camp or college health service; and any other clinic such as a board of health clinic or neighborhood health center. Excluded are telephone calls and visits by a doctor to a hospital inpatient. Person-year is defined in 40.

The mean number of physician visits for persons seeing a doctor is the mean for sample members who had at least one visit.

45. **Physician Visits, Place of**
The place of physician visit has five subcomponents:

a. *Home*—House calls.

b. *Office*—Visits to a fee-for-service physician's private office including those offices located in clinics or clinic buildings. Also includes visits to prepaid group practice physicians when these were designated "office."

c. *Outpatient Department*—Visits to an organized outpatient department of a hospital whether the patient was seen by a private physician or by salaried house staff.

d. *Emergency Room*—Visits to the emergency room of a hospital as distinct from a regular or drop-in clinic appointment.

e. *Other*—Visits to any other site, including employee and student health facilities, board of health clinics not connected with a hospital, health maintenance organizations (HMOs) and certain privately maintained union and fraternal clinics not connected with hospitals. Visits to fee for service physicians at these sites are included in office visits since the physician is then considered to maintain a private office at the site in question.

46. **Physician Visits, Prenatal**
Number of visits made to a physician in connection with a live birth occurring during the study year. Includes visits made prior to the study year and one visit post partum. Excludes physician visits in the hospital.

47. **Pregnancy, First Trimester Visit**
A visit to a physician in connection with the pregnancy by the end of the fourteenth week of the pregnancy. Women who did not see a physician until delivery are included in the analysis. Women who did not see a physician at all, even for delivery, and women who did not know what week of pregnancy they had first seen the physician are excluded from both numerator and denominator in calculating percentage of women seeing a physician by the end of the first trimester of pregnancy.

48. **Pregnancy, Terminated**
This is a pregnancy that ended during the survey year in a live birth, still birth, miscarriage or, in 1970, an abortion, whether

legal or illegal. All utilization and expenditures connected with a terminated pregnancy are included in the analysis for all survey years even if most of the utilization and expenditures took place in the previous year. To compensate for this, current pregnancies (those pregnancies that did not terminate until after the last day of the survey year) have all utilization and expenditures excluded from the analysis even though a majority of this may have taken place during the survey year. The only exception to this is that all women who had current pregnancy visits to a physician and no other physician care during the survey year were credited with seeing a physician for that year and were given one visit.

49. **Race**
Each family member is coded according to the race of the main respondent. The Census definitions of white and nonwhite are used. People of Mexican or Spanish descent are coded as white. American Indians and Orientals are coded as nonwhite. When the distinction is made between white and black, people of Mexican or Spanish descent are excluded from the white category and American Indians and Orientals from the black category.

50. **Reason for Examination**
Reason for examination is defined in answer to the question: "Which of the reasons on this card best describes why (PERSON) had the examination?: not feeling good, required, time for examination."

51. **Regular Source of Care**
Regular source of care is defined in answer to the question: "Is there a particular medical person or clinic (PERSON) usually goes to when sick or for advice about health?" The following definitions apply to the categories:

a. *General Practitioner*—Individual listed in the *AMA Directory, 1969* (AMA, 1969), with primary specialty as general practitioner, unspecified or specialty not recognized, or individual not found in the *AMA Directory* but family classifies him as "regular family doctor."

b. *Specialist*—Individual listed in the *AMA Directory, 1969* (AMA, 1969), with a recognized specialty, or individual not found in the *AMA Directory* but family classifies him as "some type of specialist."

General practitioner and specialist combine together to form the definition of MD.

c. *Clinic*—No individual doctor is initially mentioned but the name of a clinic or outpatient service is given by the family as a regular source of care. A physician's name may be mentioned as the person most often seen at the clinic.

d. *Osteopath*—Individual listed in *1970 Yearbook and Directory of Osteopathic Physicians* (AOA, 1970) or individual not found in the directory but family classifies him as "osteopath."

e. *Other*—Family classifies their regular source of care as a chiropractor or some other practitioner such as a visiting nurse, Christian Science practitioner, homeopath, podiatrist, naturopath or anyone else without a formal medical degree who gives health care.

f. *No Regular Source of Care*—The respondent indicates that there is no "particular" medical person or clinic that the individual usually goes to when sick or for advice about health.

52. **Residence**

A classification of the residence of each person in the sample was done according to U.S. Census designation of the locality in which the residence is located plus the interviewer's description of the dwelling unit and locality.

The following divisions were made exclusively for 1970:

a. *SMSA, central city*—Residence in the urban part of a Standard Metropolitan Statistical Area according to the Census which is also designated by the interviewer as "inside the largest city in the primary unit" (NORC's primary sampling units or PSUs).

b. *SMSA, other*—Defined as (a) except interviewer did not describe dwelling as "inside largest city."

c. *Urban, non-SMSA*—Residence in urban localities that are not part of an SMSA.

d. *Rural, nonfarm*—Residence in areas defined as rural by the Census that are not described as "farms" by the interviewer.

e. *Rural, farm*—Residence in areas defined as rural by the Census that are described as "farms" by the interviewer.

The following divisions apply to all studies:

a. *Large urban*—Residence in the urban areas of the ten largest SMSAs.

b. *Other urban*—All other urban residences.

c. *Rural, nonfarm*—Same as (d) for 1970.

d. *Rural, farm*—same as (e) for 1970.

53. **Severity of Illness**
    Each diagnosis or condition for which an individual was seen during 1970 was rated by a panel of five physicians according to whether the care provided was: (1) preventive or reassurance only; (2) for symptomatic relief; (3) for a condition for which a physician should be seen; (4) for a condition for which a physician must be seen. Diagnoses falling into categories (1) and (2) are classified as elective; those falling into categories (3) and (4) are classified as mandatory.

54. **Sex**
    In those few cases where the interviewer did not specify the sex of a sample member, classification was made in the office on the basis of name or other information provided in the interview or the interviewer and/or respondent was contacted again for the correct classification.

55. **Surgical-Medical Insurance**
    This is health insurance designed to pay all or part of the surgeon's bill in or outside of the hospital. In addition, the medical portion of the insurance pays for visits of a physician other than for surgery when the patient is hospitalized. Major medical insurance is considered surgical insurance. Medicare, Part B, and CHAMPUS are considered surgical medical insurance.

56. **Surgical Procedure, In-Hospital**
    Any cutting procedure (including cesarean deliveries but not normal deliveries) or setting of a dislocation or fracture performed on a hospital inpatient. Endoscopic procedures, suturing of wounds and circumcision of newborn infants, often classified as surgical procedures, are not so classified in this study. A few exceptions were made when the suturing was so extensive as to require an operating room or blood transfusions. Dentists performing inpatient procedures are included here rather than in dental care. Person-year is defined in 40.

57. **Surgical Specialty**
    This is a specialty for a physician doing surgery as reported in the *AMA Directory* (AMA, 1969). The physician need not be board-certified in his specialty and may report it as a secondary specialty rather than a primary one. Osteopaths are excluded from the analysis along with any other unidentified surgeons. The following are considered surgical specialists: general surgery, orthopedic surgery, plastic surgery, neurological surgery, thoracic surgery, colon and rectal surgery, urology, obstetrics

and gynecology, ophthalmology, and otolaryngology. All other specialties are classified as not involving surgery. General practitioners are classified as "no specialty reported."

For American board certification, the above rules apply except that the physician must be board-certified in a surgical specialty. Those physicians who claim a surgical specialty but are not board-certified in it are classified as "not certified for surgery."

Appendix IV

Questionnaire
and Verification
Forms

The questionnaire shown in this report has been altered from the one actually used in the field to the extent that answer space for more than one family member, wage earner and insurance policy does not appear in this edited version. In each case the deleted material exactly replicates that shown here. The other data collection forms included here have been reproduced in their entirety.

NORC-4106
Jan., 1971

Form approved.
OMB No. 68 - S70089

National Opinion Research Center
University of Chicago

BEGIN DECK 10

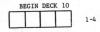

1-4

HOUSEHOLD ENUMERATION FOLDER AND SCREENER

CONFIDENTIAL

FAMILY NAME: _____

ADDRESS: _____

      (City)   (State)   (Zip Code)

Segment No.		5-11
Line No.		12-15
Sample Letter		16
Family Unit No.		17

CIRCLE ONE:

Located on farm 1   18/9

Non-farm: single family house . . . 2

Non-farm: duplex or two-family
    structure 3

Non-farm: multi-unit structure
    (e.g., apartment) . . . 4

CIRCLE ONE:

Inside largest city in the
    primary unit 5   19/9

In a suburb of the largest city
    in a primary sampling unit 6

In the outskirts (including nearby
    small towns of the primary
    sampling units) 7

In open country 8

RECORD OF ALL CALLS FOR HOUSEHOLD			
Call	Date	Time	Results
1			
2			
3			
4			
5			
6			
7			
8			

INTRODUCTION: Hello, I'm from the National Opinion Research Center. You were recently sent a letter from the Center for Health Administration Studies of the University of Chicago about the nation-wide study we are doing of health practices and the costs of medical care. To start, I'd like to know who lives here.

1. Who is the head of your household? ENTER NAME ON THE FIRST LINE IN COL. 1 OF THE TABLE BELOW.

2. Who else lives in your household?
   ENTER NAME OF EACH IN COL. 1, AND LIST RELATIONSHIP TO HEAD IN COL. 2, BEFORE GOING ON TO THE NEXT
   PERSON. LIST NAMES IN THE FOLLOWING ORDER: HEAD'S SPOUSE; UNMARRIED CHILDREN; MARRIED CHILDREN,
   THEIR SPOUSES AND OFFSPRING; OTHER RELATIVES; PERSONS UNRELATED TO ANYONE IN HEAD'S FAMILY.

   Have we missed anyone? Children or babies? Someone away for a short time--on vacation or business?
   A lodger or roomer? LIST BELOW.

3. A. ENTER "1" UNDER "FAMILY UNIT" (COL. 3) FOR HEAD, HEAD'S SPOUSE, UNMARRIED CHILDREN, AND MARRIED
      CHILDREN AND OTHER RELATIVES NOT NOW LIVING WITH THEIR SPOUSES.

   B. ENTER "2," "3," ETC. TO INDICATE ADDITIONAL FAMILY UNITS FOR:
      MARRIED COUPLES RELATED TO HEAD, WITH BOTH PARTNERS NOW LIVING IN THE HOUSEHOLD (AND THEIR
      UNMARRIED CHILDREN);
      PERSONS UNRELATED TO HEAD'S FAMILY.

   C. TRANSFER UNRELATED PERSONS TO Q. 3 TABLE ON ANOTHER FOLDER. ENTER FAMILY UNIT # GIVEN HERE ON
      COVER PAGE OF THEIR FOLDER. CONDUCT SEPARATE INTERVIEW BEGINNING WITH Q. 4. DRAW A LINE THROUGH
      THEIR NAMES ON TABLE BELOW.

PEOPLE IN HOUSEHOLD NOW OR ONLY TEMPORARILY AWAY

1. NAME		2.	3.
First	Last	Relation to HEAD	Family Unit No.
		HEAD	

4. ASK 4A AND 4B FOR EVERY HOUSEHOLD.

   A. Did any relative live with you during the past year--during 1970--who has since died, is away at
      school, or the service, or who isn't living with you now?

      Yes (ENTER NAME OF EACH RELATIVE IN
           SEPARATE COLUMN ON MIDDLE OF
           PAGE 3, AND CIRCLE "A" BEFORE NAME) . 1

      No 2

   B. Did any member of this family live with some other relative in the past year?

      Yes (ENTER NAME OF EACH "OTHER" RELA-
           TIVE IN SEPARATE COLUMN ON MIDDLE OF
           PAGE 3, AND CIRCLE "B" BEFORE NAME) . 3

      No 4

   IF "YES" TO 4A OR 4B, ASK Q. 5 FOR EACH NAME.

   IF "NO" TO BOTH 4A AND 4B, SKIP TO THE DIRECTIONS AT THE BOTTOM OF PAGE 3.

CODE RESPONSES TO QUESTIONS 5, 6, 7, 8 AND 9 IN THE APPROPRIATE NAME COLUMN BELOW.

5. How is (PERSON) related to present household head? IF NO RELATION TO <u>ANYONE IN FAMILY</u>, DRAW A LINE THROUGH NAME--GO NO FURTHER WITH PERSON. IF RELATED, ASK 6.

6. Where is this person now? IF "IN OTHER HOUSEHOLD," DRAW A LINE THROUGH NAME--GO NO FURTHER WITH PERSON. OTHERWISE ASK 7.

7. <u>Just</u> before (PERSON) (died/was institutionalized/entered the armed forces/left the U.S.) was (he/she) living with any of you who are now in this family? IF "NO," DRAW A LINE THROUGH NAME--GO NO FURTHER WITH PERSON. IF "YES," ASK 8.

8. How many months during the past year was (PERSON) in the same household as any family member(s)? ENTER NUMBER OF MONTHS. IF STUDENT IN DORMITORY, ENTER "12" WITHOUT ASKING.

9. ENTER "1," "2," ETC., GIVING THIS PERSON THE SAME FAMILY UNIT NUMBER AS THOSE HE LIVED WITH OR THOSE WHO LIVED WITH HIM.

PEOPLE NOT IN HOUSEHOLD NOW

4. A OR B. Name:	4. A OR B. Name:	4. A OR B. Name:	4. A OR B. Name:

5. Relation to
   Head (SPECIFY) . . 1
 	
   No relation (STOP). 2
	5. Relation to
	   Head (SPECIFY) . . 1
	
	   No relation (STOP). 2
		5. Relation to
		   Head (SPECIFY) . . 1
		
		   No relation (STOP). 2
			5. Relation to
			   Head (SPECIFY) . . 1
			
			   No relation (STOP). 2

6. In other house-
   hold (STOP) . . . 3
   Dead 4
   School dorm.⌉
   Institution
   Armed Forces ⌡ . . 5
   Outside U.S.
   Other, D.K.
	6. In other house-
	   hold (STOP) . . . 3
	   Dead 4
	   School dorm.⌉
	   Institution
	   Armed Forces ⌡ . . 5
	   Outside U.S.
	   Other, D.K.
		6. In other house-
		   hold (STOP) 3
		   Dead 4
		   School dorm.⌉
		   Institution
		   Armed Forces ⌡ . . . 5
		   Outside U.S.
		   Other, D.K.
			6. In other house-
			   hold (STOP) . . . 3
			   Dead 4
			   School dorm.⌉
			   Institution
			   Armed Forces ⌡ . . 5
			   Outside U.S.
			   Other, D.K.

7. Yes 1
   No . .(STOP) . . . 2
	7. Yes 1
	   No . . .(STOP) . . 2
		7. Yes 1
		   No . . .(STOP) . . 2
			7. Yes 1
			   No . . (STOP). . . 2

8. No. months: _____	8. No. months: _____	8. No. months: _____	8. No. months: _____
9. Family unit: _____	9. Family unit: _____	9. Family unit: _____	9. Family unit: _____

NOW TRANSFER TO SEPARATE ENUMERATION FOLDERS ALL MEMBERS OF ADDITIONAL FAMILY UNITS ("2" FAMILY, "3" FAMILY, ETC.) AS RECORDED IN ITEMS 3 AND/OR 9.

SEPARATE INTERVIEWS WILL BE CONDUCTED WITH EACH FAMILY UNIT BEGINNING WITH Q. 10 OF ITS ENUMERATION FOLDER.

ASK Q. 10 ON THE BACK OF <u>THIS</u> FOLDER FOR THE <u>FIRST</u> FAMILY UNIT - IDENTIFY THIS FAMILY UNIT AS "1" IN THE BOX ON THE COVER PAGE OF THE FOLDER.

IDENTIFY ADDITIONAL FAMILY UNITS ON THE COVER PAGE OF THEIR FOLDERS AS "2," "3," ETC.

0. Now I need some general information about each of the family members.
   LIST BELOW NAMES OF FAMILY UNIT MEMBERS ASSIGNED THE SAME NUMBER IN Q'S. 3 AND 9. LIST HEAD OF FAMILY UNIT FIRST.

   A. How old was (PERSON) on December 31, 1970? ENTER YEARS ONLY UNLESS INFANT UNDER ONE YEAR. ENTER MONTHS ONLY FOR INFANT UNDER ONE YEAR. INFANTS BORN IN DECEMBER 1970 ARE ONE MONTH OLD; INFANTS BORN IN 1971 ARE "00" MONTHS.

   B. RECORD SEX FOR EACH.

BEGIN DECK 20   BEGIN DECK 20

Full Name	Per.No.	A. Age 11-12 Years	13-14 Months	B. Sex 15 M F	Full Name	Per.No.	A. Age 11-12 Years	13-14 Months	B. Sex 15 M F
	5-6					5-6			
HEAD	0 1			1 2		0 7			1 2
	0 2			1 2		0 8			1 2
	0 3			1 2		0 9			1 2
	0 4			1 2		1 0			1 2
	0 5			1 2		1 1			1 2
	0 6			1 2		1 2			1 2

RECORD FAMILY'S TOTAL SIZE . . . . ☐☐

CONTINUE DECK 10
20-21

HOW TO PROCEED:

SEE FRONT OF FOLDER FOR SAMPLE LETTER ASSIGNED TO THIS LINE NUMBER.

IF SAMPLE LETTER IS . . U, A, or R . . ENTER NAME OF MAIN RESPONDENT(S) IN BOX BELOW,
                                       AND GO TO "REGULAR INTRODUCTION" ON MAIN QUESTIONNAIRE.

IF SAMPLE LETTER IS . . . . S . . . . ASK Q. 11 (SCREENING QUESTION).

11. Was the monthly income during 1970 for your family, before taxes, <u>more</u> or <u>less</u> than (MONTHLY FIGURE FOR THIS SIZE FAMILY ON CHART)? READ YEARLY OR WEEKLY INCOME FIGURES IF EASIER FOR RESPONDENT TO ESTIMATE.

Family Size	Monthly	Yearly	Weekly
1	$220	$2,600	$ 50
2	310	3,700	70
3	370	4,500	85
4	470	5,700	110
5	550	6,600	130
6	620	7,500	145
7+	760	9,100	175

More . . . . (GO TO A). 1   22/9

Less or Same (ENTER NAME OF MAIN RESPONDENT(S) IN BOX BELOW AND GO TO "REGULAR INTRODUCTION" ON MAIN QUESTIONNAIRE) 2

A. <u>IF MORE:</u> CHECK AGES IN Q. 10 ABOVE.
   IF ONE OR MORE FAMILY MEMBERS IS 66 OR OVER - ENTER NAME OF MAIN RESPONDENT(S) IN BOX BELOW AND GO TO "66+ INTRODUCTION" ON MAIN QUESTIONNAIRE 3   23/9

   IF NO MEMBER IS 66 OR OVER - END CONTACT: "There are no further questions. Thank you very much for your cooperation." 4

MAIN RESPONDENT(S)
"I'd like to talk to the person who knows the most about the health care and medical costs for (your family) (PERSON[S] 66 OR OVER) during the last year."
NAME: _____ PERSON NO. _____   24-25/
NAME: _____ PERSON NO. _____   26-27/

NORC-4106
Jan., 1971

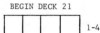

Form approved.
OMB No. 68 - S70089

National Opinion Research Center
University of Chicago

BEGIN DECK 21

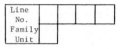

1-4

MAIN QUESTIONNAIRE

CONFIDENTIAL

TIME INTERVIEW[.]		
BEGAN: _____ AM		
PM		

Line No.				
Family Unit				

Family Name: _____

REGULAR INTRODUCTION FOR ALL HOUSEHOLDS EXCEPT "66+":

We're going to talk about the different kinds of medical care each person now in the family may have had during 1970. I want to find out about the care and expenses (READ NAME OF EACH PERSON NOW IN THE FAMILY UNIT, INCLUDING ANY STUDENT LIVING AT SCHOOL IN GROUP QUARTERS) had for the whole year 1970.

IF SOMEONE WAS IN THE FAMILY UNIT ONLY PART OF 1970: I also need to know about the medical care and expenses (READ NAME OF EACH PERSON OUT OF THE FAMILY UNIT FOR PART OF 1970) had while living with you during 1970.

INTRODUCTION FOR "66+" HOUSEHOLDS ONLY:

We're going to talk about the different kinds of medical care each person 66 or over now in the family may have had during 1970. I want to find out about the care and expenses (READ NAME OF EACH PERSON NOW IN THE FAMILY UNIT 66 OR OVER) had for the whole year 1970.

IF SOMEONE 66 OR OVER WAS IN THE FAMILY UNIT ONLY PART OF 1970: I (also) need to know about the medical care and expenses (READ NAME OF EACH PERSON 66 OR OVER OUT OF THE FAMILY UNIT FOR PART OF 1970) had while living with you during 1970.

ENTER IN SEPARATE COLUMNS NAME, PERSON NUMBER, AND AGE OF EACH FAMILY MEMBER LISTED IN Q. 10 OF ENUMERATION FOLDER <u>EXCEPT</u> BABY BORN DURING 1970 OR AFTER. RECORD INFORMATION SEPARATELY FOR EACH MEMBER.	Name: <u> </u> Per.No. 5-6

FOR "66+ HH'S" ENTER ONLY THOSE MEMBERS 66 OR OVER.	Age: <u> </u>

PRACTITIONERS	BEGIN DECK 21
1. Is there a particular medical person or clinic (PERSON) usually goes to when sick, or for advice about health? IF "NO" TO FINAL MEMBER, SKIP TO Q. 9.	Yes (ASK 2-8) . 1 $\underline{11}$ 9 No or don't know (ASK 1 NM) . 2
2. Is that a clinic, a regular family doctor, some type of specialist, an osteopath, a chiropractor, or what? CODE ONE.	Clinic (ASK A). 1 $\underline{12}$ 9 Family doctor (ASK B) . . . 2 Specialist (ASK B) . . . 3 Osteopath . . . (ASK B) . . . 4 Chiropractor (ASK B) . . . 5 Other (SPECIFY) (ASK A OR B) . 6 Don't know (GO TO 3) . . 7
A. <u>IF CLINIC</u>: Does (PERSON) go to a particular doctor at this clinic?	Yes . . . . . . 1 $\underline{13}$ 9 No 2
B. <u>IF ANY DOCTOR</u>: Is the doctor part of a clinic, or group practice?	Yes . . . . . . 3 $\underline{14}$ 9 No 4

3. A. What is the name of the (doctor and/or clinic)?
      FILL IN BOTH THE DOCTOR'S NAME AND NAME OF CLINIC OR
      GROUP IF POSSIBLE.
 	
    B. What is the address?
	
	Full Name of Doctor
	
	Name of Clinic/Group
	
	Street
	
	City
	
	State & Zip $\underline{15-24}$ 9

ENTER IN SEPARATE COLUMNS NAME, PERSON NUMBER, AND AGE OF EACH
FAMILY MEMBER LISTED IN Q. 10 OF ENUMERATION FOLDER <u>EXCEPT</u> BABY BORN
DURING 1970 OR AFTER. RECORD INFORMATION SEPARATELY FOR EACH MEMBER.

Name: Per.No.   5-6

Age: _____

FOR "66+ HH'S" ENTER ONLY THOSE MEMBERS 66 OR OVER.

4. How does (PERSON) usually get there?
CODE THE METHOD OF TRANSPORTATION USED MOST OFTEN.

DECK 21

Goes in own or family car .	. . . . 1 <u>25</u>
Goes in someone else's car	. . . . 2 9
Goes in a taxi	 3
Takes public transportation	 4
Walks	 5
Other (SPECIFY)	 6

5. How long does it usually take (PERSON) to get there from
home, the way (he/she) usually goes?

Less than 15 minutes . . .	. . . . 1 <u>26</u>
15 to 30 minutes	. . . . 2 9
Over 1/2 hour to 1 hour . .	 3
Over 1 hour to 2 hours . .	 4
Over 2 hours to 4 hours . .	 5
Over 4 hours	 6

6. Does (PERSON) usually have an appointment ahead of time
when (he/she) goes to (PLACE) or does (he/she) just
walk in?

Has an appoint-
ment (ASK 7)   1   <u>27</u>
Walks in   9
(SKIP TO 8).   2

7. Except for emergencies, how long does (PERSON) usually
have to wait to get an appointment with the doctor?

Same day	. . . . 1 <u>28</u>
1 to 2 days	. . . . 2 9
3 to 4 days	 3
5 days to 1 week	 4
Over 1 week to 2 weeks . .	 5
Over 2 weeks to 1 month . .	 6
Over 1 month	 7

8. How long does (PERSON) usually have to wait to see the
doctor, once (he/she) gets there?

Seen immediately	. . . . 1 <u>29</u>
Less than 15 minutes . . .	. . . . 2 9
15 to 30 minutes	 3
Over 1/2 hour to 1 hour . .	 4
Over 1 to 2 hours	 5
Over 2 to 4 hours	 6
Over 4 hours	 7

RETURN TO Q 1 NM

ENTER IN SEPARATE COLUMNS NAME, PERSON NUMBER, AND AGE OF EACH FAMILY MEMBER LISTED IN Q. 10 OF ENUMERATION FOLDER <u>EXCEPT</u> BABY BORN DURING 1970 OR AFTER. RECORD INFORMATION SEPARATELY FOR EACH MEMBER.

Name: Per.No. 5-6

FOR "66+ HH'S" ENTER ONLY THOSE MEMBERS 66 OR OVER.

Age: _____

DECK 21

PREGNANCIES

IF "66+ HH," SKIP TO Q. 12.

9. REVIEW QUESTION 10 ON HOUSEHOLD ENUMERATION FOLDER. IF THERE WAS A BABY BORN DURING 1970 (01-12 IN "MONTHS"), CODE "1" IN MOTHER'S COLUMN. IF INFANT BORN DURING 1971 (00 IN "MONTHS"), CODE "2" IN MOTHER'S COLUMN.

Born 1970 (GO TO PAST PREGNANCY SUPPLEMENT) . . 1

IF <u>NO</u> INFANT BORN IN 1970 OR 1971 (NO 00-12 IN "MONTHS"), CODE HERE AND GO TO INSTRUCTION BEFORE Q. 10.

No baby born in 1970 or 1971 3

Born 1971 (GO TO CURRENT PREGNANCY SUPPLEMENT) . . 2

IF THERE IS A FEMALE BETWEEN 14 AND 45 IN THE FAMILY, ASK Q. 10.

IF NO FEMALE 14-45, SKIP TO Q. 12.

10. Were there any (other) pregnancies in the family during 1970? I'm interested in <u>all</u> pregnancies including current ones and any that ended in a miscarriage or were terminated.

Yes (ASK 11) . 1

IF "YES," CODE "1" IN (EACH) MOTHER'S COLUMN AND ASK Q. 11 FOR EACH.

IF NO (OTHER) PREGNANCIES IN FAMILY, SKIP TO Q. 12.

11. Was (MOTHER) still pregnant at the end of last year, that is on December 31, 1970?

Yes (GO TO CURRENT PREG-NANCY SUP-PLEMENT). . . . 1

No (GO TO PAST PREG-NANCY

AFTER ALL PREGNANCY SUPPLEMENTS REQUIRED FOR THIS FAMILY ARE FILLED OUT, GO TO Q. 12.

SUPPLEMENT) . . 2

30/9

31/9

32-57/R

ENTER IN SEPARATE COLUMNS NAME, PERSON NUMBER, AND AGE OF EACH
FAMILY MEMBER LISTED IN Q. 10 OF ENUMERATION FOLDER EXCEPT BABY BORN
DURING 1970 OR AFTER. RECORD INFORMATION SEPARATELY FOR EACH MEMBER.

Name: ____ Per.No. 5-6

FOR "66+ HH'S" ENTER ONLY THOSE MEMBERS 66 OR OVER.

Age: ____

HOSPITALIZATION

DECK 21

12. Has (PERSON) ever been a patient in a hospital, sanatorium,
convalescent or nursing home (apart from having a baby)?

IF "NO" TO FINAL MEMBER, GO TO Q. 15.

Yes (ASK 13-
14) 1   58
No (ASK 12   9
NM) 2

13. How many times has (PERSON) been a patient in one of
these places (apart from having a baby)?

Times . [ ]   59-60
                  99

14. Was (PERSON) a patient in one of these places (apart
from having a baby) during 1970?

Yes (RET. TO
12 NM) . . . 1
No (RET. TO
12 NM) . . . 2

15. FILL OUT A HOSPITAL SUPPLEMENT (PINK) FOR EACH MEMBER CODED
"YES" IN Q. 14. CODE IN EACH MEMBER'S COLUMN WHETHER OR NOT
ANY HOSPITAL SUPPLEMENTS ARE FILLED OUT FOR THAT PERSON.

Hosp. Supp.
filled out . 1   61
No Hosp. Supp.
filled out . 2   62

MAJOR ILLNESS

16. During the last year did (PERSON) have any (other) illness,
accident, or condition for which doctors--that is, M.D.'s--
or osteopaths were seen five or more times?

Yes (ASK 16
NM) 4
No (ASK 17) . 5

17. Did (PERSON) have any (other) illness, condition or accident
for which the charges were as much as $100 altogether for
doctor's care, medicine, treatments, and so on during 1970?

Yes (RET. TO
16 NM) . . . 7
No (ASK 18) . 8

18. Did (PERSON) have any (other) one long standing medical condition for which (he/she) used regular care or medicines in the
past year (things like high blood pressure, heart condition,
arthritis, sinus trouble, or diabetes)?

Yes (RET. TO
16 NM) . . . 1
No (RET. TO
16 NM) . . . 2

19. FILL OUT MAJOR ILLNESS SUPPLEMENT(S) (BLUE) FOR EACH MEMBER
WITH A "YES" CODED IN Q'S. 16, 17, OR 18. CODE IN EACH
MEMBER'S COLUMN WHETHER OR NOT ANY MAJOR ILLNESS SUPPLEMENTS
ARE FILLED OUT FOR THAT PERSON.

Maj. Ill.
Supp(s).
filled out . 4
No Maj. Ill.
Supp. . . . 5

63-64/99

MINOR CONDITIONS

20. Did (PERSON) see a doctor, or visit any doctor's office or
clinic last year, for any (other) illness or condition? How
about for routine check-ups, shots, or tests? IF "NO" TO
FINAL MEMBER, GO TO Q. 28.

Yes (ASK 21-
24) 1   65
No (ASK 20   9
NM) 2

21. For what reason did (PERSON) see a doctor? Any other
reasons?

66-68/

69-71/

72-74/

ENTER IN SEPARATE COLUMNS NAME, PERSON NUMBER, AND AGE OF EACH
FAMILY MEMBER LISTED IN Q. 10 OF ENUMERATION FOLDER <u>EXCEPT</u> BABY BORN
DURING 1970 OR AFTER.   RECORD INFORMATION SEPARATELY FOR EACH MEMBER.

Name:	Per.No.	5-6

FOR "66+ HH'S" ENTER ONLY THOSE MEMBERS 66 OR OVER.

Age: _____

BEGIN DECK 22

22. A. What is the name of the doctor or place that
    provided the most care for (CONDITION[S] MENTIONED
    in Q. 21)?   FILL IN <u>BOTH</u> DOCTOR'S NAME AND NAME OF
    CLINIC, IF POSSIBLE.

    <u>IF SOURCE ALREADY MENTIONED</u>, ENTER NAME(S) AND GO
    TO Q. 23.
    <u>IF NEW SOURCE</u>, ASK B, AND C <u>OR</u> D.

    B. What is the address?

Full Name of Doctor
_____

Name of Clinic/Group
_____

Street
_____

City
_____

State and Zip   11-20
                    9

    C. <u>IF NEW CLINIC MENTIONED</u>: Does (PERSON) go to a
       particular doctor at the clinic?

Yes (ENTER NAME OF
   DOCTOR ABOVE). 1
No 2

    D. <u>IF NEW DOCTOR MENTIONED</u>: Is the doctor part of a
       clinic or group practice?

Yes (ENTER NAME OF
   CLINIC ABOVE). 3   21
No 4   R

23. A. At which of these
       places did visits to
       (SOURCE NAMED IN Q.22)
       take place?
       CIRCLE ALL THAT
       APPLY IN PERSON'S
       COLUMN A.

    CARD
    B

    <u>ASK B AND C FOR EACH
    PLACE CODED IN A:</u>

    B. How many visits
       were there during
       1970 at (PLACE IN
       COLUMN A)? ENTER
       VISITS IN COLUMN B.

    C. What was the cost
       for the visits at
       (PLACE IN COLUMN A),
       including anything
       that insurance paid?
       ENTER COSTS IN
       COLUMN C.

A. Place	B. Number of Visits	C. Cost $
Doctor at your home 1		22-28/9
Doctor's office or private clinic (including group practice plans) 2		29-35/9
Hospital out-patient department 3		36-42/9
Hospital emergency room . . . 4		43-49/9
Industrial, school, camp, or college health service . . 5		50-56/9
Any other clinic not connected with a hospital--such as a Board of Health clinic or a neighborhood health center . 6		57-63/9

64-70/R

24. Did (PERSON) visit any <u>other</u> doctor or clinic in
    the past year, for care we have not yet talked about?
    IF "NO" TO FINAL MEMBER, SKIP TO Q. 28.

Yes (ASK 25-27). 1   71
No (RET. TO   9
   Q.20 NM) . . 2

ENTER IN SEPARATE COLUMNS NAME, PERSON NUMBER, AND AGE OF EACH
FAMILY MEMBER LISTED IN Q. 10 OF ENUMERATION FOLDER <u>EXCEPT</u> BABY BORN
DURING 1970 OR AFTER. RECORD INFORMATION SEPARATELY FOR EACH MEMBER.

Name:	Per.No. 5-6

FOR "66+ HH'S" ENTER ONLY THOSE MEMBERS 66 OR OVER.

Age: _____

25. A. What is the name of the <u>other</u> doctor or place that (PERSON) visited? FILL IN <u>BOTH</u> DOCTOR'S NAME AND NAME OF CLINIC, IF POSSIBLE.	BEGIN DECK 23
	Full Name of Doctor
IF SOURCE ALREADY MENTIONED, ENTER NAME(S) AND GO TO Q. 26. IF NEW SOURCE, ASK B, AND C <u>OR</u> D.	Name of Clinic/Group
	Street
B. What is the address?	City
	State and Zip 11-20 9
C. IF NEW CLINIC MENTIONED: Does (PERSON) go to a particular doctor at the clinic?	Yes (ENTER NAME OF DOCTOR ABOVE). 1 No 2
D. IF NEW DOCTOR MENTIONED: Is the doctor part of a clinic or group practice?	Yes (ENTER NAME OF CLINIC ABOVE). 3 21 No . . . . 4 R

26. A. At which of these places did visits to (SOURCE NAMED IN Q.25) take place? CIRCLE ALL THAT APPLY IN PERSON'S COLUMN A.

CARD B

ASK B AND C FOR EACH PLACE CODED IN A:

B. How many visits were there during 1970 at (PLACE IN COLUMN A)? ENTER VISITS IN COLUMN B.

C. What was the cost for the visits at (PLACE IN COLUMN A), including anything that insurance paid? ENTER COSTS IN COLUMN C.

	A. Place	B. Number of Visits	C. Cost $
Doctor at your home	1		22-28/9
Doctor's office or private clinic (including group practice plans)	2		29-35/9
Hospital out-patient department	3		36-42/9
Hospital emergency room . . .	4		43-49/9
Industrial, school, camp, or college health service . .	5		50-56/9
Any other clinic not connected with a hospital--such as a Board of Health clinic or a neighborhood health center .	6		57-63/9 64-70/R

27. Did (PERSON) visit any <u>other</u> doctor or clinic in the past year, for care we have not yet talked about? IF NO TO FINAL MEMBER, GO TO Q. 28.	Yes (USE DR. CONTINU-ATION SHEET). . .1 71 No (RET.TO 20 NM).2 9

ENTER IN SEPARATE COLUMNS NAME, PERSON NUMBER, AND AGE OF EACH
FAMILY MEMBER LISTED IN Q. 10 OF ENUMERATION FOLDER <u>EXCEPT</u> BABY BORN
DURING 1970 OR AFTER. RECORD INFORMATION SEPARATELY FOR EACH MEMBER.

Name: _____

Per.No. _5-6_

Age: _____

FOR "66+ HH'S" ENTER ONLY THOSE MEMBERS 66 OR OVER.

BEGIN DECK 24

28. Apart from anything talked about so far, did anyone in the
family get care in the last year from any <u>other</u> kind of prac-
titioner--such as these? CODE EACH MEMBER'S COLUMN.
ASK Q. 29 FOR EACH MEMBER CODED "YES." THEN GO TO Q. 30.

CARD E

Yes (ASK 29) . . 1 _11_
No 2   9

29. A. What kind of practitioner
did (PERSON) see? Any
other kinds? CODE ALL
THAT APPLY, IN PERSON'S
COLUMN A.

ASK B & C FOR EACH KIND
CODED IN A:

B. How many visits
altogether did
(PERSON) have with
a (KIND OF PRAC-
TITIONER)? CODE
VISITS IN COL. B.

C. What was the cost
for (that/those)
visit(s)?
CODE COSTS IN
COL. C.

	A. Kind	B. Number of Visits	C. Cost $	
Physical therapist	1			12-18/9
Clinical psychologist . . .	2			19-25/9
Chiropractor	3			26-32/9
Chiropodist, podiatrist . .	4			33-39/9
Visiting nurse	5			40-46/9
Naturopath, naprapath . . .	6			47-53/9
Homeopath	7			54-60/9
Christian Science practitioner	8			61-67/9
Other (SPECIFY)	9			68-74/9

30. Besides what we have already talked about, did anyone get any:
medical tests (X-rays, blood tests, electrocardiograms, or
urine analysis)--special treatments (heat treatments, massages,
allergy shots, X-ray treatments)--medical appliances (hearing
aids, crutches, braces, wheel chair)? CODE EACH MEMBER'S
COLUMN. ASK 31-32 FOR EACH MEMBER CODED "YES." THEN GO TO 33.

BEGIN DECK 25
Yes (ASK 31-32) . 1 _11_
No 2   9

12-13/99
14-15/99
16-17/99
18-19/99

31. What did (PERSON) get? IF GLASSES MENTIONED,
RECORD GLASSES AND COSTS IN Q. 44.

32. How much was the cost altogether, including what you paid
and anything insurance paid?

$: ☐☐☐ 20-22
999

23-28/R

ENTER IN SEPARATE COLUMNS NAME, PERSON NUMBER, AND AGE OF EACH
FAMILY MEMBER LISTED IN Q. 10 OF ENUMERATION FOLDER <u>EXCEPT</u> BABY BORN
DURING 1970 OR AFTER. RECORD INFORMATION SEPARATELY FOR EACH MEMBER.

Name: ____   Per.No. ☐☐ 5-6

| FOR "66+ HH'S" ENTER ONLY THOSE MEMBERS 66 OR OVER. |

Age: ____

DECK 25

33. Did (PERSON) take any medicines last year that were
prescribed for (him/her) by a doctor--other than any we've
counted already?

Yes . (ASK A) . 1   29/9

No (ASK 33 NM) 2

  A. <u>IF YES</u>: What was the cost for those medicines--including
anything insurance may have paid?

$: ☐☐☐   30-32/9

34. During 1970 did (PERSON) use any medicines that were <u>not</u>
prescribed by a doctor which you have not told me about?
(I mean things like vitamins, tonics, cold pills, nose drops,
cough medicines, aspirin, and so on?)

Yes . (ASK A) . 3   33/9

No (ASK 34 NM) 4

  A. <u>IF YES</u>: About how much did these medicines cost?

$: ☐☐☐   34-36/9

35. <u>IF ANY MINOR MEDICAL EXPENSES REPORTED (FROM Q'S 20-34)</u>: Has
anyone in the family received any medical insurance benefits
in connection with any of these minor medical expenses--that
is, insurance benefits (that we haven't talked about before)
for home or office physician visits, drugs, or anything else?
CODE EACH MEMBER'S COLUMN. ASK 36-38 FOR EACH FAMILY MEMBER
CODED "YES." THEN GO TO 39.

Yes (ASK 36-38) 1   37/9

No 2

  36. Which of these expenses we've talked about did insurance
cover? RECORD ALL EXPENSES MENTIONED.

Expenses covered:
    38-39/
    40-41/

  37. What was the name of the insurance or plan that paid
the benefits? Did any other plan pay benefits?   (1)
RECORD ALL THAT ARE MENTIONED.

                                                  (2)

Name of insurance:
    42-43/9
____
    44-45/9
____

  38. About how much did (each) insurance pay on these
expenses for (PERSON)?   (1)

$: ☐☐☐☐   46-49/9

                                                  (2)

$: ☐☐☐☐   50-53/9

ENTER IN SEPARATE COLUMNS NAME, PERSON NUMBER, AND AGE OF EACH FAMILY MEMBER LISTED IN Q. 10 OF ENUMERATION FOLDER <u>EXCEPT</u> BABY BORN DURING 1970 OR AFTER. RECORD INFORMATION SEPARATELY FOR EACH MEMBER.

Name: Per. No. 5-6

Age: _____

FOR "66+ HH'S" ENTER ONLY THOSE MEMBERS 66 OR OVER.

DENTAL CARE	DECK 25

Now that we've covered medical care, I'd like to ask about other kinds of health expenses your family had in 1970.

39. Did (PERSON) have any dental care such as teeth cleaned, X-rayed, filled or pulled, or any bridge work done last year? IF "NO" TO FINAL MEMBER, GO TO Q. 44.

Yes (ASK 40-43) 1   <u>54</u>
9

No (ASK 39 NM) 2

40. How many times did (PERSON) visit a dentist's office during the past year?

Times: <u>55-56</u>
99

41. Which of the dental services shown on this card did (PERSON) receive? CODE AS MANY AS APPLY.

CARD F

a. Teeth cleaned 1   57/9

b. X-rays, examinations, or check-up 2   58/9

c. Tooth or teeth filled or inlays 3   59/9

d. Dentures, plates or bridgework made, repaired, replaced, or adjusted 4   60/9

e. Crowns (or capping) 5   61/9

f. Orthodontia (teeth straightening) 6   62/9

g. Gum treatment 7   63/9

h. Fluoride treatment 8   64/9

i. Tooth or teeth pulled 1   65/9

j. Other (SPECIFY) 2   66/9

42. About how much was (PERSON) charged for dental services last year?

$:   <u>67-70</u>
9

43. About how much, if any, of these expenses did insurance pay for?

$:   <u>71-74</u>
9

RETURN TO 39 NM

ENTER IN SEPARATE COLUMNS NAME, PERSON NUMBER, AND AGE OF EACH
FAMILY MEMBER LISTED IN Q. 10 OF ENUMERATION FOLDER <u>EXCEPT</u> BABY BORN
DURING 1970 OR AFTER. RECORD INFORMATION SEPARATELY FOR EACH MEMBER.

Name: Per.No. 5-6

FOR "66+ HH'S" ENTER ONLY THOSE MEMBERS 66 OR OVER.

Age:

OPTICAL CARE

BEGIN DECK 26

44. Did (PERSON) have any glasses made or repaired, or contact
    lenses made, or have any eye examination within the last
    year? CODE AS MANY AS APPLY.

    IF "NONE" TO FINAL MEMBER, SKIP TO Q. 50.

Glasses made
  (ASK A&B). . 1   11/9
Glasses repaired
  (ASK C) . . 2   12/9
Contacts made
  (ASK D) . . 3   13/9
Eye exam
  (ASK E) . . 4   14/9
None of these
  (ASK 44 NM). 5   15/9

ASK A-E AS APPROPRIATE:

IF GLASSES MADE: A. How many pairs did (PERSON) have
                    made last year?

A) ___ # pair   16/9

B. What was the charge for having the
   glasses made?

B) $|__|__|__| 17-20
                    9

C. IF GLASSES REPAIRED: What was the charge for
   having the glasses repaired?

C) $|__|__|__| 21-24
                    9

D. IF CONTACT LENSES MADE: What was the charge for
   the contact lenses?

D) $|__|__|__| 25-28
                    9

E. IF EYE EXAM: What was the charge for the eye
   examination?

E) $|__|__|__| 29-32
                    9

F. IF CHARGES CAN'T BE BROKEN DOWN, ENTER TOTAL HERE. ———>

F) $|__|__|__| 33-36
                    9

45. About how much, if any, of these expenses did
    insurance pay for?

$: |__|__|__|__| 37-40
                    9

46. What is the name of the individual or clinic (PERSON)
    saw for (his/her) (eye examination/glasses/lenses/etc.)?

Name of Doctor/Clinic

47. What is the address?

Street

City

State and Zip 41-50/9

48. Is this individual (clinic) an M.D. (ophthalmologist,
    oculist), an optometrist, or an optician?

M.D. 1   51
Optometrist . 2   9
Optician . . 3
Don't know . 4

49. Did (PERSON) go anywhere else for (his/her) (eye exami-
    nation/glasses/lenses/etc.)? IF YES, RECORD NAME,
    ADDRESS, AND TYPE OF PRACTIONER IN PERSON'S COLUMN.

Yes 5   52
No 6   9

RETURN TO 44 NM

ENTER IN SEPARATE COLUMNS NAME, PERSON NUMBER, AND AGE OF EACH FAMILY MEMBER LISTED IN Q. 10 OF ENUMERATION FOLDER <u>EXCEPT</u> BABY BORN DURING 1970 OR AFTER. RECORD INFORMATION SEPARATELY FOR EACH MEMBER.

Name:	Per.No. 5-6

FOR "66+ HH'S" ENTER ONLY THOSE MEMBERS 66 OR OVER.

Age:

50. IF FREE OR REDUCED RATE CARE ALREADY MENTIONED, CODE WITHOUT ASKING FOR THAT FAMILY MEMBER.

DECK 26

Aside from free samples of drugs a doctor might have given you, did anyone in the family receive any medical or dental care free of charge or at a reduced rate during 1970?

Yes (ASK
      A & B) 1   <u>53</u>
No 2   9

CODE EACH MEMBER'S COLUMN. ASK A & B FOR EACH MEMBER CODED "YES." THEN GO TO Q. 51.

A. What was the care?

54-55/

B. Which item on this card best describes the <u>main</u> reason that the care was free of charge, or at a reduced rate? CIRCLE ONE CODE ONLY, FOR MAIN REASON.

CARD
D

56-57/

On public aid (Receiving welfare payments) 01

Recipient of Medicaid (No welfare payments). 02

Went to free or part pay clinic or public hospital 03

Went to V.A. hospital for <u>non-service</u> connected
    disability 04

Private doctor or hospital didn't charge or reduced
    the bill because we couldn't pay 05

Went to V.A. hospital for <u>service</u> connected
    disability 06

Armed Forces member or dependent 07

Professional courtesy 08

Participant in medical research 09

Workmen's Compensation 10

Participant in prepaid group practice plan 11

Industrial, school, camp, or college health service 12

Other (SPECIFY) 13

<u>58-59</u>
99

ENTER IN SEPARATE COLUMNS NAME, PERSON NUMBER, AND AGE OF EACH
FAMILY MEMBER LISTED IN Q. 10 OF ENUMERATION FOLDER <u>EXCEPT</u> BABY BORN
DURING 1970 OR AFTER.   RECORD INFORMATION SEPARATELY FOR EACH MEMBER.

Name: _____   Per.No. 5-6

☐☐

| FOR "66+ HH'S" ENTER ONLY THOSE MEMBERS 66 OR OVER. |

Age: _____

FAMILY HEALTH

DECK 26

51. How long ago did (PERSON) last have a physical examination
    or check up?

Within the last 3 months	(ASK A) . . . 1
More than 3 but up to 6 months . .	(ASK A) . . . 2
More than 6 months up to 1 year .	(ASK A) . . . 3
More than 1 year up to 2 years .	(ASK A) . . . 4
More than 2 years up to 5 years	(ASK A) . . . 5
More than 5 years	(ASK A) . . . 6
Never	(ASK 51 NM) . 7

60
9

A. Which of the reasons on this card best describes why
   (PERSON) had the examination? CIRCLE ONE CODE ONLY.

CARD
 G

Not feeling good 1
Required 2
Time for examination 3

61
9

52. Would you say (PERSON)'s health, in general, is excellent,
    good, fair, or poor?

Excellent 4
Good 5
Fair 6
Poor 7

62
9

53. Over the past year has (PERSON)'s health caused a great deal
    of worry, some worry, hardly any worry, or no worry at all?

A great deal 1
Some 2
Hardly any 3
None at all 4

63
9

54. In the past year would you say (PERSON) has experienced pain
    very often, fairly often, occasionally, or not at all?

Very often 5
Fairly often 6
Occasionally 7
Not at all 8

64
9

55. As a result of illness and injury, approximately how many days
    during all of 1970 was (PERSON) kept in bed, indoors, or away
    from (his/her) usual activities?

Days: ☐☐☐

65-67
9

ENTER IN SEPARATE COLUMNS NAME, PERSON NUMBER, AND AGE OF EACH FAMILY MEMBER LISTED IN Q. 10 OF ENUMERATION FOLDER <u>EXCEPT</u> BABY BORN DURING 1970 OR AFTER. RECORD INFORMATION SEPARATELY FOR EACH MEMBER.

Name: Per.No. 5-6

| FOR "66+ HH'S" ENTER ONLY THOSE MEMBERS 66 OR OVER. | Age: |

56. Please look at the symptoms on this card, and we'll go over them together. ASK FOR EACH SYMPTOM:

CARD H

A. Did anyone have (SYMPTOM) during 1970? IF YES, ASK B FOR EACH PERSON WITH SYMPTOM. IF NO, CIRCLE "N" AND ASK ABOUT NEXT SYMPTOM.

B. <u>IF YES TO A</u>: Did (PERSON) see a doctor about it during 1970 or since the first of the year? <u>IF YES</u>, CODE "1" IN PERSON'S COLUMN. <u>IF NO OR DK</u>, ASK C.

C. <u>IF NO OR DK TO B</u>: Has (PERSON) <u>ever</u> seen a doctor about this condition or one like it? <u>IF YES</u>, CODE "2"; <u>IF NO</u>, CODE "3"; <u>IF DON'T KNOW</u>, CODE "4" IN PERSON'S COLUMN.

B.   C.   BEGIN DECK 27

OFFICE USE

		Doctor seen in 1970	Doctor seen before 1970	No doctor ever seen	DK if doctor ever seen	No answer	No symptom	
a.	Cough any time during the day or night which lasted for three weeks?	N	1	2	3	4	9	0	11/
b.	Sudden feelings of weakness or faintness?	N	1	2	3	4	9	0	12/
c.	Getting up some mornings tired and exhausted even with a usual amount of rest?	N	1	2	3	4	9	0	13/
d.	Feeling tired for weeks at a time for no special reason?	N	1	2	3	4	9	0	14/
e.	Frequent headaches?	N	1	2	3	4	9	0	15/
f.	Skin rash or breaking out on any part of the body?	N	1	2	3	4	9	0	16/
g.	Diarrhea (loose bowel movements) for four or five days?	N	1	2	3	4	9	0	17/
h.	Shortness of breath even after light work?	N	1	2	3	4	9	0	18/
i.	Waking up with stiff or aching joints or muscles?	N	1	2	3	4	9	0	19/
j.	Pains or swelling in any joint during the day?	N	1	2	3	4	9	0	20/
k.	Frequent backaches?	N	1	2	3	4	9	0	21/
l.	Unexplained loss of over ten pounds in weight?	N	1	2	3	4	9	0	22/
m.	Repeated pains in or near the heart?	N	1	2	3	4	9	0	23/
n.	Repeated indigestion or upset stomach?	N	1	2	3	4	9	0	24/
o.	Repeated vomiting for a day or more?	N	1	2	3	4	9	0	25/
p.	Sore throat or running nose with a fever as high as 100° F. for at least two days?	N	1	2	3	4	9	0	26/
q.	Nose stopped up, or sneezing, for two weeks or more?	N	1	2	3	4	9	0	27/
r.	Unexpected bleeding from any part of the body not caused by accident or injury?	N	1	2	3	4	9	0	28/
s.	Abdominal pains (pains in the belly or gut) for at least a couple of days?	N	1	2	3	4	9	0	29/
t.	Any infections, irritations, or pains in the eyes or ears?	N	1	2	3	4	9	0	30/
u.	Toothache?	N	1	2	3	4	9	0	31/
v.	Bleeding gums?	N	1	2	3	4	9	0	32/

ENTER IN SEPARATE COLUMNS NAME, PERSON NUMBER, AND AGE OF EACH FAMILY MEMBER LISTED IN Q. 10 OF ENUMERATION FOLDER <u>EXCEPT</u> BABY BORN DURING 1970 OR AFTER. RECORD INFORMATION SEPARATELY FOR EACH MEMBER.

Name: Per.No.   5-6

| FOR "66+ HH'S" ENTER ONLY THOSE MEMBERS 66 OR OVER. |

Age:

RECENT FAMILY HEALTH

DECK 27

Now, a few questions about the past <u>two weeks</u>; that is from

_____ to _____

57. Within the past two weeks, how many days did (PERSON) stay in bed all or part of the day because (he/she) was not feeling well?

Days: 33-34   99
IF 14 DAYS, SKIP TO Q. 60.

58. (Apart from the days [PERSON] stayed in bed) how many days within the last two weeks was (PERSON) not able to do the things (he/she) usually does, because (he/she) was not feeling well?

Days: 35-36   99
IF ANY NUMBER IN 57 OR 58, SKIP TO 60.

59. Within the same two weeks, how many days were there when (PERSON) was not feeling well, or when (he/she) noticed something wrong with (his/her) health?

Days: 37-38   99

60. Within the last two weeks, did (PERSON) visit or talk (on the phone) to a doctor about (his/her) health?

Yes (ASK A) . 1   39
No (RETURN TO   9
57 NM) . . 2

    A. How many times?

Times: 40-41   99
RETURN TO 57 NM

MEDICARE--INSURANCE SCREENING

I'd like to get some information about your health insurance.

<u>ASK Q'S 61-63 FOR ALL PERSONS 66 AND OVER ONLY</u>

61. Is (PERSON) covered by Medicare?

Yes (ASK 62). 1   42
             9
No (ASK 61
FOR NM 66 YRS.
OR OVER) . . 2

62. May I see (his/her) Medicare card?

Card shown
(RECORD MEDICARE   43
NUMBER). . . 3   9

#:

Card not
shown . . . 4

63. <u>IF YOU ALREADY KNOW, CODE WITHOUT ASKING</u>: Is (PERSON) covered by Part B of Medicare (the part that pays for doctors' expenses, and costs $5.30 a month)?

Yes 5   44
No 6   9

45-74
R

BEGIN DECK 11

64. IF HOSPITAL OR MEDICAL INSURANCE WAS MENTIONED EARLIER--ASIDE FROM MEDICARE-- CODE "1" AND FILL OUT INSURANCE SUPPLE-MENT.

Insurance mentioned (FILL OUT INSURANCE SUPPLEMENT) 1

No insurance men-tioned (ASK 65) . . . 2

$\underline{11}$
9

---

65. IF HOSPITAL OR MEDICAL INSURANCE HAS NOT BEEN MENTIONED: (Aside from Medicare) Do you (Does anyone here) have any kind of medical, surgical, or hospital insurance, or pre-paid health care plan that meets any part of a doctor's bill or hospital expenses; or did (any of) you have any insurance like this at any time during 1970?

Yes (FILL OUT INSURANCE SUPPLEMENT) 3

No . . (ASK 66) 4

$\underline{12}$
9

---

66. Do (any of) you belong to any organization such as a union or lodge, having a medical plan which provides for any sort of hospital care for its members--or did (any of) you belong to such an organization at any time last year?

Yes (FILL OUT INSURANCE SUPPLEMENT) 5

No . . (ASK 67) 6

$\underline{13}$
9

OTHER HEALTH EXPENDITURES

IF "66+ HOUSEHOLD," SKIP TO Q. 75.

67. Apart from any of the costs we've considered so far, did (any of) you pay any other hospital, medical or dental bills in the last year, for anyone else, either related to you or not? This would include expenses for anyone staying in a nursing home, state hospital, convalescent home, old people's home, sanatorium, or other places like that.

Yes . . (ASK 68-69) . . 1

No . . (SKIP TO 70) . . 2

$\underline{14}$
9

68. Who is this person? (What relationship to the family?) IF NOT RELATED, RECORD "FAMILY FRIEND," ETC. IF MORE THAN ONE PERSON, RECORD ALL RELATIONSHIPS.

Relationship:

$\underline{15-16}$
99
$\underline{17-18}$
99

69. How much altogether did you pay for (PERSON)'s medical bills in the last year?

A. What was the care for? _____

$ ☐☐☐☐☐

$\underline{19-23}$
9

24-25/

---

70. During the last year did anyone, either a friend or a relative--not in the family now--pay anything toward your medical expenses?

Yes . . (ASK 71-72) . . 3

No . . (SKIP TO 73) . . 4

$\underline{26}$
9

71. Who is this person? (What relationship to the family?) IF NOT RELATED, RECORD "FAMILY FRIEND," ETC. IF MORE THAN ONE PERSON, RECORD ALL RELATIONSHIPS.

Relationship:

$\underline{27-28}$
99
$\underline{29-30}$
99

72. How much did they pay toward the family's medical expenses?

A. What was the care for? _____

$ ☐☐☐☐☐

$\underline{31-35}$
9

36-37/

---

73. Do you owe anything for medical care received in 1970 or before? I mean bills that you have already gotten from hospitals, doctors, dentists, and so forth, as well as loans still to be paid that you took out to meet medical expenses?

Yes . . (ASK 74) . . . 5

No . . (SKIP TO 75) . . 6

$\underline{38}$
9

74. How much do you owe for medical expenses?

$ ☐☐☐☐☐

$\underline{39-43}$
9

FOR <u>ALL</u> HOUSEHOLDS, INCLUDING "66+ HH":
ENTER IN SEPARATE COLUMNS NAME(S) AND PERSON NO.(S) OF FAMILY MEM-
BERS 14 YEARS OF AGE AND OLDER. (IF MEMBER HAS DIED OR LEFT HOUSE-
HOLD, ASK QUESTIONS IN TERMS OF THE PERIOD IN WHICH HE OR SHE WAS
ACTUALLY IN HOUSEHOLD.)

Name:	Per.No.

Now we need a little background information on members of the
family.   BEGIN DECK 28

75. What is the highest grade or year (PERSON) has completed
     in school? IF NOT SURE OF YEAR, PROBE FOR ESTIMATE OR
     BEST GUESS.

None	 01	11-12
1-4 years	 02	99
5-6 years	 03	
7-8 years	 04	
9-11 years (some high school). .	 05	
12 years (completed high school)	 06	
13-15 (some college)	 07	
16+ (completed college or beyond)	 08	
Don't know	 09	

76. IF YOU ALREADY KNOW, CODE WITHOUT ASKING:
     Is (PERSON) currently married, separated, widowed, divorced,
     or has (PERSON) never been married?

Married . .	1	13
Separated .	2	9
Widowed . .	3	
Divorced . .	4	
Never been married .	5	

77. Which category on this card best describes (PERSON)'s
     religious preference?

CARD I			
	Catholic	 01	14-15
	Jewish	 02	99
	Baptist	 03	
	Methodist	 04	
	Presbyterian	 05	
	Episcopalian	 06	
	Lutheran	 07	
	Other Protestant (SPECIFY) . . .	 08	
	Christian Scientist	 09	
	Mormon, Seventh Day Adventist . .	 10	
	Other religion (SPECIFY)	 11	
	None	 12	
		RETURN TO 75 NM.	

FOR <u>ALL</u> HOUSEHOLDS, INCLUDING "66+ HH":
ENTER IN SEPARATE COLUMNS NAME(S) AND PERSON NO.(S) OF FAMILY MEM-
BERS 14 YEARS OF AGE AND OLDER. (IF MEMBER HAS DIED OR LEFT HOUSE-
HOLD, ASK QUESTIONS IN TERMS OF THE PERIOD IN WHICH HE OR SHE WAS
ACTUALLY IN HOUSEHOLD.)

Name: Per.No.

	EMPLOYMENT STATUS AND INCOME	DECK 28

78. Which number on this card best describes (PERSON)'s current
situation?

CARD
K

Work full time
(SKIP TO 81) . 1   <u>16</u>
Work part time   9
(SKIP TO 81) . 2
Laid off or on strike
(SKIP TO 80) . 3
Unemployed
(ASK 79) . . . 4
Retired
(ASK 79) . . . 5
Keeping house
(SKIP TO 80) . 6
Full-time
student
(SKIP TO 80) . 7
Unable to work
(ASK 79) . . . 8

79. Did (PERSON) ever have a regular job or do regular work
in (his/her) own trade, profession or business?

Yes (SKIP TO
81) 1   <u>17</u>
No (ASK 80) . . 2   9

80. Did (PERSON) earn $200 or more from working in the
last year?
     IF NO TO FINAL MEMBER, SKIP TO 88.

Yes (ASK 81-85). 3   <u>18</u>
No (RETURN TO   9
    78 NM) . . 4

81. What kind of work does (did) (PERSON) do?

Occupation: <u>19-21</u>

82. What kind of business or industry does (did) (PERSON)
work in?

Industry: <u>22-24</u>

IF RETIRED, SKIP TO 85.

83. Does (did) (PERSON) work for a private employer or
company, a government agency, or for himself?

Private employer 1   <u>25</u>
Government . . . 2   9
Own business . . 3
Other (SPECIFY) 4

84. Where does (did) (PERSON) work? RECORD NAME AND ADDRESS
OF COMPANY OR PLACE OF EMPLOYMENT.

Name

Street

City

State & Zip   <u>26-27</u>
      99

FOR <u>ALL</u> HOUSEHOLDS, INCLUDING "66+ HH":
ENTER IN SEPARATE COLUMNS NAME(S) AND PERSON NO.(S) OF FAMILY MEM-
BERS 14 YEARS OF AGE AND OLDER. (IF MEMBER HAS DIED OR LEFT HOUSE-
HOLD, ASK QUESTIONS IN TERMS OF THE PERIOD IN WHICH HE OR SHE WAS
ACTUALLY IN HOUSEHOLD.)

Name: Per.No.

85. How many weeks did (PERSON) work last year including paid vacation time? IF "0," RETURN TO 78 FOR NEXT MEMBER.

DECK 28

Weeks: <u>28-29</u>
                  99

86. About how many hours a week (does/did) (PERSON) usually
work?

Hours: <u>30-31</u>
                  99

87. How much was (PERSON)'s income from working in the past
year (after business expenses were subtracted, but) before
taxes were deducted?

$

<u>32-37/9</u>
RETURN TO 78 NM

OTHER INCOME

88. Did anyone in the family receive any income during the past
year other than what you've told me about--such as money
from any of these? CODE EACH MEMBER'S COLUMN YES OR NO.
ASK 89-90 FOR EACH MEMBER CODED "YES." THEN GO TO 91.

| CARD |
| J |

Yes (ASK
89-90) . 1   <u>38</u>
                    9
No 2

89. IF NOT VOLUNTEERED: From what source was this?
CODE AS MANY ANSWERS AS GIVEN.

a. Interest or dividends . . .	. . . . . .	1	39/9
b. Rent	. . . . . .	2	40/9
c. Social Security-Retirement .	. . . . . .	3	41/9
d. Social Security-Disabled . .	. . . . . .	4	42/9
e. Social Security-Survivors . .	. . . . . .	5	43/9
f. Private pensions	. . . . . .	6	44/9
g. Friends or relatives . . .	. . . . . .	7	45/9
h. Alimony or child support . .	. . . . . .	8	46/9
i. Armed forces allotment . . .	. . . . . .	1	47/9
j. Unemployment compensation . .	. . . . . .	2	48/9
k. Workmen's compensation . . .	. . . . . .	3	49/9
l. Public aid (Welfare)	. . . . . .	4	50/9
m. Veterans Administration . . .	. . . . . .	5	51/9
n. Other (SPECIFY)	. . . . . .	6	52/9

90. How much was (PERSON)'s income last year from these
sources? (NON-EMPLOYMENT INCOME)

$

<u>53-58/9</u>

91. <u>TOTAL ALL FAMILY INCOME (FROM Q'S 87 AND 90 EACH MEMBER). ENTER TOTAL.</u>
Then this makes the family's total income about:
Is that correct? (ADJUST WHERE REQUIRED. IF SOME
INCOME INFORMATION IS UNAVAILABLE, CHECK BOX.) ☐

$

BEGIN
DECK 12

11-16/9

17/

DECK 12

92. Do you own or rent your home?

Own . . (ASK 93) . 1 <u>18</u>
Rent . (SKIP TO 94). 2   9
Other (SPECIFY)

_____
(SKIP TO 94). 3

93. About how much is it worth today?

$: | | | | | | <u>19-24</u>
      9

| NOW SKIP TO 97. |

IF RENT OR OTHER:
94. How much is the monthly rent?

$: | | | <u>25-27</u>
   9

95. Does the rent include heating expenses?

Yes 1   <u>28</u>
No 2   9

96. Does the rent include lighting costs?

Yes 3   <u>29</u>
No 4   9

97. How long has (HEAD AND/OR SPOUSE) lived in this (neighborhood/suburb)?

Less than 6 months 1   <u>30</u>
Over 6 months, less than 1 year . . 2   9
1 to 2 years 3
Over 2 years, less than 5 years . . 4
5 years or more 5

98. May I have your telephone number, (in case my office wants to verify this interview)?
IF NO PHONE, ASK IF THERE IS A PHONE WHERE RESPONDENT CAN BE REACHED.
IF PHONE NUMBER GIVEN, CODE: PHONE LOCATED IN:

Phone No._____ 1   <u>31</u>
No phone. 2   9
Refused . 3

Respondent's home 4   <u>32</u>
Home of neighbor 5   9
 ⟵ Other (SPECIFY) 6

GIVE ONE <u>HEALTH OPINIONS</u> QUESTIONNAIRE TO EACH HOUSEHOLD HEAD AND SPOUSE.
(FOR "66+ HH" GIVE TO EACH PERSON 66 AND OVER, IF HOUSEHOLD HEAD OR SPOUSE.)
Up to this point we've been talking about <u>facts</u>. To finish the interview I'd like to ask your <u>opinion</u> about some matters related to health. Please mark your answers on this form.
BE SURE TO LEAVE A FORM FOR EACH ABSENT HEAD AND SPOUSE.

HEALTH INFORMATION PERMISSION FORM

YOU ARE TO OBTAIN A SIGNED PERMISSION FORM FOR EVERY FAMILY UNIT INTERVIEWED.
<u>ASK FOR AUTHORIZATION</u>: "Doctors, hospitals, and providers of health insurance are also interested in our study. We will be asking them a few questions about charges for medical care and insurance coverage for families in our sample. Just so they know it's all right with you, please sign this permission form. (Any information we collect is of course completely confidential and will be used for statistical purposes only.)"

Form signed 1   <u>33</u>
Will mail 2   9
Oral permission only 3
Refused permission (RECORD REASON GIVEN BELOW) 4

IN THE EVENT THAT THE RESPONDENT WILL GIVE PERMISSION FOR CERTAIN SOURCES AND NOT OTHERS, LIST BELOW THOSE SOURCES WHO SHOULD <u>NOT</u> BE CONTACTED.

Name   Q. Number

                                                            34-35/9

_____   _____   36-37/9

_____   _____   38-39/9

_____   _____

INTERVIEWER'S SUMMARY   DECK 12

TIME		AM
ENDED:	————	PM

Health Opinion   Male head . . 1
Quex <u>left</u> for: Female head . 2
                 Wife of head . 3
                 None left . . 4

Date interview completed: _____   40-43
                                           9
Total time required   44-46
  for interview: _____   9
Signature of
  interviewer: _____

1. What was the race of the main respondent?

White 1   47
Black 2   9
Oriental 3

2. Is the main respondent Puerto Rican, Mexican, or American Indian?

Puerto Rican 4   48
Mexican 5   9
American Indian 6
None of these 7

3. In general, how accurate would you say the cost data are?

Inaccurate 1   49
Fairly accurate 2   9
Very accurate 3

4. Which bills or records did the respondent(s) check to give you the cost information?

50
 9

5. Which, if any, of the cost data do you think is inaccurate and why?

51
 9

6. Apart from the cost data, is there any other information in this interview that you are doubtful about?

Yes . (ANSWER 7) 1   52
No . . (SKIP TO 8) . . . 2   9

   7. Which information are you doubtful about and why?

53
 9

8. How would you rate the overall cooperation received from the family during the interview?

Excellent 1   54
Good 2   9
Fair 3
Poor 4

9. Fill in the number of each type of completed supplements accompanying the main questionnaire.

Past Preg.		55-56/99
Current Preg. . .		57-58/99
Hospital		59-60/99
Major Illness . .		61-62/99
Insurance		63-64/99
Health Opinions .		65-66/99
Permission Form .		67-68/99

NORC-4106
January, 1971

PAST PREGNANCY SUPPLEMENT
(If pregnancy ended by
December 31, 1970)

Form approved.
OMB No. 68 - S70089

BEGIN DECK 32

Family
Name_____

Line
No.

1-4

Respondent's
Name_____

Family
Unit

Mother's
Name and
Per. No. _____

5-6

This is Mother's past pregnancy: _____ of _____
(during 1970)

7
9

IF THIS SUPPLEMENT IS BEING USED FOR A <u>CURRENT</u> PREGNANCY WITH
A HOSPITAL STAY, CODE HERE AND SKIP TO Q. 2-B.

Current
pregnancy . 1

11
9

1. IF YOU ALREADY KNOW, CODE WITHOUT ASKING: How did the
pregnancy end--was it a live birth, a stillbirth, a
miscarriage, or was it terminated?

Single live birth . 2

Twin live birth . . 3

Stillbirth 4

Miscarriage 5

Terminated
(abortion) . . . 6

2. A. Did (MOTHER) spend one night or more in a hospital
for this pregnancy?
IF BABY WAS ADOPTED, CODE HERE AND SKIP TO Q. 37.

Yes (ASK B) . . . 1
No (SKIP TO 15) . . 2
Baby adopted . . . 3

12
9

B. How many times was (MOTHER) in the hospital for this
pregnancy; up to and including time of (delivery/
termination/miscarriage)? IF MORE THAN TWO HOSPITAL-
IZATIONS, USE ANOTHER <u>PREGNANCY SUPPLEMENT</u> TO RECORD
ADDITIONAL HOSPITALIZATION, THEN COME BACK TO THIS
FORM FOR Q. 15 AND REST OF SUPPLEMENT.

Times . .

13-14
99

ASK Q.'S 3-14 SEPARATELY FOR
EACH HOSPITAL STAY.

3. What was this hospitalization
for?

BEGIN DECK 31

Stay_____ of _____   8
<u>First Hospital Stay</u>

Delivery/termina-
tion/miscar-
riage 1   11
Other (SPECIFY) . 2   9

BEGIN DECK 31

Stay_____ of _____   8
<u>Second Hospital Stay</u>

Delivery/termina-
tion/miscar-
riage 1   11
Other (SPECIFY) . . 2   9

4. What hospital was (MOTHER)
in?

12-21
9

Name

Street   City

12-21
9

Name

Street   City

5. How many days was (MOTHER)
in the hospital?

Days .

22-24
9

Days .

22-24
9

6. What were the approximate
dates? IF DATES NOT KNOWN,
RECORD TIME OF MONTH (BE-
GINNING, MIDDLE, END).

FROM_____
     Mo. Day Year

25-30
9

TO _____
     Mo. Day Year

31-36
9

FROM _____
      Mo. Day Year

25-30
9

TO _____
     Mo. Day Year

31-36
9

PP

		DECK 31	DECK 31
		First Hospital Stay	Second Hospital Stay
7.	How many beds were there in (MOTHER)'s room?	One bed . . . . . . 1 37 Two beds . . . . . 2 9 Three or more . . . 3	One bed . . . . . . 1 37 Two beds . . . . . 2 9 Three or more . . . 3
8.	How much was the <u>hospital</u> bill--<u>counting</u> anything insurance may have paid, but <u>not counting</u> what the doctor charged for delivering the baby?	$: ⬜⬜⬜⬜⬜ IF $0, SKIP TO Q. 15. 38-42/9	$: ⬜⬜⬜⬜⬜ IF $0, SKIP TO Q. 15. 38-42/9
9.	Did any kind of hospital plan or insurance cover any part of the cost of hospitalization--or will any plan, even though it hasn't paid yet?	Yes . (ASK 10-14) . 1 43 No (SKIP TO Q. 15). 2 9	Yes . (ASK 10-14) . 1 43 No (SKIP TO Q. 15). 2 9
10.	IF INSURANCE: What plans or insurance covered the hospitalization costs? MORE THAN ONE MAY BE RECORDED.	Plan (1): _____ 44-45/99 Plan (2): _____ 46-47/99	Plan (1): _____ 44-45/99 Plan (2): _____ 46-47/99

11.	ASK FOR EACH PLAN: Has the insurance [PLAN (1), PLAN (2)] paid yet? CIRCLE ONE CODE FOR EACH PLAN.	Plan (1): Yes . . 1 48
		          No . . . 2 9
		Plan (2): Yes . . . 3 49
		          No . . . 4 9
			Plan (1): Yes . . 1 48
			          No . . . 2 9
			Plan (2): Yes . . . 3 49
			          No . . . 4 9

12.	ASK FOR EACH PLAN: How much (did/will) [PLAN (1), PLAN (2)] pay on the hospitalization?	(1)
		$: ⬜⬜⬜⬜⬜
		(2) 50-54/9
		$: ⬜⬜⬜⬜⬜
		           55-59/9
			(1)
			$: ⬜⬜⬜⬜⬜
			(2) 50-54/9
			$: ⬜⬜⬜⬜⬜
			           55-59/9

13.	And how much did you yourself (the family) have to pay?	$: ⬜⬜⬜⬜⬜
		           60-64/9
			$: ⬜⬜⬜⬜⬜
			           60-64/9

14.	ADD AMOUNTS IN 12 AND 13. IF TOTAL DIFFERS FROM AMOUNTS IN 8, PROBE FOR CORRECTION.	Total $: _____
		           65-69/9
		           70-74/R
			Total $: _____
			           65-69/9
			           70-74/R

15. How many weeks had (MOTHER) been pregnant before seeing a doctor in connection with this pregnancy?

No. weeks ☐☐ $\frac{9-10}{99}$

16. A. What is the name of the doctor or place that provided the <u>most</u> care for (MOTHER) during the pregnancy? FILL IN <u>BOTH</u> DOCTOR'S NAME AND NAME OF CLINIC, IF POSSIBLE.

    IF SOURCE ALREADY MENTIONED, ENTER NAME(S) AND GO TO Q. 17.

    IF NEW SOURCE, ASK B, AND C <u>OR</u> D.

    B. What is the address?

    _____
    Full Name of Doctor

    _____
    Name of Clinic/Group

    _____
    Street

    _____
    City

    _____
    State and Zip $\frac{11-20}{9}$

    C. IF NEW CLINIC MENTIONED: Does (MOTHER) go to a particular doctor at the clinic?

    Yes (ENTER NAME OF DOCTOR ABOVE) . . 1

    No 2

    D. IF NEW DOCTOR MENTIONED: Is the doctor part of a clinic or group practice?

    Yes (ENTER NAME OF CLINIC ABOVE) . . 3

    No 4

17. Which reason on this card best describes why (MOTHER) happened to go to (PHYSICIAN/PLACE) for this pregnancy?

CARD A

    Usual doctor or clinic . . . . 1 $\frac{21}{9}$

    Referred by usual doctor 2

    Referred by another (not usual) doctor 3

    Picked by patient or family to treat this condition 4

    Recommended by other relatives or friends to treat this condition . . 5

    Referred by someone else (SPECIFY) 6

PP   DECK 33

18.

<table>
<tr>
<td rowspan="2">CARD B</td>
<td colspan="1">A.
At which of these places did visits of or to ((SOURCE NAMED IN Q. 16) take place? CODE ALL THAT APPLY IN COLUMN A BELOW.</td>
<td colspan="2">ASK B AND C FOR EACH PLACE CODED IN A.</td>
</tr>
<tr>
<td>B.
How many visits were there during the pregnancy at (PLACE IN COLUMN A)? ENTER VISITS IN COLUMN B BE-LOW.</td>
<td>C.
What was the cost for the visits at (PLACE IN COLUMN A), including anything that insurance paid? ENTER COSTS IN COLUMN C.

NOTE: IF RESPONDENT CAN'T BREAK DOWN COSTS BY KIND OF VISIT, RECORD TOTAL BILL FOR THIS SOURCE FOR PREGNANCY ON LINE D, BELOW.</td>
</tr>
<tr>
<td></td>
<td>A.   Places</td>
<td>B.   No. of Visits</td>
<td>C.   Costs</td>
</tr>
<tr>
<td></td>
<td>Doctor at your home   1</td>
<td></td>
<td>$:   22-28 / 9</td>
</tr>
<tr>
<td></td>
<td>Doctor's office or private clinic (in- cluding group practice plan)   2</td>
<td></td>
<td>$:   29-35 / 9</td>
</tr>
<tr>
<td></td>
<td>Hospital out- patient dept.   3</td>
<td></td>
<td>$:   36-42 / 9</td>
</tr>
<tr>
<td></td>
<td>Hospital emergency room   4</td>
<td></td>
<td>$:   43-49 / 9</td>
</tr>
<tr>
<td></td>
<td>Industrial, school, camp, or col- lege health service   5</td>
<td></td>
<td>$:   50-56 / 9</td>
</tr>
<tr>
<td></td>
<td>Any other clinic not connected with a hospital-- such as a board   6 of health clinic or a neighborhood health center</td>
<td></td>
<td>$:   57-63 / 9</td>
</tr>
<tr>
<td></td>
<td>In-hospital visits   7</td>
<td></td>
<td>$:   64-70 / · 9</td>
</tr>
<tr>
<td></td>
<td>D.   IF NO COST BREAKDOWN:</td>
<td>Total cost for pregnancy for this source</td>
<td>$:   71-74 / 9</td>
</tr>
</table>

IF "HOSPITALIZED CURRENT PREGNANCY," SKIP TO Q. 26.

CONTINUE DECK 32

19. ASK IF <u>LIVE OR STILLBIRTH</u>: Was this a
Caesarean delivery?

Yes . . . . 1 <u>15</u>

No 2   9

---

20. ASK IF <u>LIVE OR STILLBIRTH</u>: Did (SOURCE NAMED
IN Q. 16) do the delivery?

Yes (SKIP TO Q. 26) . . . . 3 <u>16</u>

No (SKIP TO Q. 23) 4   9

---

21. ASK IF <u>MISCARRIAGE OR TERMINATION</u>: Did (MOTHER)
have a dilation and curettage (D and C/scraping)
or other operation at the time of the (mis-
carriage/termination)?

Yes . (ASK Q. 22) . . . . . 1 <u>17</u>

No (SKIP TO Q. 26) 2   9

---

    22. Did (SOURCE NAMED IN Q. 16) perform the
        (D and C/operation)?

Yes (SKIP TO Q. 26) . . . . 3 <u>18</u>

No . (GO TO Q. 23) 4   9

---

23. A. What is the name of doctor (or place) that
(delivered the baby)(performed the D and C/
operation)? FILL IN <u>BOTH</u> DOCTOR'S NAME AND
NAME OF CLINIC, IF POSSIBLE.

IF SOURCE ALREADY MENTIONED, ENTER NAME(S)
AND GO TO Q. 24.

IF NEW SOURCE, ASK B, AND C <u>OR</u> D.

B. What is the address?

BEGIN DECK 34

Full Name of Doctor
_____

Name of Clinic/Group
_____

Street
_____

City
_____

State and Zip   11-20/9

C. IF NEW CLINIC MENTIONED: Does (MOTHER)
go to a particular doctor at the clinic?

Yes (ENTER NAME OF DOCTOR
  ABOVE) 1

No 2

D. IF NEW DOCTOR MENTIONED: Is the doctor
part of a clinic or group practice?

Yes (ENTER NAME OF CLINIC
  ABOVE) 3

No 4

---

24. Which reason on this card best describes why (MOTHER) happened to go **to**
(PHYSICIAN/PLACE) for the (delivery/D and C/operation)?

CARD
A

Usual doctor or clinic . . . . 1 <u>21</u>

Referred by usual doctor 2   9

Referred by another (not usual) doctor 3

Picked by patient or family to treat this condition 4

Recommended by other relatives or friends to treat this condition 5

Referred by someone else (SPECIFY) 6

PP

25.

CARD B	A. At which of these places did visits of or to (SOURCE NAMED IN Q. 23) take place? CODE ALL THAT APPLY IN COLUMN A BELOW.	ASK B AND C FOR EACH PLACE CODED IN A.	
		B. How many visits were there during the pregnancy at (PLACE IN COLUMN A)? ENTER VISITS IN COLUMN B BELOW.	C. What was the cost for the visits at (PLACE IN COLUMN A), including anything that insurance paid? ENTER COSTS IN COLUMN C. NOTE: IF RESPONDENT CAN'T BREAK DOWN COSTS BY KIND OF VISIT, RECORD TOTAL BILL FOR THIS SOURCE FOR PREGNANCY ON LINE D, BELOW.
	A. Places	B. No. of Visits	C. Costs

Doctor at your home 1	☐☐☐	$: ☐☐☐	22-28 / 9
Doctor's office or private clinic (including group practice plan) 2	☐☐☐	$: ☐☐☐	29-35 / 9
Hospital outpatient department 3	☐☐☐	$: ☐☐☐	36-42 / 9
Hospital emergency room 4	☐☐☐	$: ☐☐☐	43-49 / 9
Industrial, school, camp, or college health service 5	☐☐☐	$: ☐☐☐	50-56 / 9
Any other clinic not connected with a hospital--such as a board of health clinic or a neighborhood health center 6	☐☐☐	$: ☐☐☐	57-63 / 9
In-hospital visits 7	☐☐☐	$: ☐☐☐	64-70 / 9
D. IF NO COST BREAKDOWN:	Total cost for pregnancy for this source	$: ☐☐☐	71-74 / 9

CONTINUE DECK 32

26. Did (MOTHER) visit any <u>other</u> doctor or clinic in connection with this pregnancy?

Yes . (GO TO PHYS. CONTINUATION SHEET) 1 $\frac{19}{9}$

No   . . . . . (GO TO Q. 27) 2

27. ADD AMOUNTS OF ALL DOCTOR CHARGES FOR PREGNANCY (Q.'S 18, 25, AND ANY CONTINUATION SHEETS USED). ENTER TOTAL.

$: ☐☐☐☐ $\frac{20-23}{9}$

28. Did any kind of medical plan or insurance cover any part of the cost of these doctor visits--(AMOUNT IN Q.27)? Or will it, even if it hasn't paid yet?

Yes (ASK Q.'S 29-33) . . . . . 1 $\frac{24}{9}$

No . (SKIP TO Q. 34) 2

29. What insurance or plans paid (will pay) on the doctor bills? Did (Will) any <u>other</u> insurance pay part of the bills? MORE THAN ONE PLAN MAY BE LISTED.

Plan (1) _____ $\frac{25-26}{99}$

Plan (2) _____ $\frac{27-28}{99}$

30. <u>ASK FOR EACH PLAN</u>: Has the insurance paid yet? CODE FOR EACH PLAN.

(1) Yes   . . . . 1 $\frac{29}{9}$

No 2

(2) Yes . . . . 3 $\frac{30}{9}$

No 4

31. <u>ASK FOR EACH PLAN</u>: How much did (will) the insurance pay toward the doctor bill(s)? RECORD FOR EACH PLAN.

(1) $: ☐☐☐☐ $\frac{31-34}{9}$

(2) $: ☐☐☐☐ $\frac{35-38}{9}$

32. And how much did (will) you yourself (the family) have to pay?

$: ☐☐☐☐ $\frac{39-42}{9}$

33. ADD AMOUNTS IN Q.'S 31 AND 32. IF THE TOTAL DIFFERS FROM AMOUNT IN Q. 27, PROBE FOR CORRECTION.

Total: $: ☐☐☐☐ $\frac{43-46}{9}$

PP

34. ASK EVERYONE:

A. Did (MOTHER) have any other medical care connected with the pregnancy that was not included in the hospital or doctors' bills we just talked about--for things like--READ THROUGH LIST OF ITEMS; CIRCLE "YES" OR "NO" FOR EACH ONE.		ASK B-E ABOUT FIRST ITEM CIRCLED "YES" BEFORE GOING TO NEXT "YES" ITEM.			
		B. What were the total expenses for (ITEM) in connection with the pregnancy--including anything that insurance may have paid? ENTER AMOUNT BELOW. IF "0" EXPENSES, SKIP TO NEXT "YES" ITEM.	C. And how much of that was paid by insurance? ENTER AMOUNT BELOW. IF NONE, ENTER "0" AND SKIP TO NEXT "YES" ITEM.	D. What insurance paid that? ENTER NAME(S) OF INSURANCE BELOW.	E. Then that left (AMOUNT IN "B" MINUS AMOUNT IN "C") that you had to pay. Is that right? IF "YES," ENTER AMOUNT BELOW. IF "NO," MAKE NECESSARY CORRECTIONS.
Item	A. Yes No	B. Total	C. Insurance Paid	D. Name of Insurance	E. "Net"
DECK 32 Prescriptions?	1 2 _47_ 9	48-51	52-55	56-57 99	58-61
BEGIN DECK 35 Non-prescribed medicine?	1 2 _11_ 9	12-15	16-19	20-21 99	22-25
Blood tests or other laboratory work?	1 2 _26_ 9	27-30	31-34	35-36 99	37-40
An anesthetist's fee?	1 2 _41_ 9	42-45	46-49	50-51 99	52-55
A practical nurse at home?	1 2 _56_ 9	57-60	61-64	65-66 99	67-70

BEGIN DECK 36

Anything else? IF "YES," LIST BELOW:

(1)					
	1 2 _11_ 9	12-15	16-19	20-21 99	22-25
(2)					
	1 2 _26_ 9	27-30	31-34	35-36 99	37-40

35. IF FREE OR REDUCED RATE CARE ALREADY MENTIONED, CODE
    WITHOUT ASKING.

    Aside from free samples of drugs (MOTHER'S) doctor might
    have given her, was any of the care you've told me about   Yes (ASK A&B)   1   <u>41</u>
    free of charge or at a reduced rate?   No (GO TO 36)   2   9

    <u>IF YES:</u>

    A. What was the care?   _____   <u>42-43</u>

                                                             <u>44-45</u>

    B. Which item on this card best describes the <u>main</u>
       reason that the care was free of charge, or at a
       reduced rate?   CIRCLE ONE CODE ONLY, FOR MAIN
       REASON.

    | CARD C |

    On public aid (receiving welfare payments) 01   <u>46-47</u>

    Recipient of Medicaid (no welfare payments) 02   99

    Went to free or part pay clinic or public hospital 03

    Private doctor or hospital didn't charge or reduced the bill
        because we couldn't pay 05

    Armed Forces member or dependent 07

    Professional courtesy 08

    Participant in medical research 09

    Participant in prepaid group practice plan 11

    Industrial, school, camp, or college health service 12

    Other (SPECIFY) 13

                                                       <u>48-74</u>
                                                         R

36. THIS SUPPLEMENT IS BEING USED IN CONNECTION WITH:

                              A live birth (GO TO Q. 37) .   1

                              A stillbirth, miscarriage,
                              terminated pregnancy, or
                              current pregnancy (GO TO
                              INSTRUCTION BOX AFTER
                              Q. 61, P. 16)   2

PP   BEGIN DECK 21

IF TWINS, FILL OUT SEPARATE PREGNANCY SUPPLEMENTS FOR   1-4
EACH, BEGINNING WITH Q. 37.

Baby's Name: _____ Baby's Per. No.   5-6

IF BABY ADOPTED, ASK Q.'S 37-39, AND THEN SKIP TO Q. 43.

37. Now a few questions about (BABY). Is there a particular medical person or
    clinic that is (will be) the baby's regular source of care?

                                        Yes (ASK 38-39) . . . 1 $\frac{11}{9}$

                                        No or don't know
                                            (SKIP TO 40) . . . 2

---

38. Is that a clinic, a regular family doctor, some type of specialist, an
    osteopath, a chiropractor, or what? CODE ONE.

                            Clinic . . . . (ASK A) . . . 1 $\frac{12}{9}$

                            Family doctor . (ASK B) . . . 2

                            Specialist . . (ASK B) . . . 3

                            Osteopath . . . (ASK B) . . . 4

                            Chiropractor . (ASK B) . . . 5

                            Other (SPECIFY)(ASK A OR B) . 6

                            Don't know (GO TO 39) 7

    A. IF CLINIC: Does (BABY) go to a particular doctor at this clinic?

                            Yes . . . . 1 $\frac{13}{9}$

                            No 2

    B. IF ANY DOCTOR: Is the doctor part of a clinic, or group practice?

                            Yes . . . . 3 $\frac{14}{9}$

                            No 4

---

39. A. What is the name of the (doctor and/or clinic)? FILL IN BOTH THE
       DOCTOR'S NAME AND NAME OF CLINIC OR GROUP IF POSSIBLE.

                            _____
                            Full Name of Doctor

                            _____
                            Name of Clinic/Group

    B. What is the address? _____
                            Street

                            _____
                            City

                            _____ 15-24/9
                            State and Zip   25-31/R

40. Where was (he/she) born--in a hospital, at home, or somewhere else?

    IF BABY BORN HOME OR "OTHER" AND MOTHER AND BABY THEN WENT TO HOSPITAL, CODE "HOSPITAL."

    Hospital (ASK Q. 41) . . . 1   32/9

    Home (SKIP TO Q. 43) . . . 2

    Other (SPECIFY AND SKIP TO
      Q. 43) 3

---

41. Did the baby stay in the hospital one or more nights after (MOTHER) returned home?

    > IF BABY <u>DIED WHILE MOTHER STILL</u>
    > <u>IN HOSPITAL</u>, CODE HERE AND SKIP
    > TO INSTRUCTION BOX AFTER
    > Q. 61, P. 16 6

    Yes (FILL OUT HOSPITAL
      SUPPLEMENT) 4   33/9

    No (ASK Q. 42) 5

    34

ASK ONLY IF "NO" TO Q. 41:

42. Did any doctor examine (BABY) before (he/she) came home from the hospital?

    Yes (ASK A) 7   35/9
    No . (GO TO Q. 43) 8

    A. IF YES: What is that doctor's name?

       IF DOCTOR ALREADY MENTIONED, ENTER NAME AND SKIP TO D.

       IF NEW DOCTOR, ASK B-F.

       Full Name of Doctor

       Name of Clinic/Group

    B. And what is his address?

       Street

       City

       State and Zip   36-45/9

    C. Is the doctor part of a clinic or group practice?

       Yes (ENTER NAME OF CLINIC
       ABOVE) 1
       No 2

    D. How many times did doctor see (BABY) in the hospital then?

       Visits   46-47/99

    E. What was the cost for those visits, including anything insurance paid?

       $:   48-50/9

    F. Was any part of the cost of these visits paid for by any kind of medical plan or insurance?

       Yes (ASK G & H) 1   51/9
       No (GO TO Q. 43) 2

       IF YES TO F:
       G. What plan or insurance is that?   52-53/99

       H. How much did insurance pay for those visits?

          $:   54-57/9

       58-60/R

PP   DECK 21

43. Has the baby had any illness or condition for   Yes . (FILL OUT HOS-
     which (he/she) had to go to a hospital for one   PITAL SUPPLEMENT) . . 1   ☐☐
     or more nights (after being home)?   ‾‾‾‾‾
                                                        No 2   61-62
                                                                                        99

44. Has (BABY) had any (other) illness, accident,
     or condition for which doctors were seen five   Yes . (FILL OUT MAJOR
     or more times, or for which expenses amounted   ILLNESS SUPPLEMENT) . 4   ☐☐
     to $100 or more, or for which regular care or   ‾‾‾‾‾
     treatment were required during 1970?   No 5   63-64
                                                                                        99

45. Has a doctor seen the baby, or has the baby   Yes . (ASK Q.'S 45-49) 1   65
     been to a doctor's office or clinic for any   9
     illness or condition? How about for routine   No . (SKIP TO Q. 53) . . 2
     check-ups, shots, tests, or vaccination?

46. Why did (BABY) see the doctor? Any other
     reasons?)
                                                                                      66-68
                                                                                        9

                                                                                      69-71
                                                                                        9

                                                                                      72-74
                                                                                        9

47. A. What is the name of the doctor or place that   BEGIN DECK 22
         provided the most care for (CONDITION[S]
         MENTIONED IN Q. 46)? FILL IN BOTH
         DOCTOR'S NAME AND NAME OF CLINIC, IF   ‾‾‾‾‾‾‾‾‾‾‾‾‾‾‾‾‾‾‾‾‾‾‾‾‾‾‾‾‾‾
         POSSIBLE.   Full Name of Doctor

         IF SOURCE ALREADY MENTIONED, ENTER   ‾‾‾‾‾‾‾‾‾‾‾‾‾‾‾‾‾‾‾‾‾‾‾‾‾‾‾‾‾‾
         NAME(S) AND GO TO Q. 48.   Name of Clinic/Group

         IF NEW SOURCE, ASK B, AND C OR D.   ‾‾‾‾‾‾‾‾‾‾‾‾‾‾‾‾‾‾‾‾‾‾‾‾‾‾‾‾‾‾
                                                       Street
     B. What is the address?
                                                       ‾‾‾‾‾‾‾‾‾‾‾‾‾‾‾‾‾‾‾‾‾‾‾‾‾‾‾‾‾‾
                                                       City

                                                       ‾‾‾‾‾‾‾‾‾‾‾‾‾‾‾‾‾‾‾‾‾‾‾‾‾‾‾‾‾‾
                                                       State and Zip   11-20
                                                                                        9
     C. IF NEW CLINIC MENTIONED: Does (BABY) go   Yes (ENTER NAME OF DOCTOR
         to a particular doctor at the clinic?   ABOVE) 1

                                                       No 2

     D. IF NEW DOCTOR MENTIONED: Is the doctor   Yes (ENTER NAME OF
         part of a clinic or group practice?   CLINIC ABOVE) 3

                                                       No 4

                                                                                        21
                                                                                         R

48.

A.	ASK B AND C FOR EACH PLACE CODED IN A.	
At which of these places did visits of or to (SOURCE NAMED IN Q. 47) take place? CODE ALL THAT APPLY IN COLUMN A BELOW.	B. How many visits were there during the past year at (PLACE IN COLUMN A)? ENTER VISITS IN COLUMN B BELOW.	C. What was the cost for the visits at (PLACE IN COLUMN A), including anything that insurance paid? ENTER COSTS IN COLUMN C.
A. Places	B. No. of Visits	C. Costs

CARD B

Doctor at your home 1	☐☐☐	$: ☐☐☐☐ 22-28 / 9
Doctor's office or private clinic (including group practice plan) 2	☐☐☐	$: ☐☐☐☐ 29-35 / 9
Hospital out-patient department 3	☐☐☐	$: ☐☐☐☐ 36-42 / 9
Hospital emergency room 4	☐☐☐	$: ☐☐☐☐ 43-49 / 9
Industrial, school, camp, or college health service 5	☐☐☐	$: ☐☐☐☐ 50-56 / 9
Any other clinic not connected with a hospital-- such as a board of health clinic or a neighborhood health center 6	☐☐☐	$: ☐☐☐☐ 57-63 / 9 64-70 / R

49. Did (BABY) visit any <u>other</u> doctor or clinic for care that we have not yet talked about?

Yes . (ASK Q.'S 50-52) . 1
No (SKIP TO Q. 53) . . . 2

71 / 9

PP

50. A. What is the name of the other doctor or place that (BABY) visited? FILL IN BOTH DOCTOR'S NAME AND NAME OF CLINIC, IF POSSIBLE.

   IF SOURCE ALREADY MENTIONED, ENTER NAME(S) AND GO TO Q. 51.

   IF NEW SOURCE, ASK B, AND C OR D.

   B. What is the address?

Full Name of Doctor
Name of Clinic/Group
Street
City

State and Zip   11-20
                9

   C. IF NEW CLINIC MENTIONED: Does (BABY) go to a particular doctor at the clinic?

Yes (ENTER NAME OF DOCTOR ABOVE) . . . 1

No 2

   D. IF NEW DOCTOR MENTIONED: Is the doctor part of a clinic or group practice?

Yes (ENTER NAME OF CLINIC ABOVE) . . . 3

No 4   21
                                R

51. CARD B

A. At which of these places did visits of or to (SOURCE NAMED IN Q. 50) take place? CODE ALL THAT APPLY IN COLUMN A BELOW.	ASK B AND C FOR EACH PLACE CODED IN A.	
	B. How many visits were there during the past year at (PLACE IN COLUMN A)? ENTER VISITS IN COLUMN B BELOW.	C. What was the cost for the visits at (PLACE IN COLUMN A), including anything that insurance paid? ENTER COSTS IN COLUMN C.
A. Places	B. No. of Visits	C. Costs
Doctor at your home 1	☐☐☐	$: ☐☐☐ 22-28 / 9
Doctor's office or private clinic (including group practice plan) 2	☐☐☐	$: ☐☐☐ 29-35 / 9
Hospital outpatient department 3	☐☐☐	$: ☐☐☐ 36-42 / 9
Hospital emergency room 4	☐☐☐	$: ☐☐☐ 43-49 / 9
Industrial, school, camp, or college health service 5	☐☐☐	$: ☐☐☐ 50-56 / 9
Any other clinic not connected with a hospital-- such as a board of health clinic or a neighborhood health center 6	☐☐☐	$: ☐☐☐ 57-63 / 9

                                                                64-70 / 9

52. Did (BABY) visit any other doctor or clinic in the past year for care that we have not yet talked about?

Yes (USE DR. CONTINUATION SHEET) 1   71

No (GO TO Q. 53) . . . 2   / 9

53. Did (BABY) have any X-rays or laboratory tests of any kind; appliances, or equipment like braces, vaporizer, or special shoes; or anything like that?

    Yes . (ASK A) 1   11
    No 2   9
                 12-19

    A. IF YES: What was the cost altogether?

    $: ☐☐☐   R / 20-22 / 9

---

54. IF BOY BABY: Was there a separate charge for circumcision that hasn't been included in any of the charges you've told me about?

    Yes . (ASK A & B) . . 1   23
    No, included in   9
      other costs 2
    No, no circumcision . 3

    IF YES:
    A. What was the cost (including anything insurance may have paid)?

    $: ☐☐☐   24-26 / 9

    B. What doctor performed the circumcision? RECORD NAME. IF NOT DR., RECORD TYPE OF PRACTITIONER.

                 27-28/99
    Name of Doctor or Clinic

---

55. During the last year did (BABY) take any medicine prescribed for (him/her) by a doctor--other than any we've counted already?

    Yes . (ASK A) 1   29
    No 2   9

    A. IF YES: What was the cost for those medicines-- including anything insurance may have paid?

    $: ☐☐☐   30-32 / 9

---

56. During 1970 did (BABY) use any medicines which were not prescribed by a doctor? I mean things like vitamins, tonics, cold pills, nose drops, cough medicine, aspirin, and so on?

    Yes . (ASK A) 3   33
    No 4   9

    A. IF YES: What was the cost for those medicines?

    $: ☐☐☐   34-36 / 9

---

57. IF ANY MINOR MEDICAL EXPENSES REPORTED (FROM Q.'S 45-56): Have you received any medical insurance benefits in connection with any of these minor medical expenses for (BABY)? That is, insurance benefits (that we haven't talked about before) for home or office physician visits, drugs, or anything else?

    Yes . (ASK 58-60) . . 1   37
    No (SKIP TO Q. 61) . 2   9

    58. Which of these expenses we've talked about did insurance cover?

                 38-39

                 40-41

    59. What was the name of the insurance or plan that paid the benefits? MORE THAN ONE PLAN MAY BE ENTERED.

                 42-43
    Plan (1)   99

                 44-45
    Plan (2)   99

    60. About how much did the insurance pay on these expenses?

    Plan (1) $: ☐☐☐☐   46-49 / 9

    Plan (2) $: ☐☐☐☐   50-53 / 9

                 54-7 / R

?F

61. IF FREE OR REDUCED RATE CARE ALREADY MENTIONED,   11-52
     CODE WITHOUT ASKING.   R

Aside from free samples of drugs the doctor
might have given (BABY), was any of the care
you've told me about free of charge or at a   Yes (ASK A & B) . . . 1   53
reduced rate?   9
                                                     No 2

IF YES:

A. What was the care? _____   54-55
                                                                         99

                                                                        56-57
                                                                         99

B. Which item on this card best describes the <u>main</u>
    reason that the care was free of charge, or at
    a reduced rate?
    CIRCLE ONE CODE ONLY, FOR MAIN REASON.

    CARD C

    On public aid (receiving welfare payments) 01   58-59
    Recipient of Medicaid (no welfare payments) 02   99
    Went to free or part pay clinic or public hospital 03
    Private doctor or hospital didn't charge or reduced the bill
       because we couldn't pay 05
    Armed Forces member or dependent 07
    Professional courtesy 08
    Participant in medical research 09
    Participant in prepaid group practice plan 11
    Industrial, school, camp, or college health service 12
    Other (SPECIFY) 13

                                                                        60-74
                                                                          R

> NOW GO ON TO ANY OTHER PREGNANCY SUPPLEMENTS YOU KNOW ARE REQUIRED
> FOR THIS FAMILY. OTHERWISE, RETURN TO MAIN QUESTIONNAIRE, Q. 10.

NORC-4106
Jan., 1971

CURRENT PREGNANCY SUPPLEMENT
(Still pregnant at time of interview
or pregnancy ended in 1971)

Form approved.
OMB No. 68 - S70089

BEGIN DECK 30

Family
Name _____

Respondent's
Name _____

Line No.

Family
Unit

Mother's Name

and Person No.

1-4

5-6

0. Did (MOTHER) spend one or more nights in the hospital during 1970 in connection with this pregnancy?

Yes (FILL OUT A PAST PREG. SUPPLEMENT) . . . 1
No . . (ASK 1) 2

1. Did (MOTHER) see a doctor or go to a clinic in connection with this pregnancy?

Yes . . (ASK 2-7) 3
No . . (SKIP TO 11) . . . 4

11
9

2. How many times altogether did (MOTHER) see a doctor at his office in connection with this pregnancy?

Office visits:

12-14
999

3. And how many times did a doctor come to the home to see (MOTHER) in connection with this pregnancy?

Home visits:

15-17
999

4. (Besides this) did (MOTHER) go to a maternity clinic or any other kind of clinic for this pregnancy?

Yes . . . (ASK 5) . . . 5
No . . . (SKIP TO 6) . . . 6

18
9

5. How many times?

Clinic visits:

19-21
999

6. Who is the doctor who gave (MOTHER) the most care for this pregnancy?
IF CLINIC, GIVE NAME AND ADDRESS OF CLINIC.

_____
Full name of doctor/clinic

_____
Street

_____
City   State   Zip

22-31
9

7. Have you paid out anything for doctor care in connection with this pregnancy?

Yes . . (SKIP TO 8) . . . 1
No . . . . (ASK A) 2

32
9

A. IF NO: Do you expect to be billed for doctor care later, or is there no charge to you for this care?

Dr. will bill (SKIP TO 11) 3
No charge (SKIP TO 11) . . 4

33
9

8. Was this (Were these) amount(s) an advance payment on the doctor's final bill, or was the doctor billing you as you went along?

Advance payment (SKIP TO 11) 1
Billing along (ASK 9-10) . 2

34
9

9. How much did you pay out for visits to the doctor at his office or clinic for this pregnancy?

$ . . . . .

35-38
9

10. And how much have you paid out for times the doctor saw (MOTHER) at home for this pregnancy?

$ . . . . .

39-42
9

(Continued on reverse side)

CP

11. Did (MOTHER) take any medicines in connection with this pregnancy?

Yes . (ASK 12-13) . . 1

No . (SKIP TO 14) . . 2

43
9

   12. How much was spent for medicines the doctor <u>prescribed</u> for (MOTHER) in connection with this pregnancy?

$ . . ☐☐☐☐

44-47
9

   13. How much was spent for <u>non-prescribed</u> medicines for (MOTHER)'s pregnancy?

$ . . ☐☐☐☐

48-51
9

14. Did (MOTHER) get any blood tests or other laboratory tests, did she have X-rays, a practical nurse at home, special medical appliances, or anything like that in connection with the pregnancy?

Yes . . (ASK 15). . . 1

No . . (SKIP TO 16) . 2

52
9

15.

A. What did (MOTHER) have? LIST TESTS OR CARE BELOW, AND ASK "B" FOR EACH ITEM.	B. How much did (ITEM) cost? RECORD BELOW.	

(1) _____ $ . . ☐☐☐☐   53-56 / 9

(2) _____ $ . . ☐☐☐☐   57-60 / 9

(3) _____ $ . . ☐☐☐☐   61-64 / 9

16. IF <u>ANY</u> CARE, MEDICINES, OR TREATMENT MENTIONED, ASK Q. 16. OTHERWISE, SKIP TO BOTTOM OF PAGE.

IF FREE OR REDUCED RATE CARE ALREADY MENTIONED, CODE WITHOUT ASKING.
Aside from free samples of drugs (MOTHER)'s doctor might have given her, was any of the care you've told me about free of charge or at a reduced rate?

Yes . (ASK A & B) . 1

No 2

65
9

·IF YES:

A. What was the care? _____

66-69
9

B. Which item on Card C best describes the main reason that the care was free of charge, or at a reduced rate?   CIRCLE ONE CODE ONLY, FOR MAIN REASON.

| CARD C |

On public aid (Receiving welfare payments) 01

Recipient of Medicaid (No welfare payments) 02

Went to free or part pay clinic or public hospital. 03

Private doctor or hospital didn't charge or reduced the bill because we couldn't pay 05

Armed Forces member or dependent 07

Professional courtesy 08

Participant in medical research 09

Participant in prepaid group practice plan 11

Industrial, school, camp, or college health service 12

Other (SPECIFY) _____ 13

70-71
99

NOW GO ON TO ANY OTHER PREGNANCY SUPPLEMENTS YOU KNOW ARE REQUIRED FOR THIS MOTHER; OTHERWISE RETURN TO MAIN QUESTIONNAIRE, Q. 10.

NORC 4106
January, 1971

National Opinion Research Center
University of Chicago

Form approved.
OMB No. 68 - S70089

HOSPITAL SUPPLEMENT

BEGIN DECK 40

Line
No.

Family Unit

Patient's
Name

1-4

and Person Number

5-6

Hospitalized Illness ____ of ____   7

Family name: _____

Respondent's name: _____

---

1. What was the <u>main</u> reason (PATIENT) had to go to the
   hospital? ENTER KIND OF ILLNESS, ACCIDENT, OR
   CONDITION.

   $\frac{11-13}{999}$

   $\frac{14-16}{999}$

---

2. How many times was (PATIENT) in the hospital for
   this condition during 1970?
   IF MORE THAN TWO HOSPITALIZATIONS, USE ANOTHER
   HOSPITAL SUPPLEMENT FOR Q'S. 3-16, ABOUT THIRD,
   FOURTH, ETC. HOSPITALIZATIONS.

   Times . . .

   $\frac{17-18}{99}$

BE SURE TO IDENTIFY EACH
HOSPITAL STAY BY NUMBER.

ASK Q'S 3-16 (AND 17-26 IF AP-
PLICABLE) FOR FIRST HOSPITAL
STAY BEFORE GOING ON TO NEXT.

HS

	BEGIN DECK 50	BEGIN DECK 50
	Stay ____ of ____ 8 First Hospital Stay $\frac{11-20}{9}$	Stay ____ of ____ 8 Second Hospital Stay $\frac{11-20}{9}$

3. What hospital was
   (PATIENT) in?

   What is its
   address?

	First Hospital Stay	Second Hospital Stay
Full Name of Hospital:	_____	_____
Street:	_____	_____
City & State:	_____	_____

4. How many days was (PATIENT)
   in the hospital?

Days . . . ☐☐☐ $\frac{21-23}{9}$	Days . . . ☐☐☐ $\frac{21-23}{9}$

5. What were the approximate
   dates? IF DATES NOT KNOWN,
   RECORD TIME OF MONTH (BEGIN-
   NING, MIDDLE, END).

From _____ $\frac{24-29}{9}$
     Mo. Day Year
To _____ $\frac{30-35}{9}$
     Mo. Day Year
	From _____ $\frac{24-29}{9}$
	     Mo. Day Year
	To _____ $\frac{30-35}{9}$
	     Mo. Day Year

6. How many beds were there in
   (PATIENT)'s room?

One bed . . . . . . 1 $\frac{36}{9}$ Two beds . . . . . . 2 Three or more . . . 3	One bed . . . . . 1 $\frac{36}{9}$ Two beds . . . . . 2 Three or more . . . 3

7. How much was the <u>hospital</u>
   bill--<u>counting</u> anything
   insurance may have paid, but
   <u>not counting</u> doctor's bills
   or any surgeon's fees?

$: ☐☐☐☐☐ $\frac{37-41}{9}$	$: ☐☐☐☐☐ $\frac{37-41}{9}$

8. Did any kind of hospital plan
   or insurance cover any part
   of the cost of hospitalization
   --or will any plan, even though
   it hasn't paid yet?

Yes . (ASK 9-14) . . 1 $\frac{42}{9}$ No . (SKIP TO 15). . 2	Yes . (ASK 9-14) . . 1 $\frac{42}{9}$ No . (SKIP TO 15). . 2

9. <u>IF INSURANCE</u>: What plans
   or insurance covered the
   hospitalization costs?
   RECORD ALL PLANS
   MENTIONED.

Plan (1): $\frac{43-44}{99}$	Plan (1): $\frac{43-44}{99}$
Plan (2): $\frac{45-46}{99}$	Plan (2): $\frac{45-46}{99}$

10. ASK FOR EACH PLAN:
    Has the insurance [PLAN (1),
    PLAN (2)] paid yet?
    CIRCLE ONE CODE FOR EACH
    PLAN.

Plan (1): Yes . . . 1 $\frac{47}{9}$
          No . . . 2
Plan (2): Yes . . . 3 $\frac{48}{9}$
          No . . . 4
	Plan (1): Yes . . . 1 $\frac{47}{9}$
	          No . . . 2
	Plan (2): Yes . . . 3 $\frac{48}{9}$
	          No . . . 4

	DECK 50	DECK 50
	Stay ___ of ___	Stay ___ of ___
	First Hospital Stay	Second Hospital Stay

11. ASK FOR EACH PLAN:

How much (did/will) [PLAN (1), PLAN (2)] pay on the hospitalization?

(1) $: [ ][ ][ ][ ][ ] 49-53 / 9   (1) $: [ ][ ][ ][ ][ ] 49-53 / 9

(2) $: [ ][ ][ ][ ][ ] 54-58 / 9   (2) $: [ ][ ][ ][ ][ ] 54-58 / 9

Total of (1) & (2) $: [ ][ ][ ][ ][ ] 59-63 / 9 $: [ ][ ][ ][ ][ ] 59-63 / 9

12. IF TOTAL IN Q. 11 IS MORE THAN TOTAL IN Q. 7, ENTER DIFFERENCE HERE AND SKIP TO Q. 15.

$: [ ][ ][ ][ ][ ] 64-68 / 9 $: [ ][ ][ ][ ][ ] 64-68 / 9

13. And how much did you (your family) have to pay for the hospital bill that was not covered by any insurance?

$: [ ][ ][ ][ ][ ] 69-73 / 9 $: [ ][ ][ ][ ][ ] 69-73 / 9

14. ADD AMOUNTS IN Q'S. 11 (TOTAL) AND 13. IF TOTAL DIFFERS FROM AMOUNT IN 7, PROBE FOR CORRECTION.

BEGIN DECK 51   BEGIN DECK 51

TOTAL: _____ 11-15 / 9   TOTAL: _____ 11-15 / 9

15. Did (PATIENT) have any kind of operation or have any broken or dislocated bones set while in the hospital that time?

Yes . .(ASK 16) . . . 1 16 / 9
No (RETURN TO Q.3 FOR NEXT HOSPITAL STAY. IF LAST STAY, SKIP TO 27) 2

Yes . . (ASK 16) . . 1 16 / 9
No (RETURN TO Q.3 FOR NEXT HOSPITAL STAY. IF LAST STAY, SKIP TO 27) 2

16. How many times was (PATIENT) on the operating table during this hospital stay?

Operations: [ ][ ] 17-18 / 99   Operations: [ ][ ] 17-18 / 99

IF MORE THAN TWO OPERATIONS, USE ANOTHER SUPPLEMENT FOR Q'S 17-26, ABOUT THIRD, FOURTH, ETC. OPERATION.

BE SURE TO IDENTIFY OPERATION AND HOSPITAL STAY BY NUMBER.

ASK Q'S. 17-26 FOR FIRST OPERATION BEFORE GOING TO NEXT.

During hospital stay ___ of ___ BEGIN DECK 60 8   During hospital stay ___ of ___ BEGIN DECK 60 8

Operation ___ of ___ 9   Operation ___ of ___ 9

Operation: Operation:

17. What kind of operation or bone setting was it?

11-12 / 99   11-12 / 99

18. Who was the doctor who performed the operation (or set the broken bones)?

What is his address?

13-22 / 9   13-22 / 9

Full Name of Doctor   Full Name of Doctor

Street   Street

City   State   Zip   City   State   Zip

		During hospital stay ____ of ____	DECK 60	During hospital stay ____ of ____	DECK 60
		Operation ____ of ____		Operation ____ of ____	
19.	How much was the <u>surgeon's</u> total bill for the operation --including anything that insurance paid, as well as what you paid?	$: ☐☐☐☐☐	23-27 9	$: ☐☐☐☐☐	23-27 9
20.	Did any kind of surgical plan or insurance cover any part of the cost of the operation --or will any plan, even though it hasn't paid yet?	Yes (ASK 21-26) . 1 No (SKIP TO 27) . 2	28 9	Yes (ASK 21-26) . 1 No (SKIP TO 27) . 2	28 9
21.	IF INSURANCE: What insurance or plans covered the operation? RECORD ALL PLANS MENTIONED.	First Plan: Second Plan:	29-30 99 31-32 99	First Plan: Second Plan:	29-30 99 31-32 99
22.	ASK FOR EACH PLAN: Has the insurance [PLAN (1), PLAN (2)] paid yet?	Plan (1): Yes . . 1 No . . 2 Plan (2): Yes . . 3 No . . 4	33 9 34 9	Plan (1): Yes . . 1 No . . 2 Plan (2): Yes . . 3 No . . 4	33 9 34 9
23.	How much (did/will) the insurance [PLAN (1), PLAN (2)] pay on the (NAME OF OPERATION IN Q. 17)?	(1) $ ☐☐☐☐ (2) $ ☐☐☐☐	35-39 9 40-44 9	(1) $ ☐☐☐☐ (2) $ ☐☐☐☐	35-39 9 40-44 9
	Total of (1) & (2)	Total $ ☐☐☐☐	45-49 9	Total $ ☐☐☐☐	45-49 9
24.	IF TOTAL IN Q. 23 IS MORE THAN TOTAL IN Q.19, ENTER DIFFERENCE HERE AND SKIP TO Q. 27.	$ ☐☐☐☐☐	50-54 9	$ ☐☐☐☐☐	50-54 9
25.	How much of the charge for (NAME OF OPERATION) did you (your family) have to pay that was not covered by insurance?	$ ☐☐☐☐☐	55-59 9	$ ☐☐☐☐☐	55-59 9
26.	ADD AMOUNTS IN Q'S. 23 (TOTAL) AND 25. IF TOTAL DIFFERS FROM AMOUNT IN Q.19, PROBE FOR CORRECTIONS.	Total: $_____	60-64 9	Total: $_____	60-64 9

DECKS 40-42

27. ASK EVERYONE:	ASK B-E ABOUT FIRST ITEM CODED "YES." THEN GO ON TO NEXT "YES" ITEM.				
A. Did (PATIENT) have any other expenses in the hospital that were <u>not</u> covered on the hospital bill, for which (he/she) was billed separately--expenses for things like--READ EACH ITEM CODING "YES" OR "NO" FOR EACH.	**B.** What were the total charges for (ITEM) <u>including</u> anything insurance paid, as well as what you paid? ENTER AMOUNT BELOW.	**C.** And was anything paid on (ITEM) by insurance? ENTER AMOUNT BELOW. IF MORE THAN ONE PLAN PAID, RECORD AMOUNTS SEPARATELY. IF NOTHING, ENTER "0" AND SKIP TO NEXT "YES" ITEM.	**D.** What insurance plan paid this amount? ENTER NAME(S) OF INSURANCE PLAN(S) BELOW.	**E.** Then that left (AMOUNT IN "B" MINUS AMOUNT IN "C") that you had to pay... is that right? IF YES: ENTER AMOUNT BELOW. IF NO: MAKE NECESSARY CORRECTIONS.	
Item	A. Yes No	B. Total	C. Insurance Paid	D. Name of Insurance	E. "Net"
CONTINUE DECK 40 An anesthesiologist's fee that was not charged on the hospital bill?	1　2 <u>19</u> 9	☐☐☐☐ 20-23	☐☐☐☐ 24-27 ☐☐☐☐ 28-31	<u>32-33</u> 99 <u>34-35</u> 99	☐☐☐☐ 36-39
A pathologist's <u>separate</u> charge for laboratory tests?	1　2 <u>40</u> 9	☐☐☐☐ 41-44	☐☐☐☐ 45-48 ☐☐☐☐ 49-52	<u>53-54</u> 99 <u>55-56</u> 99	☐☐☐☐ 57-60
BEGIN DECK 41 A radiologist's <u>separate</u> charge for X-ray tests or treatments?	1　2 <u>11</u> 9	☐☐☐☐ 12-15	☐☐☐☐ 16-19 ☐☐☐☐ 20-23	<u>24-25</u> 99 <u>26-27</u> 99	☐☐☐☐ 28-31
Private duty nursing?	1　2 <u>32</u> 9	☐☐☐☐ 33-36	☐☐☐☐ 37-40	<u>41-42</u> 99	☐☐☐☐ 43-46
Oxygen?	1　2 <u>47</u> 9	☐☐☐☐ 48-51	☐☐☐☐ 52-55	<u>56-57</u> 99	☐☐☐☐ 58-61
BEGIN DECK 42 Ambulance?	1　2 <u>11</u> 9	☐☐☐☐ 12-15	☐☐☐☐ 16-19	<u>20-21</u> 99	☐☐☐☐ 22-25
Anything else that was charged for <u>separately</u>? (IF YES: SPECIFY)	1　2 <u>26</u> 9	☐☐☐☐ 27-30	☐☐☐☐ 31-34 ☐☐☐☐ 35-38	<u>39-40</u> 99 <u>41-42</u> 99	☐☐☐☐ 43-46

28. A. What is the name of the doctor or place that gave
       (PATIENT) the <u>most</u> care for (CONDITION)?
       FILL IN <u>BOTH</u> DOCTOR'S NAME AND NAME OF CLINIC,
       IF POSSIBLE.   _____
                                                                 Full Name of Doctor
       <u>IF SOURCE ALREADY MENTIONED</u>, ENTER NAME(S) AND GO
       TO Q. 29.   _____
                                                                 Name of Clinic/Group
       <u>IF NEW SOURCE</u>, ASK B, AND C <u>OR</u> D.
                                                                 _____
    B. What is the address?   Street

                                                                 _____
                                                                 City

                                                                 _____
                                                                 State and Zip   <u>11-20</u>
                                                                                        9

    C. <u>IF NEW CLINIC MENTIONED</u>: Does (PATIENT) go
       to a particular doctor at the clinic?   Yes (ENTER NAME OF
                                                                   DOCTOR ABOVE) . . 1

                                                                 No 2

    D. <u>IF NEW DOCTOR MENTIONED</u>: Is the doctor part of a
       clinic or group practice?   Yes (ENTER NAME OF
                                                                   CLINIC ABOVE) . . 3

                                                                 No 4

---

29. Which reason on this card best describes why (PATIENT) happened to go to (PHYSICIAN/
    PLACE) for (CONDITION)?

    | CARD |
    | A |

        Usual doctor or clinic 1   <u>21</u>
        Referred by usual doctor 2   9
        Referred by another (not usual) doctor 3
        Picked by patient or family to treat this condition 4
        Recommended by other relatives or friends to treat this condition . 5
        Referred by someone else (SPECIFY) 6

30.

CARD B

A. At which of these places did visits of or to (SOURCE NAMED IN Q. 28) take place? CODE ALL THAT APPLY IN COLUMN A BELOW.	ASK B AND C FOR EACH PLACE CODED IN A.	
	B. How many visits were there during the past year at (PLACE IN COLUMN A)? ENTER VISITS IN COLUMN B BELOW.	C. What was the cost for the visits at (PLACE IN COLUMN A), including anything that insurance paid? ENTER COSTS IN COLUMN C.
A. Places	B. No. of Visits	C. Cost
Doctor at your home 1	☐☐☐	$: ☐☐☐☐ 22-28 / 9
Doctor's office or private clinic (including group practice plan) 2	☐☐☐	$: ☐☐☐☐ 29-35 / 9
Hospital out-patient department 3	☐☐☐	$: ☐☐☐☐ 36-42 / 9
Hospital emergency room 4	☐☐☐	$: ☐☐☐☐ 43-49 / 9
Industrial, school, camp, or college health service 5	☐☐☐	$: ☐☐☐☐ 50-56 / 9
Any other clinic not connected with a hospital--such as a board of health clinic or a neigh-borhood health center 6	☐☐☐	$: ☐☐☐☐ 57-63 / 9
In-hospital visits 7	☐☐☐	$: ☐☐☐☐ 64-70 / 9

D. IF THIS DOCTOR IS THE SURGEON (Q. 18), AND NO COSTS ARE REPORTED FOR VISITS ABOVE, ASK:

Are costs for these visits included in (SURGEON)'s bill?

Yes 1   71 / 9
No   2

31. Did (PATIENT) see any <u>other</u> doctor or visit any <u>other</u> doctor's office or clinic about this condition in the past year?

Yes (ASK Q'S 32-35). 3   72 / 9
No (SKIP TO Q. 36) . 4

32. A. What is the name of the other doctor
       whom (PATIENT) saw, or place that
       (PATIENT) visited?
       FILL IN <u>BOTH</u> DOCTOR'S NAME AND NAME
       OF CLINIC, IF POSSIBLE.   _____
                                                      Full Name of Doctor

       <u>IF SOURCE ALREADY MENTIONED</u>, ENTER
       NAME(S) AND GO TO Q. 33.   _____
       <u>IF NEW SOURCE</u>, ASK B, AND C <u>OR</u> D.   Name of Clinic/Group

    B. What is the address?   _____
                                                      Street

                                                      _____
                                                      City

                                                      _____
                                                      State and Zip
                                                                          11-20
    C. <u>IF NEW CLINIC MENTIONED</u>: Does (PATIENT)   9
       go to a particular doctor at the clinic?   Yes (ENTER NAME OF
                                                          DOCTOR ABOVE) . . . 1

                                                      No 2

    D. <u>IF NEW DOCTOR MENTIONED</u>: Is the doctor
       part of a clinic or group practice?   Yes (ENTER NAME OF
                                                          CLINIC ABOVE) . . . 3

                                                      No 4

---

33. Which reason on this card best describes why (PATIENT) happened to go to
    (PHYSICIAN/PLACE) for (CONDITION)?

    ┌────────┐
    │ CARD   │ Usual doctor or clinic 1   21
    │ A   │   ──
    └────────┘ Referred by usual doctor 2   9

                Referred by another (not usual) doctor 3

                Picked by patient or family to treat this condition 4

                Recommended by other relatives or friends to treat this
                    condition 5

                Referred by someone else (SPECIFY) 6

34.	A. At which of these places did visits of or to (SOURCE) NAMED IN Q. 32) take place? CODE ALL THAT APPLY IN COLUMN A BELOW.	ASK B AND C FOR EACH PLACE CODED IN A.	
CARD B		B. How many visits were there during the past year at (PLACE IN COLUMN A)? ENTER VISITS IN COLUMN B BELOW.	C. What was the cost for the visits at (PLACE IN COLUMN A), including anything that insurance paid? ENTER COSTS IN COLUMN C.
	A. Places	B. No. of Visits	C. Cost
	Doctor at your home 1	☐☐☐	$: ☐☐☐ 22-28 / 9
	Doctor's office or private clinic (including group practice plan) 2	☐☐☐	$: ☐☐☐ 29-35 / 9
	Hospital out-patient department 3	☐☐☐	$: ☐☐☐ 36-42 / 9
	Hospital emergency room 4	☐☐☐	$: ☐☐☐ 43-49 / 9
	Industrial, school, camp, or college health service 5	☐☐☐	$: ☐☐☐ 50-56 / 9
	Any other clinic not connected with a hospital--such as a board of health clinic or a neighborhood health center 6	☐☐☐	$: ☐☐☐ 57-63 / 9
	In-hospital visits 7	☐☐☐	$: ☐☐☐ 64-70 / 9

	D. IF THIS DOCTOR IS THE SURGEON (Q. 18), AND NO COSTS ARE REPORTED FOR VISITS ABOVE, ASK:	Are costs for these visits included in (SURGEON)'s bill?	Yes . . . . 1 No 2	71 / 9

35. Did (PATIENT) visit any <u>other</u> doctor or clinic about this condition in the past year?

Yes (USE DR. CONTINU-ATION SHEET) . . . 3   72 / c

No   (GO TO Q. 36) . 4

36. Do you have any medical insurance that helped (will help) pay any of these doctor bills?

Yes   .(ASK 37-38) . . . 1 $\frac{17}{9}$

No . (SKIP TO 39) . . . 2

---

37. What insurance or plan helped?

RECORD AS MANY PLANS AS MENTIONED.

Plan (1):

_____ $\frac{18-19}{99}$

Plan (2):

_____ $\frac{20-21}{99}$

---

38. How much did (will) insurance pay for . . . (ITEM)? READ EACH ITEM THAT APPLIES TO PATIENT.

MAKE SURE AMOUNTS ARE NOT ALREADY RECORDED IN INSURANCE FOR SURGEON'S FEE.

IF INSURANCE PAID NOTHING, RECORD "0" IN APPROPRIATE BOXES.

In-hospital visits $: \boxed{\ \ | \ \ | \ \ }$ $\frac{22-25}{9}$

Home visits $: \boxed{\ \ | \ \ | \ \ }$ $\frac{26-29}{9}$

Care in doctor's office $: \boxed{\ \ | \ \ | \ \ }$ $\frac{30-33}{9}$

Clinic visits (including hospital out- patient or emer- gency room) $: \boxed{\ \ | \ \ | \ \ }$ $\frac{34-37}{9}$

39. ASK EVERYONE:

ASK B-D FOR EACH ITEM CODED "YES." THEN GO TO NEXT "YES" ITEM.

A. During 1970 did (PATIENT) have any other medical care for this condition--that is not counting what you've already told me about? Things like ....READ THROUGH LIST, CODING "YES" OR "NO" FOR EACH ITEM.	B. What were (PATIENT'S) total expenses for (ITEM)--including anything insurance paid, as well as what you paid? ENTER AMOUNT BELOW.	C. And was anything paid on (ITEM) by insurance? ENTER AMOUNT BELOW. IF NONE, ENTER "0" AND SKIP TO NEXT "YES" ITEM.	D. Then that left (AMOUNT IN "B" MINUS AMOUNT IN "C") that you had to pay. Is that right? IF YES: ENTER AMOUNT BELOW. IF NO: MAKE NECESSARY CORRECTIONS.
Expenses	A. Yes No	B. Total	C. Insurance Paid	D. "Net"

DECK 45

Expenses	A. Yes No	B. Total	C. Insurance Paid	D. "Net"
Medicines the doctor or hospital prescribed for this condition?	1 2 <u>38</u> 9	39-42	43-46	47-50
Other non-prescribed medicines for this condition?	1 2 <u>51</u> 9	52-55	56-59	60-63
BEGIN DECK 46. X-ray tests?	1 2 <u>11</u> 9	12-15	16-19	20-23
Other special tests like blood tests, electrocardiograms, urine analyses, and so on?	1 2 <u>24</u> 9	25-28	29-32	33-36
Special treatments like X-ray treatments, heat or diathermy treatments, massages, and so on?	1 2 <u>37</u> 9	38-41	42-45	46-49
Home nursing care?	1 2 <u>50</u> 9	51-54	55-58	59-62
BEGIN DECK 47. Any medical equipment or appliances like braces, crutches, wheel chair, vaporizer, or anything like that?	1 2 <u>11</u> 9	12-15	16-19	20-23
Anything else? IF "YES," LIST:	1 2 <u>24</u> 9	25-28	29-32	33-36

IF INSURANCE PAID PART OF EXPENSES IN Q. 39:

40. What insurance plan paid on the expenses? RECORD AS MANY AS GIVEN.

37-38 / 99
39-40 / 99
41-42 / 99

41. IF FREE OR REDUCED RATE CARE ALREADY MENTIONED, CODE WITHOUT ASKING.

Aside from free samples of drugs the doctor might have given (PATIENT), was any of the care you've told me about received free of charge or at a reduced rate?

Yes . . (ASK A&B) 1		43
No . . (GO TO 42) . . . 2		9

IF YES:

A. What was the care? _____   44-45

B. Which item on this card best describes the <u>main</u> reason that the care was free of charge or at a reduced rate?   CIRCLE ONE CODE ONLY FOR MAIN REASON.   46-47

CARD D

On public aid (Receiving welfare payments).	01
Recipient of Medicaid (No welfare payments)	02
Went to free or part-pay clinic or public hospital.	03
Went to V.A. hospital for <u>non-service</u>-connected disability	04
Private doctor or hospital didn't charge, or reduced the bill because we couldn't pay	05
Went to V.A. hospital for <u>service</u>-connected disability	06
Armed Forces member or dependent	07
Professional courtesy	08
Participant in medical research	09
Workmen's Compensation	10
Participant in pre-paid group practice plan	11
Industrial, school, camp, or college health service	12
Other (SPECIFY) _____	13

48-49
99

---

42. Now, was (PATIENT) in a hospital for one night or more for any <u>other</u> illness, accident, or condition during 1970?

Yes (FILL OUT ANOTHER HOSPITAL SUPPLEMENT) . 1	50
No (RETURN TO MAIN QUESTIONNAIRE Q. 16 OR PAST PREGNANCY SUPPLEMENT, Q. 44) . . 2	9

NORC 4106
January, 1971

Form approved.
OMB No. 68 - S70089

National Opinion Research Center
University of Chicago

MAJOR ILLNESS SUPPLEMENT

BEGIN DECK 70

| Line No. | | | | |
| Family Unit | |

Patient's Name   1-4

and Per. No.   5-6

Illness ____ of _____   7/

Family name: _____

Respondent's name: _____

---

1. What was the condition (injury/illness) (PATIENT) had?

11-13/

14-16/

17-19/

---

2. Did this condition involve any kind of surgery (or bone-setting) during 1970, that was performed when (PATIENT) was not an overnight patient in a hospital?

Yes 1   20/9

No 2

MI

3. A. What is the name of the doctor or place that
(provided the most care for this condition)
(performed [OPERATION IN Q 2])? FILL IN
BOTH DOCTOR'S NAME AND NAME OF CLINIC, IF
POSSIBLE. IF NO PHYSICIAN SEEN OR CLINIC
VISITED, CIRCLE CODE AND SKIP TO Q 11.

BEGIN DECK 71

Full Name of Doctor

No Dr./Place visited (SKIP TO Q 11) . . X

Name of Clinic/Group

IF SOURCE ALREADY MENTIONED, ENTER NAME(S) AND GO TO Q.4.

Street

IF NEW SOURCE, ASK B, AND C OR D.

B. What is the address?

City

State and Zip   11-20/9

C. IF NEW CLINIC MENTIONED: Does (PATIENT) go to
a particular doctor at the clinic?

Yes (ENTER NAME
OF DOCTOR
ABOVE) 1

No 2

D. IF NEW DOCTOR MENTIONED: Is the doctor part of a
clinic or group practice?

Yes (ENTER NAME
OF CLINIC
ABOVE) 3

No 4

4. Which reason on this card best describes why (PATIENT) happened to go to (PHYSICIAN/
PLACE) for (CONDITION)?

CARD
A

Usual doctor or clinic 1   21/9

Referred by usual doctor 2

Referred by another (not usual) doctor 3

Picked by patient or family to treat this condition 4

Recommended by other relatives or friends to
treat this condition 5

Referred by someone else (SPECIFY) 6

5. CARD B	A. At which of these places did visits of or to (SOURCE NAMED IN Q 3) take place? CODE ALL THAT APPLY IN COLUMN A. BELOW.	ASK B. AND C. FOR EACH PLACE CODED IN A.	
		B. How many visits were there during the past year at (PLACE IN COLUMN A.)? ENTER VISITS IN COLUMN B. BELOW.	C. What was the cost for the visits at (PLACE IN COLUMN A.), including anything that insurance paid? ENTER COSTS IN COLUMN C.
	A. Place	B. No. of Visits	C. Cost
	Doctor at your home 1	☐☐☐	$ ☐☐☐☐ 22-28/9
	Doctor's office or private clinic (including group practice plan) 2	☐☐☐	$ ☐☐☐☐ 29-35/9
	Hospital out-patient dept. 3	☐☐☐	$ ☐☐☐☐ 36-42/9
	Hospital emergency room 4	☐☐☐	$ ☐☐☐☐ 43-49/9
	Industrial, school, camp, or college health service 5	☐☐☐	$ ☐☐☐☐ 50-56/9
	Any other clinic not connected with a hospital--such as a board of health clinic or a neighborhood health center 6	☐☐☐	$ ☐☐☐☐ 57-63/9
			64-70/R

6. Did (PATIENT) see any <u>other</u> doctor or visit any <u>other</u> doctor's office or clinic about this condition in the past year?

Yes (ASK Q'S 7-10) . . . 1   71/9

No (SKIP TO Q 11) . . . 2

MI

7. A. What is the name of the other doctor or place that (PATIENT) visited? FILL IN <u>BOTH</u> DOCTOR'S NAME AND NAME OF CLINIC, IF POSSIBLE.

<u>IF SOURCE ALREADY MENTIONED, ENTER NAME(S) AND GO TO Q. 8.</u>

<u>IF NEW SOURCE</u>, ASK B., AND C. <u>OR</u> D.

Full Name of Doctor

Name of Clinic/Group

B. What is the address?

Street

City

State and Zip	11-20/9

C. <u>IF NEW CLINIC MENTIONED</u>: Does (PATIENT) go to a particular doctor at the clinic?

Yes (ENTER NAME OF
   DOCTOR ABOVE) . . 1

No 2

D. <u>IF NEW DOCTOR MENTIONED</u>: Is the doctor part of a clinic or group practice?

Yes (ENTER NAME OF
   CLINIC ABOVE) . . 3

No 4

---

8. Which reason on this card best describes why (PATIENT) happened to go to (PHYSICIAN/ PLACE) for (CONDITION)?

CARD
A

Usual doctor or clinic 1 21/9

Referred by usual doctor 2

Referred by another (not usual) doctor 3

Picked by patient or family to treat this condition . . 4

Recommended by other relatives or friends to treat
   this condition 5

Referred by someone else (SPECIFY) 6

DECK 72

9. CARD B	A. At which of these places did visits of or to (SOURCE NAMED IN Q. 7) take place? CODE ALL THAT APPLY IN COLUMN A. BELOW.	ASK B. AND C. FOR EACH PLACE CODED IN A.	
		B. How many visits were there during the past year at (PLACE IN COLUMN A.)? ENTER VISITS IN COLUMN B. BELOW.	C. What was the cost for the visits at (PLACE IN COLUMN A.), including anything that insurance paid? ENTER COSTS IN COLUMN C.

A. Place		B. No. of Visits	C. Cost	
Doctor at your home	1	☐☐☐	$ ☐☐☐	22-28/9
Doctor's office or private clinic (including group practice plan)	2	☐☐☐	$ ☐☐☐	29-35/9
Hospital outpatient dept.	3	☐☐☐	$ ☐☐☐	36-42/9
Hospital emergency room	4	☐☐☐	$ ☐☐☐	43-49/9
Industrial, school, camp, or college health service	5	☐☐☐	$ ☐☐☐	50-56/9
Any other clinic not connected with a hospital--such as a board of health clinic or a neighborhood health center	6	☐☐☐	$ ☐☐☐	57-63/9
				64-70/R

10. Did (PATIENT) visit any <u>other</u> doctor or clinic about this condition in the past year?

Yes (USE DR. CONTINU-
ATION SHEET) . . . 1   71/9

No (GO TO Q. 11) . . 2

I

l1.

A. Did (PATIENT) have any (other) medical care for this condition last year--things like. . . READ THROUGH LIST, CODING "YES" OR "NO" FOR EACH ITEM.				B. ASK ABOUT EACH ITEM CODED "YES": What were (PATIENT'S) total expenses for (ITEM)--including anything that insurance may have paid? ENTER AMOUNTS BELOW.
	A. Yes No			B. Expense
Medicines the doctors prescribed for this condition?	1	2	11/9	$ \boxed{\quad\quad\quad\quad}$ 12-15/9
Other non-prescribed medicines?	1	2	16/9	$ \boxed{\quad\quad\quad\quad}$ 17-20/9
X-ray tests?	1	2	21/9	$ \boxed{\quad\quad\quad\quad}$ 22-25/9
Other special tests--like blood tests, electrocardiograms, urine analyses, and so on?	1	2	26/9	$ \boxed{\quad\quad\quad\quad}$ 27-30/9
Special treatments--like X-ray treatments, massages, heat or diathermy treatments, or any other kind of treatment?	1	2	31/9	$ \boxed{\quad\quad\quad\quad}$ 32-35/9
Home nursing care?	1	2	36/9	$ \boxed{\quad\quad\quad\quad}$ 37-40/9
Any medical equipment or appliances like braces, crutches, wheelchair, a vaporizer, or anything like that?	1	2	41/9	$ \boxed{\quad\quad\quad\quad}$ 42-45/9
Anything else? IF "YES," SPECIFY:	1	2	46/9	$ \boxed{\quad\quad\quad\quad}$ 47-50/9

12. IF ANY CARE REPORTED (Q'S 3-11), WITH ANY COSTS REPORTED: Did any kind of insurance or medical care plan cover any part of these costs--or will it, even though it hasn't paid yet?

Yes (ASK 13-14) . 1   51/9

NO (SKIP TO 15) . 2

    13. What is the name of the insurance? RECORD ALL THAT ARE MENTIONED.

Plan (1) _____   52-53/99

Plan (2) _____   54-55/99

BEGIN DECK 74

14. How much (did/will) insurance pay on . . .
READ EACH ITEM THAT APPLIES:

(a) Doctor visits to your home: $ [| |]   11-14/9

(b) Visits to doctor's office or clinic: $ [| |]   15-18/9

(c) Drugs and medicine: $ [| |]   19-22/9

(d) Other medical expenses (tests, treatments, nursing care, medical appliances): $ [| |]   23-26/9

15. IF FREE OR REDUCED RATE CARE ALREADY MENTIONED, CODE WITHOUT ASKING.

Aside from free samples of drugs the doctor might have given (PATIENT), was any of the care you've told me about received free of charge or at a reduced rate?

Yes (ASK A & B) . 1   **27**
No (GO TO 16) . . 2   9

28-29

A. What was the care? _____

B. Which item on this card best describes the main reason that the care was free of charge, or at a reduced rate? CIRCLE ONE CODE ONLY, FOR MAIN REASON.   30-31

CARD D

On public aid (receiving welfare payments) 01   **32-33**
Recipient of Medicaid (no welfare payments) 02   99
Went to free or part pay clinic or public hospital 03
Went to V.A. hospital for <u>non-service</u> connected disability 04
Private doctor or hospital didn't charge or reduced the bill because we couldn't pay 05
Went to V.A. hospital for <u>service</u> connected disability 06
Armed Forces member or dependent 07
Professional courtesy 08
Participant in medical research 09
Workmen's Compensation 10
Participant in prepaid group practice plan 11
Industrial, school, camp, or college health service 12
Other (SPECIFY) 13

16. Has (PATIENT) had any <u>other</u> illness, accident or condition for which expenses amounted to $100 or more, or for which a doctor was seen five or more times, or for which regular care or treatment was required during 1970?

Yes (FILL OUT ANOTHER MAJOR ILLNESS SUPPLEMENT) 1   **34**
9

No (RETURN TO Q 20, MAIN QUESTION- NAIRE OR Q 45, PAST PREGNANCY SUPPLEMENT) 2

NORC-4106
Jan., 1971

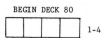

Form approved.
OMB No. 68 - S70089

National Opinion Research Center
University of Chicago

INSURANCE SUPPLEMENT

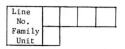

BEGIN DECK 80

1-4

Line No.				
Family Unit				

Family Name: _____

Respondent's Name: _____

	DECK 80	
	Plan ____ of ____	5

1. As well as you remember, what is the full name of each of your health insurance policies or health care plans? ENTER NAME OF EACH PLAN MENTIONED AT HEAD OF A SEPARATE COLUMN (EXCEPT: ENTER BLUE CROSS/BLUE SHIELD IN SAME COLUMN, IF FAMILY HAS BOTH).

Name of Plan or Insurance:

Do you (or anyone in the family) have any <u>other</u> hospital or medical insurance or plans, or did (any of) you have one during the last year, even if you don't have it now? Do you have any separate policy that pays <u>only for dental care</u>? ENTER ADDITIONAL POLICIES AT COLUMN HEADS. IF MORE THAN FIVE, USE ANOTHER SUPPLEMENT.

11-12

2. CLASSIFY EACH PLAN LISTED AS DENTAL ONLY, "BLUE" PLAN, OR OTHER. THEN ASK Q'S 3-15, AS APPROPRIATE, FOR FIRST PLAN BEFORE GOING ON TO SECOND, ETC. ASK FOR <u>ALL</u> PLANS BEFORE GOING ON TO Q. 16.

Dental only (GO TO NEXT PLAN) . . 1
Blue Plan (SKIP TO 7) 2
Other (ASK 3) . . 3

13
9

3. IF "OTHER": Does (NAME OF PLAN) cover expenses in the case of <u>accident only</u> or does it cover expenses of medical care <u>for illness too</u>? IF "ACCIDENT ONLY," DRAW "X" THROUGH NAME OF POLICY; ASK <u>NO MORE</u> QUESTIONS ABOUT IT.

Accident only (STOP) 4
Illness too (ASK 4) 5

14
9

4. IF "ILLNESS TOO": Does this plan pay you a flat amount of weekly benefits or does it pay according to the amount of medical care used?

Flat amount (ASK 5) 6
According to medical care (SKIP TO 6) . . 7

15
9

5. IF "FLAT AMOUNT": Does this plan pay: <u>only</u> when you are in the hospital; <u>more</u> when you are in the hospital; or whenever you are ill and can't work? IF "PAYS WHEN CAN'T WORK," DRAW "X" THROUGH NAME OF POLICY. ASK <u>NO MORE</u> QUESTIONS ABOUT IT.

Only in hospital (ASK 6) . 1
More in hospital (ASK 6) . 2
When can't work (STOP) 3

16
9

6. IF "ACCORDING TO MEDICAL CARE" (Q.4), OR "ONLY IN HOSPITAL" OR "MORE IN HOSPITAL" (Q.5): Does this policy pay <u>only</u> on expenses connected with some serious or rare diseases, such as cancer, or does it pay on <u>any</u> kind of illness?

Rare diseases (RETURN TO Q 2, NEXT PLAN) . . 5
Any illness (ASK 7) 6

17
9

ASK FOR "BLUE PLANS" (Q 2) AND "ANY ILLNESS" (Q 6):

7. Would this plan cover any part of the hospital charges if someone had to go to the hospital?

Yes 1
No 2

18
9

8. Would (NAME OF PLAN) cover any part of the surgical expenses if someone had to have an operation?

Yes 3
No 4

19
9

	DECK 80
	Plan ____ of ____ <u>5</u>
	Name of Plan or Insurance:
	11-12

9. Would this plan cover any doctor bills in the hospital other than for surgery?

Yes . . . . 5 $\frac{20}{9}$
No 6

10. Would it pay any part of bills for visits to a doctor at a doctor's office, or provide free office visits to certain doctors?

Yes . . . . 7 $\frac{21}{9}$
No 8

11. Would it pay any part of the doctor's charges for house calls?

Yes . . . . 1 $\frac{22}{9}$
No 2

12. Would it cover any charges for prescribed medicines taken outside the hospital?

Yes . . . . 3 $\frac{23}{9}$
No 4

13. Would this plan cover <u>any</u> charges for dental care, outside of a hospital?

Yes . . . . 5 $\frac{24}{9}$
No 6

14. Is this plan a Major Medical or Master Medical type plan?

Yes . (ASK 15). . 1 $\frac{25}{9}$
No (RETURN TO Q 2, NEXT PLAN) 2
DK (RETURN TO Q 2, NEXT PLAN) 3

15. IF "MAJOR MEDICAL" OR "MASTER MEDICAL": Is this insurance <u>only</u> Major Medical, or is it part of a basic plan that also gives you regular hospital and/or surgical coverage?

NOW RETURN TO Q.2, NEXT PLAN. IF LAST PLAN, GO ON TO Q. 16.

Only Major Medical . . . . 4 $\frac{26}{9}$
Also regular plan 5
DK 6

ASK 16 FOR <u>ALL</u> PLANS AND FILL IN INFORMATION A-C. THEN ASK 17-24 AS APPROPRIATE, FOR FIRST PLAN BEFORE GOING ON TO SECOND, ETC.

16. Do you happen to have a copy of the (NAME) policy or a membership card from it?

FILL IN AS MUCH OF THE FOLLOWING INFORMATION ABOUT EACH POLICY AS IS READILY ACCESSIBLE.

A. Full name of Insurance Company or Underwriter:

Yes (ASK A-C) . . 7 $\frac{27}{9}$
No (ASK FOR NEXT PLAN. IF LAST PLAN GO TO 17) . 8
Name:

28-32

B. Policy or Certificate Number (FOR BLUE PLANS: Contract No., which is also Subscriber No. on Membership Card):

Policy No.:

C. Type of policy or certificate (IF BLUE CROSS <u>AND</u> BLUE SHIELD, RECORD BOTH TYPES, IF DIFFERENT):

Type Policy:

	DECK 80	
Plan ____ of ____		5
Name of Plan or Insurance:		
		11-12

17.	How many months during 1970 was this plan in effect? IF "ALL YEAR," CODE 12, AND SKIP TO Q 19.	Months: ☐☐ 33-34/99 IF LESS THAN 12 MONTHS, ASK Q 18.
	18. Was this plan in effect December 31, 1970?	Yes . . . . . 1 35/9 No, dropped (SKIP TO 20) 2

19. ENTER ON SEPARATE LINES NAMES OF ALL FAMILY MEMBERS FROM Q 10 OF THE HOUSEHOLD FOLDER. BE SURE PERSON NO. CORRESPONDS TO CORRECT NAME.

ASK FOR EACH POLICY, UNLESS DROPPED (Q 18).

ASK FOR EACH PERSON LISTED:

Was (PERSON) covered by (NAME OF PLAN) on December 31?

[IF PERSON DIED OR LEFT FAMILY UNIT BEFORE DEC. 31, ASK: Was (PERSON) covered at the time (he/she) (died/left the household)?]

NAME OF PERSON	PER.NO.	COVERED ON DEC. 31? Yes No	
Name:	01	1 2	36/9
Name:	02	1 2	37/9
Name:	03	1 2	38/9
Name:	04	1 2	39/9
Name:	05	1 2	40/9
Name:	06	1 2	41/9
Name:	07	1 2	42/9
Name:	08	1 2	43/9
Name:	09	1 2	44/9
Name:	10	1 2	45/9

ASK Q'S 20-21 FOR EACH POLICY:

20.	In whose name is (was) this policy or plan membership--that is, which person is (was) the main subscriber?	Name: Per.No. ☐☐ 46-47
21.	How does (did) (SUBSCRIBER) carry this insurance--through work or a union, through membership in some other kind of group (Grange, Farm Bureau, Medical Society, etc.), directly through the insurance company, or what?	Work or union (ASK 22) . . . . 1 48/9 Other group (SKIP TO 24) . 2 Directly (SKIP TO 24) . 3 Other (SKIP TO 24) . 4
22.	Does (did) the employer pay all of the cost of this insurance, a part of the cost, or none of the cost?	ALL (RET. TO 17, NEXT POLICY) . 1 49/9 Part (ASK 23-24) 2 None (ASK 23-24) 3
23.	Is the amount that (SUBSCRIBER) pays (paid) for this insurance deducted from his salary or pay check by the employer?	Yes . . . . . . 5 50/9 No . . . . . . 6 DK 7
24.	(Outside of what the employer pays) How much does (did) this insurance cost the family itself per year?	$: ☐☐☐☐ 51-54 9

WHEN ALL QUESTIONS HAVE BEEN ASKED FOR ALL POLICIES, RETURN TO Q 67, MAIN QUESTIONNAIRE.

NORC-4106
Jan., 1971

Form approved.
OMB· No. 68 - S70089

National Opinion Research Center
University of Chicago

HEALTH OPINIONS QUESTIONNAIRE

BEGIN DECK 90

1-4

Person No. . . . .

5-6

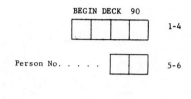

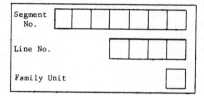

Segment No.

Line No.

Family Unit

Filled in by: (CIRCLE ONE)

Male head with spouse in household 1
Male head without spouse in household . . 2
Female head without spouse in household . 3
Wife of head 4
Other: (SPECIFY) _____ 5

11/9

(CIRCLE ONE)

Filled out in presence of interviewer . . 7
Filled out alone 8

12/9

HO

1. As you probably know, Medicare is the government-sponsored health insurance for people 65 and over. It is paid for mainly through Social Security taxes on workers and employers. By increasing the taxes that workers and employers have to pay, Medicare could cover other people in the population as well.

   Do you favor . . . (CIRCLE ONE ONLY)

Keeping it as it is . . (SKIP TO Q. 3) 1	13
Extending it to cover people under 65 who cannot afford their own health insurance 2	9
Extending it to cover all people in the country 3	
Doing away with the program (SKIP TO Q.. 4) . . . 4	

2. What, in your opinion, is the best way to pay for covering more people under Medicare? (CIRCLE ONE ONLY)

By increasing the Social Security taxes paid by workers and their employers 5	14
By raising income taxes 6	9
By charging premiums to the people getting the coverage, as is now done for supplementary medical bills (where people over 65 pay $5.30 a month for doctor bill coverage) 7	

3. Medicare currently pays for a large part of hospital bills and some doctors' bills for people 65 and over. It could pay for all their medical care, including prescribed drugs and dental care, by increasing Social Security or income taxes or by charging extra premiums.

   Are you in favor of . . . (CIRCLE ONE ONLY)

Keeping Medicare benefits as they are now . . . 1	15
Increasing benefits to include all hospital and doctor expenses and also drug and dental expenses 2	9
Cutting back on what Medicare now pays for . . . 3	

4. An alternative to extending Medicare to other groups in the population is for the government to reimburse families for what they spend themselves on health insurance, say up to $500 a year. The lower the family income the more the government would contribute.

   Do you favor . . . (CIRCLE ONE ONLY)

The government paying families for health insurance costs 4	16
Extending Medicare 5	9
Do not support either approach 6	

HO   DECK 90

5. Do you think doctors will provide better medical care for everyone if they
    are paid . . . (CIRCLE ONE ONLY)

                 A flat monthly salary 1   17
                                                                        ──
                 According to the amount of treatment   9
                 they give their patients. 2

                 How a doctor is paid doesn't affect the
                 kind of care he provides 3

---

6. Do you agree or disagree with each of the following statements about universal govern-
    ment health insurance (extending Medicare to everyone): (CIRCLE ONLY ONE NUMBER FOR
    EACH STATEMENT).

		Strongly agree	Agree	Disagree	Strongly disagree	
A.	It will allow people of low or moderate income to get more or better health care.	1	2	3	4	$\frac{18}{9}$
B.	It will interfere with the right of each doctor to treat his patients as he sees fit.	5	6	7	8	$\frac{19}{9}$
C.	It will result in too much government regulation of health care.	1	2	3	4	$\frac{20}{9}$
D.	It is necessary because private health insurance has not done an adequate job.	5	6	7	8	$\frac{21}{9}$
E.	It will keep the costs of medical care from going up so fast.	1	2	3	4	$\frac{22}{9}$
F.	It will result in overuse of medical care.	5	6	7	8	$\frac{23}{9}$
G.	It will provide all people with access to high-quality care.	1	2	3	4	$\frac{24}{9}$
H.	It will mean a longer wait to see a doctor.	5	6	7	8	$\frac{25}{9}$

---

7. Some people say one way to provide more medical care at reasonable costs is
    to allow a nurse or specially-trained doctor's assistant to do some of the
    less complicated work doctors now do. Others feel that allowing non-M.D.'s
    to do some of the doctor's work reduces the quality of medical care. Would
    you be willing to let a nurse or doctor's assistant . . . (CIRCLE ONE FOR
    EACH STATEMENT)

		Yes	No	Undecided	
A.	Do the preliminaries of a medical examination before the doctor comes in, including medical history taking, blood pressure, and so on.	1	2	3	$\frac{26}{9}$
B.	Decide whether or not you need to see a doctor when you go to a doctor's office or clinic when you are not feeling well.	5	6	7	$\frac{27}{9}$
C.	Provide follow-up care and treatment after a physician has diagnosed your condition and prescribed treatment.	1	2	3	$\frac{28}{9}$
D.	See pregnant women and babies on their regular visits when nothing seems to be wrong.	5	6	7	$\frac{29}{9}$

HO

8. Thinking over the medical care you and those close to you have received over
    the past few years from doctors and hospitals, how satisfied have you been with
    each of the following: (CIRCLE ONE FOR EACH STATEMENT):

		Very satis-fied	Satis-fied	Unsatis-fied	Very unsatis-fied	
A.	Overall quality of the medical care received.	1	2	3	4	$\frac{30}{9}$
B.	Waiting time in doctor's offices or clinics.	5	6	7	8	$\frac{31}{9}$
C.	Availability of medical care at night and on weekends.	1	2	3	4	$\frac{32}{9}$
D.	Ease and convenience of getting to a doctor from where you live.	5	6	7	8	$\frac{33}{9}$
E.	The out-of-pocket costs of the medical care received.	1	2	3	4	$\frac{34}{9}$
F.	The information given to you about what was wrong with you.	5	6	7	8	$\frac{35}{9}$
G.	The information given to you about what you should do at home to treat illness.	1	2	3	4	$\frac{36}{9}$
H.	The courtesy and consideration shown you by doctors.	5	6	7	8	$\frac{37}{9}$
I.	The courtesy and consideration shown you by nurses.	1	2	3	4	$\frac{38}{9}$
J.	The follow-up care received after an initial treatment or operation.	5	6	7	8	$\frac{39}{9}$
K.	Concern of doctors for your overall health rather than just for an isolated symptom or disease.	1	2	3	4	$\frac{40}{9}$
L.	Getting all of your medical care needs taken care of at the same location.	5	6	7	8	$\frac{41}{9}$
M.	Information you have been able to obtain to help you choose a physician.	1	2	3	4	$\frac{42}{9}$

9. Here are some things people sometimes say about health care, doctors, hospitals and also about other people you might turn to for help, like lawyers. Do you agree or disagree with each statement? Please circle the number under the phrase which best describes your own feeling toward each statement. (CIRCLE ONLY ONE NUMBER FOR EACH STATEMENT.)

	Strongly Agree	Tend to Agree	Tend to Disagree	Strongly Disagree	
A. If you wait long enough, you can get over most any disease without getting medical aid.	1	2	3	4	$\frac{43}{9}$
B. Good personal health depends more on an individual's strong will power than on vaccinations, shots, and vitamins.	5	6	7	8	$\frac{44}{9}$
C. Some home remedies are still better than prescribed drugs for curing illness.	1	2	3	4	$\frac{45}{9}$
D. No matter how well a person follows his doctor's orders, he has to expect a good deal of illness in his lifetime.	5	6	7	8	$\frac{46}{9}$
E. A person understands his own health better than most doctors do.	1	2	3	4	$\frac{47}{9}$
F. Modern medicine can cure most any illness.	5	6	7	8	$\frac{48}{9}$
G. The medical profession is about the highest calling a man can have in this country.	1	2	3	4	$\frac{49}{9}$
H. Most doctors are more interested in their incomes than in making sure everyone receives adequate medical care.	5	6	7	8	$\frac{50}{9}$
I. Choosing your own doctor is about the most important thing in getting good medical care.	1	2	3	4	$\frac{51}{9}$
J. The care I have generally received from doctors in the last few years was excellent.	5	6	7	6	$\frac{52}{9}$
K. There is a crisis in health care today in the United States.	1	2	3	4	$\frac{53}{9}$
L. Lawyers usually charge reasonable fees.	5	6	7	8	$\frac{54}{9}$
M. If you have a good lawyer, he can get you out of trouble if he really tries.	1	2	3	4	$\frac{55}{9}$
N. All people have a right to good medical care whether they can pay for it or not.	5	6	7	8	$\frac{56}{9}$

HO

10. People react in various ways to their medical conditions. Please look at each condition and circle the number under the phrase which best describes what <u>you</u> would do if <u>you</u> had the condition. (CIRCLE ONLY ONE NUMBER FOR EACH SYMPTOM.)

	Call ambulance at once	Go to hospital emergency room same day	See my doctor within three days	See my doctor within one month	Do nothing (treat it myself)	
A. You have a sharp chest pains for the first time.	1	2	3	4	5	$\frac{57}{9}$
B. Your wrist swells two hours after a fall.	1	2	3	4	5	$\frac{58}{9}$
C. You have a sore throat or running nose with a fever as high as 100° F. for at least two days.	1	2	3	4	5	$\frac{59}{9}$
D. You have your third severe headache in as many days.	1	2	3	4	5	$\frac{60}{9}$
E. You cut your finger deeply with a dirty knife.	1	2	3	4	5	$\frac{61}{9}$

11. Read each statement below about what symptoms may be early signs of various common diseases. Circle the number under agree, disagree, or undecided depending on your opinion about each statement. (CIRCLE ONLY ONE NUMBER FOR EACH STATEMENT.)

	Agree	Disagree	Undecided	
A. Shortness of breath after light exercise may be a sign of cancer.	1	2	3	$\frac{62}{9}$
B. Shortness of breath after light exercise may be a sign of heart disease.	6	7	8	$\frac{63}{9}$
C. Coughing or spitting up of blood may be a sign of tuberculosis.	1	2	3	$\frac{64}{9}$
D. Coughing or spitting up of blood may be a sign of diabetes.	6	7	8	$\frac{65}{9}$
E. Open sores or ulcers that do not heal may be a sign of cancer.	1	2	3	$\frac{66}{9}$
F. Open sores or ulcers that do not heal may be a sign of heart disease.	6	7	8	$\frac{67}{9}$
G. Unexplained loss of weight may be a sign of tuberculosis.	1	2	3	$\frac{68}{9}$
H. Unexplained loss of weight may be a sign of diabetes.	6	7	8	$\frac{69}{9}$
I. Pains in the chest may be a sign of heart disease.	1	2	3	$\frac{70}{9}$
J. Pains in the chest may be a sign of tuberculosis.	6	7	8	$\frac{71}{9}$

NORC-4106
Jan., 1971

National Opinion Research Center
University of Chicago

PERMISSION FORM

Form approved.
OMB No. 68 - S70089

1-4

Segment No.

Line No.

Family Unit

The National Opinion Research Center of the University of Chicago has my permission to obtain information on charges and insurance benefits for medical care received during 1970 by myself and members of my family listed below. I understand that this information will be completely confidential and will be used for statistical purposes only.

DATE: _____

SIGNED: _____

ADDRESS: _____

_____

Per. No.

NORC 4130
December, 1971

HOSPITAL RECORD FORM

Calendar Year 1970

Form approved.
OMB No. 68-S70089
DECK 57

Illness ☐☐ 14-15

Admission ☐☐ 16-17

Supplement ☐ 18

Patient's Name _____

Street Address _____

FOR NORC
USE ONLY

City _____ State _____

PATIENT'S AGE: _____ ☐☐ 19-20

PATIENT'S SEX: _____ ☐ 21

1. Number of times person was in your hospital from January 1, 1970, through
   December 31, 1970: . . . . ☐☐ ☐ 22-23
   IF "0" SKIP TO ITEM 9 ON REVERSE OF FORM.

2. IF MORE THAN ONE HOSPITAL STAY DURING 1970, PLEASE USE A SEPARATE FORM FOR EACH HOSPITAL-
   IZATION, AND STAPLE ALL FORMS FOR THE SAME PATIENT TOGETHER.
   This form is for hospital stay number: ☐ ☐ 24-25

3. Date of Admission: _____ Date of Discharge: _____ ☐ 26-28
   (Month, Day, Year)   (Month, Day, Year)   ☐ 29

   IN THE EVENT THAT THE STAY FOR A HOSPITALIZATION BEGAN BEFORE JANUARY 1, 1970, OR EXTEND-
   ED BEYOND DECEMBER 31, 1970, INCLUDE ONLY THOSE CHARGES INCURRED AND OPERATIONS PER-
   FORMED DURING 1970.
   ☐☐☐☐☐ 30-34

Item	Total hospital charges (IF NONE, ENTER "0")	Amount paid to hospital directly by insurance or other third-party payer. (Include assignments taken by the hospital for commercial insurance.) (IF NONE, ENTER "0")	Name of insurance or other third-party payer(s) (Such as Medicare or Public Aid)
Room and Board, Number of days: ___ Daily rate: $_____ FOR MATERNITY STAYS, INCLUDE CHARGE FOR BABY HERE.	$	$	
Operating or delivery room	$	$	
All other charges (drugs, X-rays, lab., anesthesia, other)	$	$	
GRAND TOTAL	$	$	

☐☐☐☐ 35-38

☐☐☐☐☐ 39-43

☐☐☐☐☐☐ 44-49

☐☐ 50-51

☐☐☐☐☐☐ 52-57

☐☐ 58-59

☐☐☐☐☐☐ 60-65

☐☐ 66-67

Total paid by patient (exclusive of
payments to hospital by third-party
payers) . . . . $ _____

IF AMOUNT HERE PLUS AMOUNT
PAID BY THIRD-PARTY PAYERS
DOES NOT EQUAL TOTAL,
PLEASE EXPLAIN BELOW.

☐☐☐☐☐ 68-72

☐☐ 73-74

_____

-Side two-

4. Please list here the name of any insurance policies that did <u>not</u> pay the hospital directly but which may have paid the patient or his family for hospital care.

FOR NORC
USE ONLY

_____

_____   □□   19-20

_____   □□   21-22

5. Was there any special billing by: (CIRCLE ONE NUMBER FOR EACH.)

	Yes	No	
Anesthesiologist?	1	2	23
Pathologist?	3	4	24
Radiologist?	5	6	25
Private duty nurse?	7	8	26

6. Admitting diagnoses: _____

                  _____

		27-29
		30-32
		33-35

   Discharge diagnoses: _____

		36-38
		39-41
		42-44

7. Name of doctor mainly in charge of patient's care while patient was in the hospital:

_____
(First)   (Last)   □□□□□ 45-49

    Is this doctor a . . . . (CIRCLE APPROPRIATE NUMBER.)

              private physician? 1   50

              salaried staff doctor (including
              interns and residents)? 2

8. Was there a surgical procedure performed?
   (CIRCLE ONE NUMBER.)   Yes . . (ANSWER A, B, & C) . . 3   51

   IF YES: No . . (IF NO, SKIP TO 9) . . 4

   A.   Name of surgical procedure: _____

	52-53
	54-55

   B.   Name of surgeon: _____
                (First)   (Last)   □□□□□ 56-60

   C.   Is this doctor a . . . . (CIRCLE APPROPRIATE NUMBER.)

              private physician? 5   61

              salaried staff doctor (including
              interns and residents)? 6

9. FOR PATIENTS NOT HOSPITALIZED IN 1970, PLEASE CIRCLE APPROPRIATE NUMBER BELOW:

       This person has <u>no record</u> of being hospitalized here at any time . . 1   62

       This person has been hospitalized here, but <u>prior to</u> 1970 2

       This person has been hospitalized here <u>since</u> December 31, 1970 3

	63		67

10. Name of person preparing this report: _____

	64		68

   Title: _____ Date: _____

	65		69
	66		70

   Phone: _____
        (Area Code)

Form Approved.				
OMB No. 68-S70089				

HEALTH INSURANCE RECORD FORM
Non-group Insurance
Calendar Year 1970

BEGIN DECK 87

NORC-4129
1/72

Family ⬚⬚⬚ 1-4

Member ⬚⬚ 5-6

Plan ⬚⬚ 7-8

9-12

Member's Name:

Address:

City-State:

FROM OUR RECORDS:

Name of Insurance Company:

Type of Policy:

Identification Number:

13-14/R

1. Was the person listed above covered by health or sickness insurance through your company or plan during any part of the calendar year 1970? (Circle one number below.)

Yes . . (Go to Item 2) . . . 1   15/9

No . (If no, skip to Item 10) . 2

Answer A and B:

2. A. What types of coverage did person have during 1970? (Circle a number under "Yes" or "No" in Column A for each type of coverage listed.)

   B. For each type of coverage person had during 1970: Under what type of contract was the coverage provided? (Circle a number in Column B for each coverage in effect.)

	A. Covered during 1970		B. Type of Contract		
	Yes	No	One Person	Family	
Basic hospital	1	2	3	4	16-17
Basic surgical-medical	5	6	7	8	18-19
Major medical or comprehensive	1	2	3	4	20-21
Flat rate per week when hospitalized	5	6	7	8	22-23
Prepaid group practice	1	2	3	4	24-25
Other (SPECIFY TYPE SUCH AS SUPPLEMENTARY TO MEDICARE, RARE DISEASE, ETC.)	5	6	7	8	26-27

3. How much was the annual premium for this coverage for the calendar year 1970?   28-53/R

Total annual premium: $ ⬚⬚⬚⬚   54-57

4. If Basic Hospital and/or Surgical-Medical Insurance included, enter following amounts:

Maximum per day room and board payment:
(If no limit, or if most common semi-private, please write in.) $ ☐☐☐   58-60

_____

Number of days covered: ☐☐☐   61-63

Payment for appendectomy (indemnity plan): . . . . $ ☐☐☐   64-66

Per cent of reasonable and customary charges (service plan): . . . . ☐☐ %   67-68

5. If Major Medical or Comprehensive insurance included, enter following amounts: BEGIN DECK 88

13-14/R

Deductible: . . . . $ ☐☐☐   15-17

Co-insurance (Per cent paid by individual): . . . . ☐☐ %   18-19

Maximum payment: $ ☐☐☐☐☐☐   20-25

6. If flat rate policy, enter following amounts, then skip to Item 8.

Amount paid per week when hospitalized: . . . . $ ☐☐☐☐   26-29

Day of hospitalization on which payment starts: . . . . . ☐☐   30-31

For all insurance except flat rate policies:

7. A. Does this insurance provide benefits for the services listed below? (Circle a number under "Yes" or "No" in Column A for each service listed.)

For each type of service circled "Yes" in A below, answer B.

B. Is this service covered under Basic coverage, Major medical or comprehensive coverage, both, or some other kind of coverage? (Circle appropriate number for each benefit provided in Column B.)

Service	A. Service provided?		IF YES TO A: B. Type of Coverage				
	Yes	No	Basic	Major Medical/ Compre- hensive	Both	Other	
Inpatient hospital care	1	2	3	4	5	6	32-33
Treatment in outpatient department or emergency room of hospital	1	2	3	4	5	6	34-35
In-hospital surgery	1	2	3	4	5	6	36-37
Surgery in a doctor's office	1	2	3	4	5	6	38-39
Doctor visits in a hospital	1	2	3	4	5	6	40-41
Doctor visits in a private office, clinic, or patient's home	1	2	3	4	5	6	42-43
X-rays and lab tests	1	2	3	4	5	6	44-45
Nursing home care	1	2	3	4	5	6	46-47
Out-of-hospital prescribed drugs	1	2	3	4	5	6	48-49
Dental care outside of a hospital	1	2	3	4	5	6	50-51

☐☐   52-53

8. Please list separately each family member who received any services during <u>calendar year 1970</u> paid for by this insurance. Enter total paid (to the nearest dollar) for each service received in person's column. If you are unable to give the amount paid by insurance, simply indicate which services the person received which were covered by insurance.

	Office only	Office only	Office only	Office only	Office only	
	Name	Name	Name	Name	Name	13-14
Inpatient hospital care	$	$	$	$	$	15-20
Treatment in out-patient department or emergency room of hospital	$	$	$	$	$	21-24
In-hospital surgery	$	$	$	$	$	25-29
Surgery in a doctor's office	$	$	$	$	$	30-33
Doctor visits in a hospital	$	$	$	$	$	34-37
Doctor visits in a private office, clinic, or patient's home	$	$	$	$	$	38-41
X-rays and lab tests	$	$	$	$	$	42-45
Nursing home care	$	$	$	$	$	46-50
Out-of-hospital prescribed drugs	$	$	$	$	$	51-54
Dental care outside of a hospital	$	$	$	$	$	55-58
Other (Describe):	$	$	$	$	$	59-62
Total	$	$	$	$	$	63-68

CONTINUE DECK 88

9. <u>Please list identifying numbers, letters, and names of health insurance policies, riders, and endorsements in the space below:</u>

54/R

10. <u>If no record of health insurance for this person during 1970, circle one number for appropriate statement</u>:

Person was covered <u>during 1969</u> 1   55/9

Person was covered <u>since January 1, 1971</u> . . . 2

No record of policy holder with this name . . 3

11. <u>Please use this space for any comments which might clarify information in this form:</u>

13. Name of person completing form: _____

56/9

Position: _____

Business Phone: _____
(Area Code)

Mailing Address: _____

Thank you very much.

57	58	59	60	61
62	63	64	65	66

HEALTH INSURANCE RECORD FORM
Group Insurance
Calendar Year 1970

BEGIN DECK 87

NORC-4129
1/72

Form Approved.
OMB No. 68-S70089

Family ☐☐☐ 1-4

Member ☐☐ 5-6

Plan ☐☐ 7-8

9-12

Member's Name:

Address:

City-State:

Employer's Name:

FROM OUR RECORDS:

Name of Insurance Company:

Type of Policy:

Identification Number:

13-14/R

1. Was the person listed above covered by health or sickness insurance through your company or plan during any part of the calendar year 1970? (Circle one number below.)

Yes . . . . (Go to Item 2) . . . 1

No . . (If no, skip to Item 11) 2

15/9

Answer A and B:

2. A. What types of coverage did person have during 1970? (Circle a number under "Yes" or "No" in Column A for each type of coverage listed.)

B. For each type of coverage person had during 1970: Under what type of contract was the coverage provided? (Circle a number in Column B for each coverage in effect.)

	A Covered During 1970		B Type of Contract		
	Yes	No	One Person	Family	
Basic hospital	1	2	3	4	16-17
Basic surgical-medical	5	6	7	8	18-19
Major medical or comprehensive	1	2	3	4	20-21
Flat rate per week when hospitalized	5	6	7	8	22-23
Prepaid group practice	1	2	3	4	24-25
Other (SPECIFY TYPE SUCH AS SUPPLEMENTARY TO MEDICARE, RARE DISEASE, ETC.)	5	6	7	8	26-27

3. How much did the employer pay and how much did the employee pay per year for these policies? Do not include payment for group life insurance, annuities, or disability insurance.

	Premiums for Employee's Coverage	Premiums for Dependents' Coverage	Total	
Employee contribution	$	$	$	28-37
Employer contribution	$	$	$	38-47
Total cost	$	$	$	48-57

4. If Basic Hospital and/or Surgical-Medical Insurance included, enter following amounts:

Maximum per day room and board payment:
(If no limit, or if most common semi-private, please write in.) $ ☐☐☐   58-60

Number of days covered: ☐☐☐   61-63

Payment for appendectomy (indemnity plan): . . . . $ ☐☐☐   64-66

Per cent of reasonable and customary charges (service plan): . . . . ☐☐ %   67-68

---

5. If Major Medical or Comprehensive insurance included, enter following amounts: BEGIN DECK 88

                                                                   13-14/R

Deductible: . . . . $ ☐☐☐   15-17

Co-insurance (Per cent paid by individual): . . . . ☐☐ %   18-19

Maximum payment: $ ☐☐☐☐☐☐   20-25

---

6. If flat rate policy, enter following amounts, then skip to Item 8.

Amount paid per week when hospitalized: . . . . $ ☐☐☐☐   26-29

Day of hospitalization on which payment starts: . . . . . ☐☐   30-31

For all insurance except flat rate policies:

7. A. Does this insurance provide benefits for the services listed below? (<u>Circle a number</u> under "Yes" or "No" in Column A for each service listed.)

For each type of service circled "Yes" in A below, answer B.

B. Is this service covered under Basic coverage, Major medical or comprehensive coverage, both, or some other kind of coverage? (<u>Circle appropriate number for each benefit</u> provided in Column B.)

Service	A. Service provided?		IF YES TO A: B. Type of Coverage				
	Yes	No	Basic	Major Medical/ Compre- hensive	Both	Other	
Inpatient hospital care	1	2	3	4	5	6	32-33
Treatment in outpatient department or emergency room of hospital	1	2	3	4	5	6	34-35
In-hospital surgery	1	2	3	4	5	6	36-37
Surgery in a doctor's office	1	2	3	4	5	6	38-39
Doctor visits in a hospital	1	2	3	4	5	6	40-41
Doctor visits in a private office, clinic, or patient's home	1	2	3	4	5	6	42-43
X-rays and lab tests	1	2	3	4	5	6	44-45
Nursing home care	1	2	3	4	5	6	46-47
Out-of-hospital prescribed drugs	1	2	3	4	5	6	48-49
Dental care outside of a hospital	1	2	3	4	5	6	50-51

☐☐   52-53

8. Please list separately each family member who received any services during <u>calendar year 1970</u> paid for by this insurance. Enter total paid (to the nearest dollar) for each service received in person's column. If you are unable to give the amount paid by insurance, simply indicate which services the person received which were covered by insurance.

	Office only	Office only	Office only	Office only	Office only	
	Name	Name	Name	Name	Name	13-14
Inpatient hospital care	$	$	$	$	$	15-20
Treatment in out-patient depart-ment or emergency room of hospital	$	$	$	$	$	21-24
In-hospital surgery	$	$	$	$	$	25-29
Surgery in a doctor's office	$	$	$	$	$	30-33
Doctor visits in a hospital	$	$	$	$	$	34-37
Doctor visits in a private office, clinic, or patient's home	$	$	$	$	$	38-41
X-rays and lab tests	$	$	$	$	$	42-45
Nursing home care	$	$	$	$	$	46-50
Out-of-hospital prescribed drugs	$	$	$	$	$	51-54
Dental care outside of a hospital	$	$	$	$	$	55-58
Other (Describe):	$	$	$	$	$	59-62
Total	$	$	$	$	$	63-68

CONTINUE DECK 88

9. <u>Please list identifying numbers, letters, and names of health insurance policies, riders, and endorsements in the space below</u>:

10. Approximately how many main subscribers or policy holders were covered under this group contract as of December 31, 1970? Circle the number indicating the group's size.

Less than 5 1	50-99 5
5-9 2	100-499 6
10-24 3	500-999 7
25-49 4	1000 and over 8

54/9

11. <u>If no record of health insurance for this person during 1970, circle one number for appropriate statement</u>:

Person was covered <u>during 1969</u> 1   55/9

Person was covered <u>since January 1, 1971</u> 2

<u>Employer</u> has policy with us, but cannot locate <u>employee</u> with this name 3

No record of <u>employer</u> of this name 4

12. <u>Please use this space for any comments which might clarify information in this form</u>:

13. Name of person completing form: _____   56/9

Position: _____

Business Phone: _____
(Area Code)

Mailing Address: _____

Thank you very much.

57	58	59	60	61
62	63	64	65	66

NORC 4128
August, 1971

PATIENT RECORD FORM

CALENDAR YEAR 1970

Form approved.
OMB No. 68-S70089

DECK 97

Patient's Name

Street Address

City   State

PATIENT'S AGE: _____ 12-13

PATIENT'S SEX: _____ 14

1. Was the above patient seen at least once during 1970? (CIRCLE ONE)

Yes . . . (ANSWER Q'S. 2 THROUGH 7) . 1   15/9

No . (ANSWER Q'S. 6 & 7 ON REVERSE) . 2

2. PLEASE ANSWER BOTH A AND B:

   A. What were this patient's "chief complaints" during 1970?

   B. What were the diagnoses?

   16-17
   18-19
   20-21
   22-23
   24-25
   26-27

3. On what basis were you (the doctor) compensated for care given this patient? (CIRCLE ONE)

Fee for service 1	Retainer 3 28/9
Salary 2	Other (SPECIFY) _____ 4

4. Who paid for the care this patient received in 1970? (CIRCLE ALL THAT APPLY)

Patient paid directly 1 29/	Professional courtesy 3	36/
Medicare 2 30/	Free or part-pay clinic or hospital 4	37/
Blue Cross/Blue Shield 3 31/	Prepaid group practice 5	38/
Private Insurance (SPECIFY) 4 32/	Veteran's Administration 1	39/
_____	Armed Forces 2	40/
Public aid--Medicaid 5 33/	Employer or school 3	41/
Workmen's Compensation 1 34/	Other (DESCRIBE) _____ 4	42/
Reduced rate or no charge--hardship . 2 35/		

OVER

-2-   DECKS 97-99

RECORD OF TREATMENT FOR CALENDAR YEAR 1970

5. For each kind of service performed, enter the total number of patient visits made during the year (where applicable); the charges; and the amount(s) of insurance or other third-party payment. Please include <u>only</u> services provided during 1970, and round amounts to the nearest dollar.

Services	A. Number of Visits	B. Total Doctor Charge for Service	C. Amount paid to doctor by insurance or other third-party for specific service
Visits at patient's home Deck 97	43-45	46-49	50-53
Visits at the doctor's own office or clinic	54-56	57-60	61-64
Visits at an emergency room Deck 98	12-14	15-18	19-22
Visits at a hospital outpatient department	23-25	26-29	30-33
Visits at other outpatient site (DESCRIBE)	34-36	37-40	41-44
Visits to inpatient in hospital	45-47	48-51	52-55
Outpatient surgery (DESCRIBE)			
Hospitalized surgery (DESCRIBE) 56/ Deck 99		57-60	61-64
12-13 14-15		16-19	20-23
Drugs		24-27	28-31
Tests, special treatments, medical equipment or appliances		32-35	36-39
Other services (SPECIFY)		40-43	44-47
TOTAL		48-51	52-55

6. CIRCLE ALL OF THE FOLLOWING THAT APPLY: The patient was (also) seen . . .

    before January 1, 1970 1   56/9

    since December 31, 1970 2

    at no time that we can determine 4

7. NAME, TITLE, AND PHONE NUMBER OF PERSON FILLING OUT FORM (PLEASE PRINT):

    NAME: _____ TITLE: _____   57/9

    PHONE: _____
           (Area Code)

Thank you very much for your cooperation.

Appendix V

Uses of the 1970 Data

The following lists indicate books, articles, reports, presentations and hearings, doctoral dissertations, and organizations that used the 1970 data; these lists suggest the range of uses and dissemination of the data and study findings. The data have been used for discussions of public policy issues in federal and state government and in business, as well as for disciplinary research. The broad scope of the survey has provided these groups with health utilization, expenditure and attitude information for discussion of the wide range of topics shown in the papers listed below, including health care regulation, national health insurance, costs of catastrophic illness, distribution of health care services, international comparisons of national health systems, children's health care, access to and continuity of medical care, and control of health care costs.

PUBLISHED BOOKS AND PAPERS

Aday, Lu Ann. 1975. "Economic and non-economic barriers to the use of needed medical services." *Medical Care* 13 (June):447–56.

Aday, Lu Ann and Ronald Andersen. 1975. *Development of Indices of Access to Medical Care.* Ann Arbor, Michigan: Health Administration Press.

Andersen, Ronald. 1975. "Health service distribution and equity," In *Equity in Health Services: Empirical Analyses in Social Policy.* Andersen et al., eds. Cambridge, Massachusetts: Ballinger Publishing Co.

——. 1975. "The effect of measurement error on differences in the use of health services." In *Equity in Health Services: Empirical Analyses in Social Policy.* Andersen et al., eds. Cambridge, Massachusetts: Ballinger Publishing Co.

Andersen, Ronald; Richard Foster; and Peter Weil. 1976. "Rates and correlates of expenditure increases for personal health services in periods before and after Medicare and Medicaid." *Inquiry.* In press.

Andersen, Ronald and Judith D. Kasper. 1973. "The structural influence of family size on children's use of physician services." *Journal of Comparative Family Studies* 4 (Spring):116–30.

Andersen, Ronald; Joanna Kravits; and Odin W. Anderson. 1971. "The public's view of the crisis in medical care: an impetus for changing delivery systems?" *Economic and Business Bulletin* 24:44–52.

Andersen, Ronald; Joanna Kravits; Anita Francis; and Virginia Daughety. 1976. "Psychologically-related illness and health services utilization." *Medical Care.* Supplement. In press.

Andersen, Ronald and John F. Newman. 1973. "Societal and individual determinants of medical care utilization in the United States." *Milbank Memorial Fund Quarterly* 51 (Winter):95–124.

Andersen, Ronald and Bjorn Smedby. 1975. "Changes in response to symptoms of illness in the United States and Sweden." *Inquiry* 12. Supplement.

Benham, Lee. 1972. "The effect of advertising on the price of eyeglasses." *Journal of Law and Economics* 15 (October):337–52.

———. "Women's economic returns from college, graduate education, and nurses' training through earnings and marriage." In *Sex Discrimination and the Division of Labor.* Cynthia Lloyd, ed. New York: Columbia University Press. Forthcoming.

Benham, Lee and Alexandra Benham. 1975. "Regulating through the professions: a perspective on information control." *Journal of Law and Economics* 18 (October).

———. 1975. "The impact of incremental medical services on health status, 1963–1970." In *Equity in Health Services: Empirical Analyses in Social Policy.* Andersen et al., eds. Cambridge, Massachusetts: Ballinger Publishing Co.

———. 1975. "Utilization of physician services across income groups, 1963–1970." In *Equity in Health Services: Empirical Analyses in Social Policy.* Andersen et al., Cambridge, Massachusetts: Ballinger Publishing Co.

Diehr, Paula; Kathleen O. Jackson; and M. Vickie Boscha. 1975. "Access to medical care: the impact of outreach services on enrollees of a prepaid health insurance program." *Journal of Health and Social Behavior* 16 (September):326–40.

Kasper, Judith D. 1975. "Physician utilization and family size." In *Equity in Health Services: Empirical Analyses in Social Policy.* Andersen et al., eds. Cambridge, Massachusetts: Ballinger Publishing Co.

Kravits, Joanna. 1975. "The relationship of attitudes to discretionary physician and dentist use by race and income." In *Equity in Health Services: Empirical Analyses in Social Policy.* Andersen et al., eds. Cambridge, Massachusetts: Ballinger Publishing Co.

Kravits, Joanna and John Schneider. 1975. "Health care need and actual use by age, race and income." In *Equity in Health Services: Empirical Analyses in Social Policy.* Andersen et al., eds. Cambridge, Massachusetts: Ballinger Publishing Co.

Marmor, Theodore R.; Don A. Wittman; and Thomas C. Heagy. 1976. "The politics of inflation." *Journal of Health Politics, Policy and Law.* In press.

May, J. Joel. 1975. "Utilization of health services and the availability of resources." In *Equity in Health Services: Empirical Analyses in Social Policy.* Andersen et al., eds. Cambridge, Massachusetts: Ballinger Publishing Co.

Mitchell, Bridger and Charles E. Phelps. 1975. "Health and taxes: an assessment of the medical deduction." *Southern Economic Journal* (April).

Newhouse, Joseph P., Phelps, Charles E.; and William B. Schwartz. 1974. "Policy options and the impact of national health insurance." *New England Journal of Medicine* 290 (June 13).

Newman, John F. 1975. "Age, race and education as predisposing factors in physician and dentist utilization." In *Equity in Health Services: Empirical Analyses in Social Policy.* Andersen et al., eds. Cambridge, Massachusetts: Ballinger Publishing Co.

——. 1975. "Health status and utilization of physician services." In *Equity in Health Services: Empirical Analyses in Social Policy.* Andersen et al., eds. Cambridge, Massachusetts: Ballinger Publishing Co.

Phelps, Charles E. 1975. "Effects of insurance on demand for medical care." In *Equity in Health Services: Empirical Analyses in Social Policy.* Andersen et al., eds. Cambridge, Massachusetts: Ballinger Publishing Co.

Roos, Noralou. 1975. "Evaluating health programs: where do we find the data?" *Journal of Community Health* 1 (Fall):39–51.

Schwartz, Barry. 1975. *Queuing and Waiting: Studies in the Social Organization of Access and Delay.* Chicago: University of Chicago Press.

Shortell, Stephen M. 1975. "The effects of patterns of medical care on utilization and continuity of services." In *Equity in Health Services: Empirical Analyses in Social Policy.* Andersen et al., eds. Cambridge, Massachusetts: Ballinger Publishing Co.

——. 1976. "Continuity of medical care: conceptualization and measurement." *Medical Care.* In press.

Taylor, D. Garth; Lu Ann Aday; and Ronald Andersen. 1975. "A social indicator of access to medical care." *Journal of Health and Social Behavior* 16 (March):39–49.

REPORTS AND CURRENT RESEARCH

Abt Associates. 1976. "Characteristics of catastrophic illness in the U.S.—national profile." Cambridge, Massachusetts. In preparation.

——. 1976. "The impact of the 1974 recession on health insurance coverage and medical care utilization." Cambridge, Massachusetts. In preparation.

Aday, Lu Ann. 1975. "The impact of health policy on access to medical care." Center for Health Administration Studies, University of Chicago.

Aday, Lu Ann et al. 1973. "Development of a framework for the study of access to medical care." Preliminary report to the Robert Wood Johnson Foundation. Center for Health Administration Studies, University of Chicago.

Andersen, Ronald; Rachel McL. Greeley; Joanna Kravats; and Odin W. Anderson. 1972. *Health Service Use: National Trends and Variations, 1953–1971.* DHEW Publication No. (HSM) 73–3004 (October).

Andersen, Ronald; Joanna Kravits; Odin W. Anderson; and Joan Daley. 1973. *Expenditures for Personal Health Services: National Trends and Variations, 1953–1970.* DHEW Publication No. (HRA) 74-3105 (October).

Andersen, Ronald; Judity Kasper; and Martin Frankel (eds.). 1976. *Total Survey Error: Bias and Random Error in Health Survey Estimates.* In preparation.

Butler, John A. 1975. "Improving the organization of children's health care services." Harvard Child Health Care Project, Harvard University.

Council of Economic Advisors. 1976. *Economic Report of the President.* Executive Office of the President. Washington, D.C.: United States Government Printing Office (January).

Council on Wage and Price Stability. 1976. "The Problem of Rising Health Costs." Executive Office of the President. Washington, D.C.

Croner, Charles M. 1976. *Report on the Nation's Use of Health Resources.* Division of Health Resources Utilization Statistics, National Center for Health Statistics. In preparation.

Department of Health, Education and Welfare. 1974. *Report of Catastrophic Illness Conference.* Public Health Service, Health Resources Administration, Bureau of Health Services Research. Annapolis, Maryland (December).

Department of Health, Education and Welfare; Office Management and Budget; and Department of Defense. 1975. *Military Health Care Study.* Washington, D.C.

Eichhorn, Robert L. and Andrew M. Kulley. 1972. *Health Services Data System: The Family Health Survey.* Health Services Research and Training Program, Purdue University.

Ellwood, David. 1975. "The spend-down participation rate denominator." DHEW Contract No. SRS-74-58. Medical Spend-Down Study. Urban Systems Research and Engineering, Inc. Cambridge, Massachusetts.

Grossman, Michael. 1976. "The production and demand for children's health." National Bureau of Economic Research. In preparation.

Keeler, Emmett B.; David A. Relles; and John Rolph. 1975. "Family and individual deductibles." No. R-1393-OEO/HEW, Rand Corporation.

Mitchell, Bridger M. and Charles E. Phelps. 1975. "Employer-paid group health insurance and the costs of mandated national coverage." No. R-1509-NC/OEO, Rand Corporation (August).

National Center for Health Statistics. 1976. *Health: United States, 1975.* DHEW Publication No. (HRA) 76-1232.

Newhouse, Joseph P. and Dan Morrow. 1976. "Will consumers supplement a national health insurance plan?" Rand Corporation. In preparation.

Newhouse, Joseph P. and Maureen Murphy, 1976. "An estimate of the impact of a deductible on demand for medical care services." Rand Corporation. In preparation.

Office of the Governor (Washington). 1975. *Report of the Governor's Task Force on Catastrophic Health Care Costs.* Office of Community Development, Olympia, Washington (January).

Phelps, Charles E. 1974. "Private health insurance: what's good about it?

what's not so good? and what lessons can we learn?" *AMA Update*, American Medical Association (October).

———. 1976. "Tax-caused distortions in the health insurance market." Rand Corporation. In preparation.

Shephard, Donald. 1975. "An econometric model of variation in the incidence of surgery." Center for the Analysis of Health Practices, Harvard School of Public Health.

Sloan, Frank. 1976. "Impact of national economic conditions on health care for the poor: access to primary care." University of Florida, Gainesville. In preparation.

Ware, John E.; M. K. Snyder; and W. R. Wright. 1975. "Development and validation of scales to measure patient satisfaction with health services: volume 1 of the final report." Contract No. HSM 110-72-299, Southern Illinois University, School of Medicine (December).

Weinstein, Milton C. and William Stason. 1976. "The cost effectiveness of treatment for hypertension." Center for the Analysis of Health Practices, Harvard School of Public Health. In preparation.

PRESENTATIONS AND HEARINGS

Aday, Lu Ann. 1976. "Consumer behavior in the health marketplace: emphasis on access to medical care." Presented at the Steinhart Conference, University of Nebraska, Lincoln (March 10).

Aday, Lu Ann and Ronald Andersen. 1976. "Economic and non-economic barriers to the use of needed medical services." Presented at the Congressional Staff Briefing, National Association of Manufacturers, Washington, D.C. (January 19).

Andersen, Ronald. 1973. Testimony before the U.S. House of Representatives, Subcommittee on Public Health and Environment. Oversight Hearings on National Health Insurance (December).

Andersen, Ronald; Judith D. Kasper; and Martin Frankel. 1975. "The effect of measurement error on differences in hospital expenditures." Presented at the American Public Health Association Annual Meeting, Chicago (November).

Fleming, Gretchen V. 1975. "Measuring access to medical care: the use of consumer evaluations." Presented at the Illinois Medical Care Section, American Public Health Association Meeting (March).

Fleming, Gretchen V. and Ronald Andersen. 1976. "Health beliefs of the U.S. population: implications for self-care." Presented at the Conference on Consumer Self-Care in Health, National Center for Health Services Research, Washington, D.C. (March 25).

Harden, Stephen D. 1975. "Simulation study in the evaluation of social security programs." Presented at the Research Conference on Methods of Evaluating the Effectiveness of Social Security Programs, sponsored by the International Social Security Association, Vienna, Austria (September).

Kravits, Joanna. 1974. "Attitudes toward and use of discretionary physician and dental services by race controlling for income." Presented at the American Public Health Association Annual Meeting, New Orleans (October).

———. 1975. "Sex Differences in health care social survey research methods." Presented at the Conference on Women and Their Health: Research Implications for a New Era, University of California, San Francisco (August).

Marmor, Theodore R. 1975. "The politics of national health insurance proposals: what's in it for kids?" Presented at the Sun Valley Health Forum, Sun Valley, Idaho (August).

———. 1976. Testimony submitted to the U.S. House of Representatives, Committee on Ways and Means (February).

Marquis, Kent; M. Susan Marquis; and Joseph P. Newhouse. 1975. "The measurement of medical care utilization and expenditures: preliminary findings from the health insurance study." Presented at the American Public Health Association Annual Meeting, Chicago (November).

McClure, Walter. 1974. Testimony before the U.S. House of Representatives, Committee on Ways and Means (May).

———. 1974. Testimony before the Minnesota Senate Subcommittee on Health Care Costs (September).

———. 1975. "The medical care system under national health insurance." Presented at the American Political Science Association Meeting, San Francisco (September).

Newman, John F. 1973. "Demographic prerequisites in the development of indices of health status." Presented at the meeting of the Population Association of America, New Orleans (April).

Phelps, Charles E. 1973. Testimony before the U.S. House of Representatives, Subcommittee on Public Health and Environment. Oversight Hearings on National Health Insurance (December).

DISSERTATIONS AND THESES

Aday, Lu Ann. 1973. "Economic and non-economic barriers to the use of needed medical services." Ph.D. dissertation, Purdue University.

Colle, Ann Dukes. 1976. "Effects of wife's schooling on efficiency in health production." Ph.D. dissertation, Graduate Center of the City University of New York. In preparation.

Dawkins, Cecilia. 1976. "Occupation and income effects of utilization of health services for England and Wales and the United States." Ph.D. dissertation, University of Chicago. In preparation.

Fleming, Gretchen V. 1976. "Patient satisfaction as an expression of legitimacy of the health services system." Ph. D. dissertation, University of Chicago. In preparation.

Guzick, David. 1976. "The market for physicians' services: a monopolistic competition approach." Ph. D. dissertation, New York University. In preparation.

Kasper, Judith D. 1976. "The effects of family size on children's use of physician services." Ph.D. dissertation, University of Chicago.

Kravits, Joanna, 1974. "Attitudes toward and use of discretionary physician and dental services by race controlling for income and age." Ph.D. dissertation, University of Chicago.

Kulley, Andrew M. 1974. "The validity of survey measurement of health services utilization: a verification study of respondent reports of hospitalization." Ph.D. dissertation, Purdue University.
Mirabito, Madeline. 1974. "Access to medical care in rural areas." Master's thesis, University of Chicago.
Wayne, John D. 1976. "Four studies on the effects of Medicaid." Ph.D. dissertation, University of Florida, Gainesville. In preparation.
Weiss, Gregory L. 1972. "The influence of need for care and selected socio-demographic characteristics on the utilization of physicians' services." Master's thesis, Purdue University.
———. 1975. "The utilization of needed medical services by blacks and whites: an evaluation of structural models." Ph.D. dissertation, Purdue University.

DATA USERS: INSTITUTIONS AND ORGANIZATIONS

Blue Cross Association
Chicago, Illinois

Department of Health, Education and Welfare
Washington, D.C.
        Bureau of Health Resources Development
        Resource Analysis Staff

        Office of the Deputy Assistant Secretary for
          Health Planning and Analysis
        Office of Health Analysis

        National Center for Health Services Research
        Office of Policy Development and Planning

        National Center for Health Statistics
        Health Status and Demographic Analysis Branch

        Social Security Administration
        Bureau of Health Services Research
        National Health Insurance Modelling Group

Eli Lilly and Co.
Indianapolis, Indiana

Interstudy
Health Services Research Center
Minneapolis, Minnesota

National Urban League
Washington, D.C.

U.S. Congress
Washington, D.C.
      House of Representatives
        Ways and Means Committee

      Senate
        Finance Committee

        Committee on Labor and Public Welfare
        Subcommittee on Health

References

Aday, Lu Ann and Ronald Andersen. 1975. *Development of Indices of Access to Medical Care.* Ann Arbor, Michigan: Health Administration Press.

Aday, Lu Ann and Robert Eichhorn. 1972. *The Utilization of Health Services: Indices and Correlates.* DHEW Pub. No. (HSM) 73-3003.

American Hospital Association. 1971. Guide Issue. *Hospitals, Journal of the American Hospital Association* 45 (August 1).

American Medical Association. 1969. *1969 American Medical Directory.* Chicago.

American Osteopathic Association. 1970. *1970 Yearbook and Directory of Osteopathic Physicians.* Chicago.

Andersen, Ronald. 1975. "The effect of measurement error on differences in the use of health services." In Ronald Andersen et al., eds., *Equity in Health Services: Empirical Analyses in Social Policy:* 229–55. Cambridge, Mass.: Ballinger Publishing Co.

Andersen, Ronald and Odin W. Anderson. 1967. *A Decade of Health Services.* Chicago: University of Chicago Press.

Andersen, Ronald; Richard Foster; and Peter Weil. 1976. "Rates and correlates of expenditure increases for personal health services in periods before and after Medicare and Medicaid." *Inquiry.* In press.

Andersen, Ronald; Rachel McL. Greeley; Joanna Kravits; and Odin W. Anderson. 1972. *Health Service Use: National Trends and Variations, 1953–1971.* DHEW Pub. No. (HSM) 73-3004 (October).

Andersen, Ronald; Judith Kasper; and Martin Frankel. 1975. "The effect of measurement error on differences in hospital expenditure." Paper delivered at the American Public Health Association Meeting, Chicago, Illinois (November).

———., eds. 1976. *Total Survey Error: Bias and Random Error in Health Survey Estimates.* Research Series. Chicago: Center for Health Administration Studies. In preparation.

Andersen, Ronald and Joanna Kravits. 1971. "Disability days and physician contact for the two-week period preceding the interview date by age, sex, race, and family income." Preliminary Report No. 1. Center for Health Administration Studies.

Andersen, Ronald; Joanna Kravits; and Odin W. Anderson. 1971. "The public's view of the crisis in medical care: An impetus for changing delivery systems?" *Economic and Business Bulletin* 24:44–52.

——, eds. 1975. *Equity in Health Services: Empirical Analyses in Social Policy.* Cambridge, Mass.: Ballinger Publishing Co.

Andersen, Ronald; Joanna Kravits; Odin W. Anderson; and Joan Daley. 1973. *Expenditures for Personal Health Services: National Trends and Variations: 1953–1970.* DHEW Pub. No. (HRA) 74-3105 (October).

Andersen, Ronald, Björn Smedby; and Odin W. Anderson. 9170. *Medical Care Use in Sweden and the United States—A Comparative Analysis of Systems and Behavior.* Research Series No. 27. Chicago: Center for Health Administration Studies.

Andersen, Odin W.; Patricia Collette; and Jacob J. Feldman. 1963. *Changes in Family Medical Care Expenditures and Voluntary Health Insurance.* Cambridge, Mass.: Harvard University Press.

Anderson, Odin W. and Jacob J. Feldman. 1956. *Family Medical Costs and Voluntary Health Insurance: A Nationwide Survey.* New York: McGraw-Hill Book Co., Inc.

Barclay, G. 1958. *Techniques of Population Analysis.* New York: John Wiley and Sons, Inc.

California Medical Association. 1969. *1969 California Relative Value Studies.* San Francisco: Six Ninety Three Sutter Publications, Inc.

Cooper, Barbara S. and Nancy L. Worthington. 1972. "Medical care spending for three age groups." *Social Security Bulletin* 35 (May):3–16.

Falk, Isadore S.; Margaret C. Klem; and Nathan Sinai. 1933. *The Incidence of Illness and the Receipt and Costs of Medical Care among Representative Families: Experiences in Twelve Consecutive Months during 1928–31.* Committee on the Costs of Medical Care, Report No. 26. Chicago: University of Chicago Press.

Firestone, J. M. 1970. *Trends in Prescription Drug Prices.* Washington, D.C.: American Enterprise Institute for Public Policy Research.

Flook, Evelyn and Paul J. Sanazaro, eds. 1973. *Health Services Research and R&D.* Ann Arbor, Michigan: Health Administration Press.

Goodman, Leo. 1969. "Ransacking cross-classification tables." *American Journal of Sociology* 75 (July):1–40.

Hansen, Morris; William Hurwitz; and William Madow. 1953. *Sample Survey Methods and Theory.* Vol. 1. New York: John Wiley and Sons, Inc.

Health Insurance Institute. 1976. *Source Book of Health Insurance Data, 1975-76.* New York.

Kish, Leslie. 1965. *Survey Sampling.* New York: John Wiley and Sons, Inc.

Klarman, H. E., et al. 1970a. *Sources of Increase in Selected Medical Care Expenditures, 1929-1969.* Office of Research and Statistics Staff Paper No. 4. Washington, D.C.: Social Security Administration.

——. 1970b. "Accounting for the rise in selected medical care expenditures, 1929–1969." *American Journal of Public Health* 60 (June):1023–39.

National Center for Health Statistics. 1963. *Measurement of Personal Health Expenditures.* Series 2, No. 2 (June).

——. 1965a. *Reporting of Hospitalization in the Health Interview Survey.* Series 2, No. 6 (July).

——. 1965b. *Volume of Dental Visits, United States, July 1963–June 1964.* Series 10, No. 23.

——. 1972a. *Current Estimates from the Health Interview Survey: United States—1970.* Series 10, No. 72 (May).

——. 1972b. "Hospital and surgical insurance coverage among persons under 65 years of age in the United States, 1970." *Monthly Vital Statistics Report,* Vol. 21, No. 9, supplement 2 (December 18).

——. 1974. *Personal Out-of-pocket Health Expenses: United States, 1970.* Series 10, No. 91 (June).

——. 1975. *Current Estimates from the Health Interview Survey: United States—1974.* Series 10, No. 100 (September).

Phelps, Charles E. 1975. "Effects of insurance on demand for medical care." In Ronald Andersen et al., eds., *Equity in Health Services: Empirical Analyses in Social Policy:* 105–30. Cambridge, Mass.: Ballinger Publishing Co.

Social Security Administration. 1973. "National health expenditures, calendar years 1929–71." *Research and Statistics Notes,* No. 3 (March 3).

Taylor, D. Garth; Lu Ann Aday; and Ronald Andersen. 1975. "A social indicator of access to medical care." *Journal of Health and Social Behavior* 16 (March):39–49.

U.S. Bureau of the Census. 1971a. *Current Population Reports.* Series P-60, No. 80 (October). Washington, D.C.

——. 1971b. *Statistical Abstract of the United States: 1971.* Washington, D.C.

——. 1974. *Standards for Discussion and Presentation of Errors in Data.* Technical Paper No. 32. Washington, D.C.

U.S. Department of Labor. 1973. *Handbook of Labor Statistics.* Washington, D.C.

Index

About the Authors

Ronald Andersen is a research associate in the Center for Health Administration Studies, and associate professor in the Graduate School of Business and Department of Sociology, University of Chicago. He was study director on the nationwide social survey and verification which produced the data for this book. His major research interests include utilization of health services and international comparisons of health service systems. He has authored or co-authored: *A Decade of Health Services* (1967); *A Behavioral Model of Families' Use of Health Services* (1968); *Medical Care Use in Sweden and the United States* (1970); *Development of Indices of Access to Medical Care* (1975); and *Equity in Health Services: Empirical Analyses in Social Policy* (1975). He received his Ph.D. in Sociology from Purdue University in 1968.

Joanna Lion is director of information Services, Massachusetts Hospital Association. At the time this book was written, she was research associate in the Center for Health Administration Studies and assistant study director on the nationwide survey. Her major research interests include racial differences in the delivery of health care and comparisons of health care delivery systems, as well as practical applications of hospital planning. Among her publications are *Health Services in the Chicago Area—A Framework for Use of Data* (1969); "The Public's View of the Crisis in Medical Care: An Impetus for Changing Delivery Systems?" (1971); and *Equity in Health Services: Empirical Analysis in Social Policy* (1975) (published under the name of Joanna Kravits). She received her Ph.D. in Human Development from the University of Chicago in 1974.

Odin W. Anderson, is Professor of Sociology in the Graduate School of Business and the Department of Sociology, and Director of the Center for Health Administration Studies, University of Chicago. His entire professional career since 1942, beginning at the University of Michigan, School of Public Health, has been devoted to research and teaching in the organization and financing of health services. In later years he has become interested in cross-national comparisons of health services systems, particularly the United States, Sweden, and Great Britain and in the study of public policy formulation. He has authored or co-authored: *A Decade of Health Services: Social Survey Trends in Use and Expenditures* (1967); *The Uneasy Equilibrium: Private and Public Financing of Health Services in the United States, 1875–1965* (1968); *Health Care: Can There Be Equity? The United States, Sweden, and England* (1972). *Blue Cross Since 1929: Accountability and the Public Trust* (1975); and *Equity in Health Services: Empirical Analyses in Social Policy* (1975). He received his Ph.D. in Sociology from the University of Michigan in 1948.